A Handbook for Veterinary Physician

17th Revised and Enlarged Edition

V. A. Sapre

M.V.Sc. (Hon.) Medicine, Ph.D.
Professor and Head (Retd.)
Department of Veterinary Medicine
Nagpur Veterinary College,
Seminary Hills, Nagpur, Maharashtra

N. P. Dakshinkar

M.V.Sc. (Med.), Ph.D., F.N.A.V.S., F.I.S.V.M.
Head
Department of Clinics
Nagpur Veterinary College,
Seminary Hills, Nagpur, Maharashtra

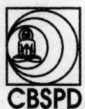

CBSPD

CBS Publishers & Distributors Pvt Ltd

New Delhi • Bengaluru • Chennai • Kochi • Kolkata • Lucknow • Mumbai
Gujarat • Hyderabad • Jharkhand • Nagpur • Patna • Pune • Uttarakhand

A Handbook for Veterinary Physician

ISBN: 978-81-239-2974-3

17th Revised and Enlarged Edition: 2013

First CBS Reprint: 2016

Reprint: 2018, 2020, 2022, 2023, **2025**

Published by **Satish Kumar Jain** and produced by **Varun Jain** for

CBS Publishers & Distributors Pvt Ltd

4819/XI Prahlad Street, 24 Ansari Road, Daryaganj, New Delhi 110 002, India
Ph: 011-23289259, 23266838
Website: www.cbspd.com
e-mail: delhi@cbspd.com

Corporate Office: 204 FIE, Industrial Area, Patparganj, Delhi 110 092
Ph: 011-4934 4934   Fax: 011-4934 4935   e-mail: publishing@cbspd.com; publicity@cbspd.com

Branches

- **Bengaluru:** Seema House 2975, 17th Cross, K.R. Road, Banasankari 2nd Stage, Bengaluru 560 070 Karnataka, India
  Ph: +91-80-26771678/79   Fax: +91-80-26771680   e-mail: bangalore@cbspd.com
- **Chennai:** 18/8B, Subbarayan Street, Shenoy Nagar, Chennai 600 030, Tamil Nadu, India
  Ph: +91-44-42032115, 26681266   e-mail: chennai@cbspd.com
- **Kochi:** 42/1325, 1326, Power House Road, Opp KSEB, Power House, Ernakulam 682 018, Kerala, India
  Ph: +91-484-4059061-65   Fax: +91-484-4059065   e-mail: kochi@cbspd.com
- **Kolkata:** 147, Hind Ceramics Compound, 1st Floor, Nilgunj Road, Belghoria, Kolkata-700056 West Bengal, India
  Ph: 033-25633055, 033-25633056   e-mail: kolkata@cbspd.com
- **Lucknow:** Basement, Khushnuma Complex, 7-Meerabai Marg (Behind Jawahar Bhawan) Lucknow 226001, India
  Ph: 0522-4000032   e-mail: tiwari.lucknow@cbspd.com
- **Mumbai:** PWD Shed. Gala no. 25/26, Ramchandra Bhatt Marg, Next to JJ Hospital Gate no. 2 Opp. Union Bank of India Noorbaug, Mumbai-400009, Maharashtra, India
  Ph: 022-66661880/89   e-mail: mumbai@cbspd.com

Representatives

- **Gujarat** 0-9879558667 • **Hyderabad** 0-9885175004 • **Jharkhand** 0-9811541605 • **Nagpur** 0-8692091830
- **Patna** 0-9334159340 • **Pune** 0-9664372571 • **Uttarakhand** 0-9716462459

Printed at SRK Graphics, Delhi, India

*This humble work is
dedicated
to All those Veterinarians
who love their profession
and
are proud of
Being a Veterinarian
With a pledge
to
serve the farmer.*

Preface to the 17th Edition

It gives immense pleasure to bring out this 17th Revised & Enlarged edition of this Handbook to day. We are very much thankful for various suggestions received through letters and telephones for incorporating latest drugs now available in the market and deleting the old remedies that are not currently prescribed as outdated.

Development participation of youth and women in rural areas is essential for rapid progress in India which has immense potentials for developments and prosperity. During our recent visits to rural areas in course of helping families in which suicides have caused enormus damage to families, we have observed that farmers are in real need of advise and guidance for undertaking profitable dairy and poultry farming particularly with active participation of women folk in the family.

We are sure that contribution of veterinarians will be duly recognised in times to come and Dairy - Poultry. Sheep - Goat rearing will be recognised as profitable side industries in this nation.

Hope that this revised & enlarged edition will meet the expectations of veterinarians & the students.

1 May 2012   **V.A. Sapre**

(Maharashtra Day)   **N.P. Dakshinkar**

Preface to the 16th Edition

We are pleased to present the Sixteenth fully updated and enlarged edition of our very popular book. From this edition, Dr N.P. Dakshinkar is associated with this work as co-author. Dr Dakshinkar was a student and co-worker of Dr Sapre; and has over 2 decades of clinical and research experience. Besides being a skilled and careful veterinarian, he has written many a book on rearing and economic exploitation of various domestic animals. This edition adds chapters of Ostrich and Dairy farming.

The past decade has seen tremendous advances in veterinary technology, hand-in-hand with medical technology. Highly sensitive an easy to use kits for a variety of serological and pathological tests, endoscopy, electrocardiography. ultrasonography, computerised asseys, microsurgical procedures etc. have made inroads in veterinary medicine and are becoming available to veterinarians in cities and selected towns. Now it is upto our veterinarians to avail of these modern technologies and provide precise and state-of-art service to clients. We have no doubt that the present day veterinarian who is highly professional and competitive, will not let these opportunities pass over his/her head!

While looking forward to such bright future for veterinary science, we cannot forget the sad state of affairs of our marginal and mainly dry-land farmers, hundred after hundreds of failed farmers are committing suicides in many states like Maharasthra, Andhra Pradesh, Karnataka and even in the co-called rich state of Punjab. Why is this happening? Simply because when their agricultural crops fail, these farmers have no other income to support their families and repay loans. If they had access to supplementary income through animal husbandry; they could have managed to carry through hard days and didn't have to drink pesticides or hang themselves from trees: Why have they not been introduced to supplementary animal husbandry industries such as Milk, Meat, Poultry production or even to upcoming highly lucrative activities like Ostrich, Rabbit, Pig farming. Dog breeding and management of Kennels or even Hay Making and marketing?

It is only a veterinary graduate who is systematically trained in all these productive technologies but sadly the full potential of veterinarians' education is not put to use at present. Veterinarians are not only animal doctors but almost half of their expertise is in production of wealth from animal sources. They should, therefore, be used as advisors, guides and even practical demonstrators to the entire animal based industry. Is it so, at present? The answer, sadly, is no.

We urge all practicing veterinarians to be more than just disease treating doctors but to get involved in the economic activities of small farmers as well as urban and semi-urban deprived people, especially their women folk who could gainfully earn income from rearing animals. Veterinarians must encourage people to exploit the vast economic potential of all species of domestic animals in a country like India which is endowed by Mother Nature with rich natural resources. What is required is dedication, patriotic spirit and hard work by our veterinarian brothers and sisters, with the dream of making India topmost developed country before the year 2020:

Wishing our readers Good Luck and best results.

4th June, 2007   **V.A. Sapre**
"Sankashti Chaturthi"   **N.P. Dakshinkar**

Preface to the 15th Edition

It is more than four decades, since I started my career as a Veterinarian and during this period I had the privilege to work in various branches of the profession.

I remember the way we practice veterinary medicine at the beginning of my career. Now, I find sea change in the material and methods used in the profession. There has been considerable progress in the veterinary science and animal husbandry, much improvement in veterinary education and spectacular developments in physical facilities available to veterinarians. Number of veterinarians has also increased many folds. At least 3 states in India, Maharashtra being the latest, have underlined importance of Veterinary Science by establishing Veterinary Universities.

All these changes have now created much impact of veterinarians on general public and have made veterinarians almost indispensable for welfare of the society. Veterinarians have successfully eradicated the dreaded rinderpest amongst ruminants by producing potent vaccines and using them on mass scale under the national rinderpest eradication campaign. Most of the common infectious disease of livestock are now under control. Livestock owners are now assured of rewarding livestock industry, thanks to safe and dependable veterinary help. "White Revolution" has come of age and milk and eggs are available in every town and city at all times and in any quantity required.

Although per capita availability of milk due to high population is low, India is ranked number one in the world as per the latest report of Food and Agriculture Organization as the highest milk producing nation in the world because of 74 million tons of milk produced in 1998, as against 71 million tons by U.S.A. Should we not be proud of this distinction?

Can anyone deny the invaluable contribution of field veterinarians who tour remote and inaccessible villages in sun and rain to render service to poor farmers and livestock keepers without expecting much in return?

Veterinarians have also laid solid foundations of animal husbandry in the fields of dairying, poultry, sheep and goat rearing, piggery, rabbit raising, horse and mule breeding, dog breeding and kennels besides being clinicians and researchers in life sciences and pharmaceutical industry and marketing. Even banking and insurance sectors fall in the sphere of veterinarian's activity. No other profession can infect, boast of such wide spectrum of active involvement.

A methodical, alert and sincere veterinarian cannot fail to create an impressive image of his profession on people and win their hearts.

Having been a teacher of veterinary medicine for more than twenty five years and having had opportunity to meet and discuss problems with so many past students, as well as colleagues during numerous work camps, I am very optimistic about future of our profession in the hands of young vets who are now better trained and equipped with modern facilities than what we had in the beginning of our careers. It has however, come to notice that during busy working day, a veterinarian has no time or access to text books on clinical subjects and he badly needs a reference book wherein he can get quick answers to his problems in brief. An up-to-date, easy to read, ready reckoner can help young vets in dealing with confronting situations with confidence and without having to consult some experienced senior, for mostly there is none available.

With the purpose of providing such a easy to use, up-to-date and concise book to assist practicing vets, I wrote this handbook many years ago. It is essentially meant to be used by students, registered veterinary physicians and field workers. Of course, it does not claim to be a substitute for standard text books nor does it profess to replace experienced and qualified veterinarians.

It gives me immense pleasure to see some veterinarians conducting high quality sophisticated work such as embryo transfer and performing skillful surgery and carrying out investigations to diagnose metabolic disorders and detecting micromineral deficiencies to give precise treatment in the field. Many are progressing towards branch specialization on human lines as in USA which I recently visited.

It is high time when a strong leadership is awaited for this profession so as to create a desirable impact on Government who must divert sizeable funds necessary for conducting quality research and launch projects to eradicate important diseases like Brucellosis, Leptospirosis and Rabies all of which form an important zoonoses.

Since 1977, when the book was first published, on popular demand, many revised and up-dated editions were released. At every edition, I have added new material to the contents, in response to suggestions from professional colleagues.

I am happy to release this Fifteenth edition today. This edition is updated in all aspects with additions in relevant pages, incorporates coloured photographs of common breeds of dogs in India and a new chapter on Rabbit Farming. The chart on vaccinations in Poultry has also been updated with latest vaccines released in market. Hope this edition will meet the expectations of readers.

(V.A. Sapre)

Contents

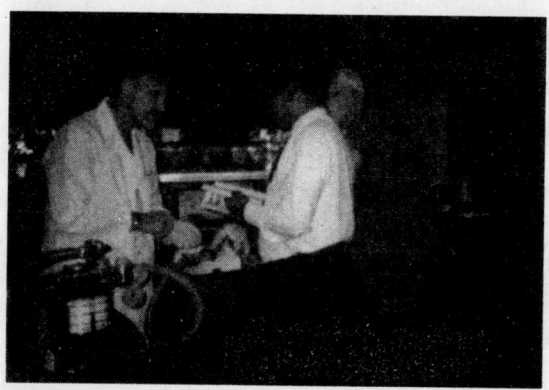

A Copy of Handbook Presented by Author Dr. Sapre.

Chapter 1

Introduction

Diagnosis of disease in an animal that cannot describe its complaints is an interesting job comparable to solving a puzzle and will be enjoyed by those who are sincere, interested in the profession and pledged for the service to the dumb.

Number of species of animals required to be dealt with, limitations in diagnostic facilities underfiled conditions, cost of treatment, utility value of animal in question, public health aspect and such other considerations render the job of a veterinary physician extremely difficult.

Quickness and accuracy in diagnosis is most important while dealing with an outbreak so as to take proper preventive measures and save a large number of animals at risk. Responsibility becomes still more while dealing with zoonotic infections.

It is with these practical difficulties that a veterinary physician has to perform his duty and only a sound knowledge of physiology, pathology, microbiology, nutrition, pharmacology, medicine and its related fields together with skill of observation and interpretation that a veterinary physician can attain proficiency and reputation.

Diagnosis of Disease

Accurate diagnosis and understanding of the disease is essential for adopting proper line of treatment. One must observe the normal behaviour and habits of animals in health and develop an ability to identify the sick animal.

Veterinary clinician has to depend on the objective symptoms observed, information about the history of a case and finally on the various methods of examination.

1

General signs of Illness

A sick animal looks dull in appearance and expression, either takes only a little feed or may be completely off-feed; rumination is suspended in case of bovines; lactating animal may reduce its production.

If the animal has fever, in addition to the above signs, the muzzle becomes dry, body surface warm and rough due to erect hair, breath is hot, dung usually hard, urine scanty and deep in colour, respiration accelerated and there may be redness of eyes and lacrymation.

General inspection of the patient is the first step in the diagnostic approach to form an overall impression of the animal initially by observing the animal from a distance and this can be done while the patient is entering the hospital or you are viewing the patient while visiting for it's treatment

Consider the Following —

(i) **Species of Animal:** Some diseases are species specific

e.g., Rinderpest, H.S., B.Q.,	*(Bovines)*
Glanders, S.A.H.S. ; Strangles	*(Equines)*
Distemper, Infectious Canine Hepatitis.	*(Canines)*

(ii) **Breed**

Milk fever, Ketosis, Mastitis.

(Common in high yielding breeds)

Theileriasis ; F.M.D.

(more severe in exotic breeds)

(iii) **Age**

Black Quarter	*(a disease of young bovines)*
Distemper, Rickets	*(disease of young pups)*
Tuberculosis	*(seen in old animals)*

(iv) **Sex:** Mastitis, Metritis, Metabolic disorders and post parturient diseases are seen only in females.

Steps in Clinical Examination

(A) History of a Case (*Anamnesis*)

A tactful enquiry of history by taking the owner or the animal attendant into confidence and by judicious and discrete questioning is the first step and a key to accurate diagnosis.

Previous History: Information about previous illness if any and it's relation with the present condition.

for example

(a) Panting in bovines as an after effect of FMD.

(b) Breeding problems due to previous history of metritis.

(c) Chorea as an after effect of Distemper in dogs.

(d) Past history of dog bite to support diagnosis of rabies.

(e) Herd history of abortions in Brucellosis.

(f) History of recent parturition for metabolic disorders.

History Pertaining to Present Illness:

The history in any case refers only to a single animal but frequently in veterinary medicine the history should extend to the other animals of the herd , flock or stud in order to find out general nature of the malady.

(a)	Duration of illness	*To know the nature of the disease i.e., whether per acute, acute or chronic, Categorization of disease is based on the duration of illness and not on the severity of illness.* *Peracute --few hours to 2 days,* *Acute --3 to 7 days* *Subacute --2 to 4 weeks* *Chronic-- more than 4 weeks.*
(b)	How are the normal functions of body and behaviour.	*(rumination, lactation, defecation, urination)* History of recent change in behaviour is a very important sign suggestive of rabies

3

(c)	First symptoms noticed	*To know what system is primarily involved.*
(d)	Appetite and water intake	*Whether feed is changed*
(e)	Circùmstances, under which disease occurred	*Azoturia(in horses) after rest period, access to pastures sprayed with inseticide consumption of grains or human food.* (In cattle).
(f)	Whether any other animals in the herd or vicinity are affected	*Possibility of common cause or infectious disease.*
(g)	Whether any treatment given earlier	*Drenching pneumonia due to faulty drenching, drug resistance due to incomplete treatment, possibility of reaction to other drugs.*

(i) General Inspection: Is the first step wherein you should observe general health, skin, bodily condition, behaviour, expression, respiration, posture etc.

General health, bodily condition, appearance of skin and coat	Stunted growth, malnutrition, oedema, rickets, chronic diseases, skin diseases, deficiency diseases can be diagnosed
Behaviour, expression, posture and gait (Habitus)	Diseases of C.N.S. paralysis, specific disease like rabies, trypanosomiasis, milk fever, tetanus, grass tetany, Colic, Traumatic pericardits can be diagnosed
Respiration	Observe change in rate, depth, character of respiration, adventitious sounds, type of nasal discharge. These abnormalities are seen in primary respiratory disease or secondarily due to cardiac involvement, allergic conditions
Abdomen	Distention of abdomen may occur in tympany, impaction, ascties, intestinal obstruction, tumors and advanced pregnancy

N.B. Inspection of the patient and history taking should not be undertaken simultaneously. because it is likely that you may miss some important lesion.

General Appearance and Behaviour

Attitude	Possible Diagnosis
Frenzied restlessness, butting, weakness of hindquarters, hoarse voice	Rabies
Pressing head against wall or hard object,circling movements	Trypanosomiasis
Localised or generalized muscle tremors, tonic or clonic contractions, stumbling gait	Grass tetany
Cow lying down, recumbency, subnormal temperature, history of recent calving	Milk Fever
Moving to and fro, lifting the feet, Kicking at the belly & anxious look	Colic

Expressions — Postures — Gait etc

Anxious expressions of face, extended neck, elbows set apart, arching of thorax, shallow breathing	Traumatic pericarditis (or Acute chest pain)
Stiffness of posture , stiff walking, locked jaw, protrusion of third eyelid, hypersensitivity when approached or touched	Tetanus

General Examination

This needs approaching and handling the animal. By the time general observation and history is completed you get the idea about the general behaviour and temperament of the animal

Restraint

The animals have to be handled routinely for the purpose of clinical examination and administration of medicines. Animals vary in their behaviour and temperament from highly docile to extremely ferocious. Each animal's behavioural pattern has to be studied while approaching and handling.

One must protect himself from accidental injuries, kicks in case of large animals and bites in case of dogs and cats. The owner or animal attendant usually knows about the habits of animal and one must explore the temperature of animal by asking appropriate questions. Sometimes animals behave in unpredictable manner due to change of place and in presence of unfamiliar persons. Proper restraint by rope jacket in large animal and by tape muzzle in dogs is always necessary. In case of horse, lifting of one of the forelimbs or twitch is necessary. While handling the mouth parts and examination of buccal cavity one must be more particular and the remotest, possibility of rabies should be ruled out. Never examine the buccal cavity without wearing hand gloves in case of any slightest injuries on your fingers.

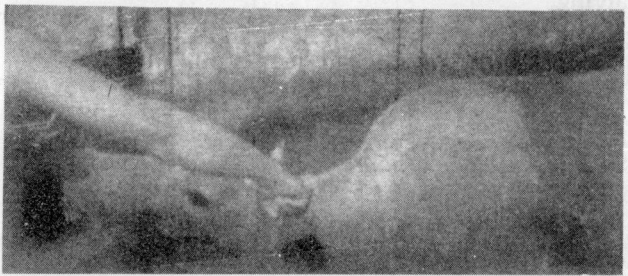

Fig. 1. Securely holding a cow for inoculation.

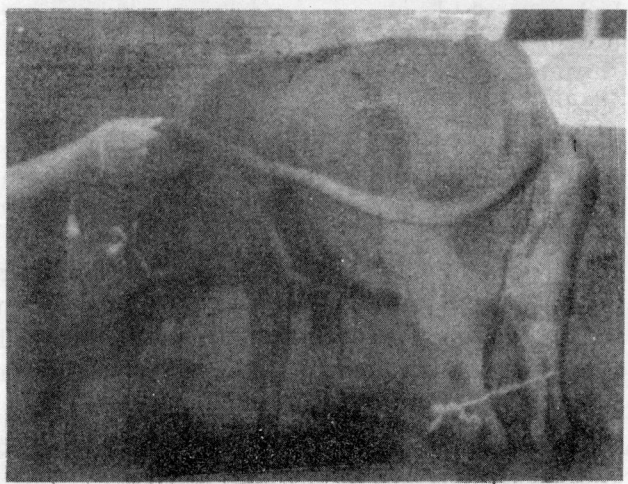

Fig. 2. Tieing hind legs to prevent kicking while the exam of udder & Rectal exam.

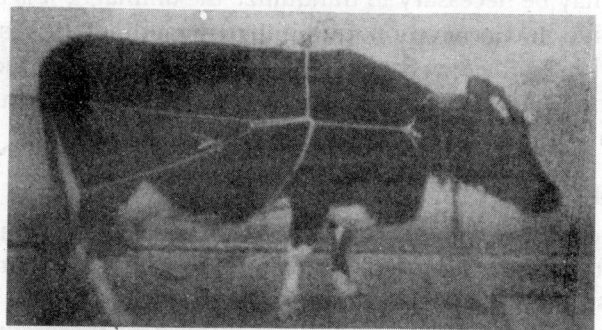

Fig. 3. Rope jacket for examination of animal.

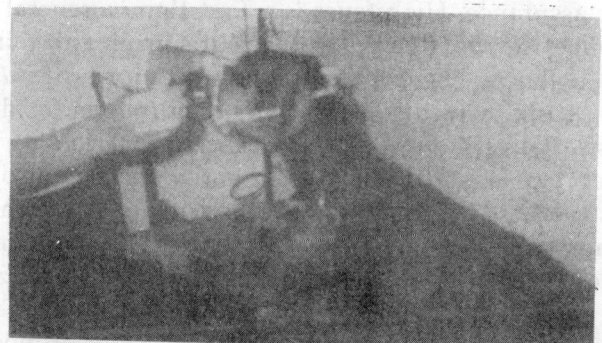

Fig. 4. Tieing a Tape muzzle to prevent biting.

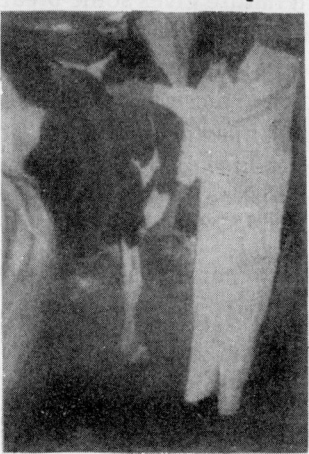

Fig. 5. Lifting one foreleg in a horse for taking temperature & other examinations.

7

It may be necessary to tranquilize the animal, if it is a very aggressive and non co-operating. Cruel methods of restraint should be avoided as they may cause accidents like fractures and sometimes strangulation and asphyxia. Always handle animals in presence of their owner.

General Clinical Examination

Recording Temperature: Record temperature while animal is at rest. Eliminate effect of high atmospheric temp., in summer. For this, dip the mercury bulb of thermometer in cold water *immediately after* recording and before reading the theromometer. Let the pet animal become quiet on the examination table. Pat him for assurance. High fever is a first sign in several acute infectious diseases. Record temperature twice a day in sick animal to know the type of fever (*continuous, recurrent, intermittent etc.*) which is a very important criteria for disease diagnosis. Range of fever is also an important deciding factor to suspect a peracute condition such as acute infectious disease like **H.S., B,Q., Anthrax, Rinderpest, Trypanosomiasis, Piroplasmosis, Acute peritonitis, Traumatic Pericarditis, Heatstroke etc.** all of which are the conditions characterized by a very high range of fever (**above 106 °F or 41 °C**) and necessisates immediate remedial measures. Fever of moderate range or intermittent nature gives some breathing time to arrive at proper diagnosis and treatment. *(In fact this is a very good guideline for the owner to decide as to how urgently the veterinary aid should be sought for only if he can record the temperature. **This is the modern trend which a livestock owner must adopt for himself to save his precious livestock).** Fever is only the symptom and other associated symptoms need however to be considered by the efficient Veterinary clinician.

Pulse : *site-Cattle* : External maxillary artery, Median artery, or Ventral coccygeal artery under the tail.

Horse :   External maxillary artery.

Dog :   Femoral artery on the inside of thigh.

Examine pulse at rest because excitement and exercise will affect its rate and character. One can know about the condition of heart, peripheral, circulation and certain diseases like chronic

8

interstitial nephritis in old dogs and endocarditis by examining pulse, irregularity and loss of rhythm is common in dogs of nervous or excitable temperament. In case of horses missing of 4th or 5th beat of pulse is common. It gets restored on exercise. **Arrhythmia in bovines is a sign of abnormality and indicates pulmonary and cardiac involvement which warrents caution.**

Type of pulse	Possible disease condition
Weak pulse	Myocardial asthenia, or Mitral incompetence
Strong pulse	Hypertension
Wiry pulse	Acute pleurisy, Pericarditis and Peritonitis.
Thready pulse	Fatal condition
Large bounding and water hammer pulse	Anaemia, Insufficiency of aortic semilunar valve or patent ductous arteriosus.

Respiration: Count respirations while animal is at rest. Note the type (*costal, abdominal, intercostal, jerky etc.*) Resp. rate increases in fevers, in summer, after exercise, and in resp. distress due to disease. It also increases due to nervous excitement and in acute painful condition. There is a ratio 1:3 between resp. and pulse in healthy animal. This ratio is altered to 1:1 in respiratory diseases. Note the type of dyspnoea.

Examining the Visible Mucous Membranes

Visible m.m. can be examined at conjunctiva, buccal or nasal mucosa and inside of vulva in females. Examine in bright natural day light. In normal healthy animal the mucous membrane is moist and rosy coloured. Examine at both so as to rule out local conditions.

Look for

Congestion	Sign in fever and inflammation
Paleness	Sing of anaemia, internal haemorrage and shock

Yellow Colouration	Sign of jaundice and liver disease
Petecheal Haemorrhages	Seen in septicemias and surra
Blue Colouration	Sign. of cyanosis observed in hypoxia, dyspnoea and congestive cardiac failure
Pink Colouration	Sign. in Infectious Euquine anaemia "Pink Eye".
Ulceration	Typical ulcers on buccal m.m. are seen in Rinderpest, F.M.D., Mucosal disease: Ulcerated nasal spetrum is seen in glanders

Examination of Eyes

Sunken Appearance	Sign. of Chr. wasting disease and dehydration.
Pupilar Response	Loss of pupilar response to light seen in toxaemias, shock, some poisoning and C.N.S. diseases.
Corneal Opacity, Ulcers	Usually due to injuries but also seen in some diseases like Distemper, Mucosal Disease Complex (*cattle*)
Protrusion of Third Eyelid	An important earlier sign of tetanus in horses

External Body Surface and Skin

One can get idea about body temperature, provided external atmospheric influences are ruled out. Look for general lustre, pliability of skin, oedema, skin disease, loss of hair, loss of pigmentation. Degree of dehydration can be assessed by pulling a fold of skin at parts where it is loose.

10

Methods of Physical Examination

A systematic approach must be developed and used on every physical examination. The initial and often the most important step in diagnostic approach to the sick animal is the physical examination. A complete examination should always be performed, even though the complaint with which the animal appears is one easily recognizable.

Each one of the following methods has its own importance when judiciously employed. An experienced clinician can note several important points simply by careful observation of the patient from distance and this has already been discussed under *"General Inspection"*.

(1) Palpation:-

By palpation or laying hand with gentle pressure on a part of a clinician can feel the consistency of organ or tissues (*fibrous, induration*) whether the part is hot and or painful (abscess, actinonbacillosis) or cold and painless (*tumour, cyst*) whether swollen and distended part of abdomen contains gases (*tympany*) or dry impacted feed (*Impaction*) or fluid (*ascites, oedema*), B.Q. can be diagnosed by palpating the typical cripitating swelling, we can palpate ruminal movements and also do rectal palpation of some organs in large animals. By deep palpation in small animals a clinician can feel the abdominal tumors, intestinal obstruction, gravid uterus, cystic calculus etc. Per rectal palpation of internal genitalia in large animals is the most valuable aid in diagnosis of pregnancy and several other ovarian and uterine diseases.

(2) Percussion:

A useful diagnostic aid and can be recognized by striking on a part of body with finger tips (*immediate percussion*) or by use of plexor (*a rubber hammer*) and pleximeter a circular disc (*mediate percussion*) the organ underneath is set into vibration and from the sounds produced, a clinician can get an idea about the contents and consistency (e.g., drum like resonance in ruminal rympany, dull resonance in impaction, consolidation of lungs). This method is more useful in small animals.

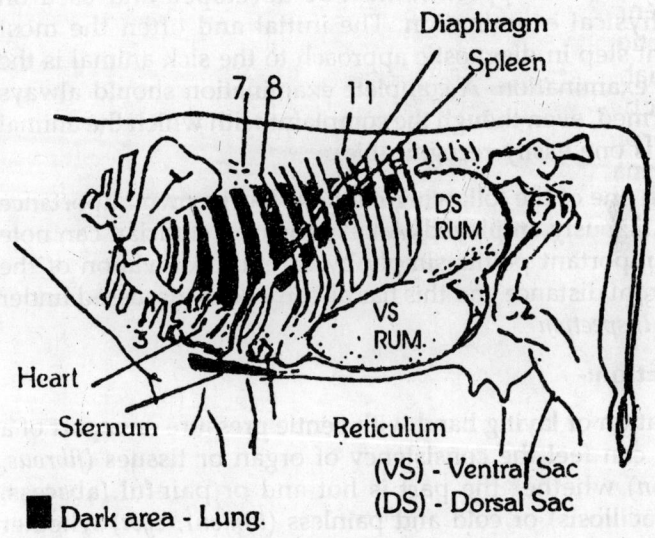

Fig. 6. Bovine Left Side.

(Labels in figure: Diaphragm, Spleen, 7, 8, 11, DS RUM, VS RUM, Heart, Sternum, Reticulum, (VS) - Ventral Sac, (DS) - Dorsal Sac, ■ Dark area - Lung, 3)

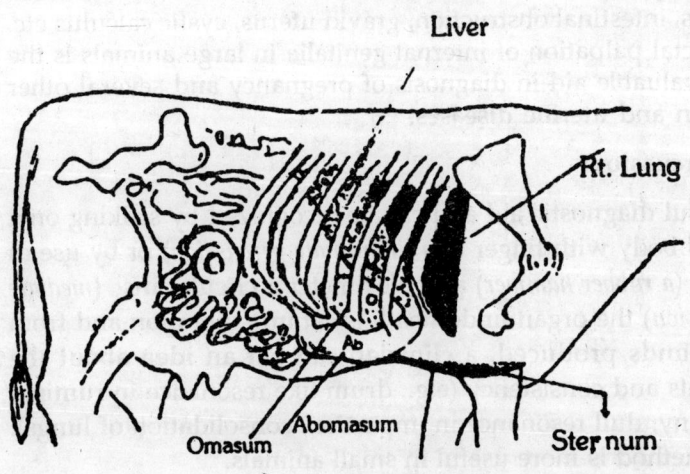

Fig. 7. Bovine Right Side.

(Labels in figure: Liver, Rt. Lung, Omasum, Abomasum, Sternum)

(3) Auscultation:-

Listening of sounds produced in course of normal physiological functioning of certain vital organs by use of stethoscope is very valuable method of clinical examination and needs considerable practice and patience to attain proficiency for correct interpretations. Useful for hearing peristaltic sounds during ruminal as well as intestinal contraction, knowing the functional state of respiratory tract and lungs : (*prominent vesicular murmur in congestion, moist rales when exudate is present*) cardiac sounds (*friction sounds in early pericarditis, cardiac murmrs in valvular diseases, splashing sounds in pericarditis with effusion and hydropericardium etc.*). It is possible to diagnose respiratory and cardio vascular diseases by auscultation by an expert physician.

It is necessary to eliminate unrelated sounds from surroundings, sounds due to movements of skin, friction sounds produced due to rubbing of hair. The animals should be properly restrained, quiet and in case of long haired animals the coat should be moistened so as to eliminate due to hair friction.

Sound knowledge of topographical anatomy is an essential prerequistite for percussion and auscultaion.

(4) Other Diagnostic Aids

In addition to the above methods various other specialized methods are now available in veterinary practice as are routinely practiced in human medicine. Branch specialization such as Gastroenerology, Nephrology, Cardiology, Neurology Dermatology, Surgery, Gynaecology, Opthalmology and so on are gradually developing in animal pactice in India. For developing such specialized consultation and sophisticated therapy there must be enough number of references made by the general practioners spread over in moffusil areas. These specialities have already developed in western countries like America where specific facilities are available. General practitioners refer specific cases to these speciality hospitals where cases are examined by subject matter specialist and the required investigations performed in certain cases for confirmation of the tentative diagnosis. X-ray examination, rectal examination, exploratory puncture, exam. of urine, milk, bacteriological exam., serological tests, allergic tests, biopsy,

13

biochemical tests and several other types of diagnostic tests, including E.C.G., which has been found very useful in small animal practice. Laproscopic exam. is also possible to visualise the visceral organs. Recent developments in diagnostics such as Endoscopy, Magnetic Resonance Imaging (MRI). Computerised Tomography Scanning (CT Scan) and ultra sonography are some of the recent diagnostic techniques which could be used in small animal practice. These diagnostic facilities need costly equipments and trained technical staff to operate and interpret the findings. Presently these facilities are available in Veterinary college hospitals and some district level Veterinary polyclinics.

Indiscriminate use of antibiotics, incomplete and delayed treatment in cases of mastitis, metritis and urogenital infections has created problems of resistant bacterial strains. In such situations cultural examination and antibiotic sensitivity tests have become valuable diagnostic aids in the successful management of mastitis, metritis and urinary tract infections.

Inference from General Clinical Examination

After careful consideration of the circumstances, tactful enquiry of the history and completion of general examination of the patient a clinician can arrive at the following reasonable conclusion:

(1) Whether the disease is restricted to a single animal or it is a herd problem (*Contagious or Otherwise*)

(2) Which system of patient is affected and needs further detailed examination.

This is, therefore, followed by the examination of individual systems of body.

> *"Personally I have always felt that the best doctor in the world is a Veterinarian.. He can't ask his patients what is the matter. He's just got to know".*
>
> **Will Rogers**
> SENATOR

14

Chapter 2

Digestive System (Bovine)

igestive disorders are the commonest conditions in bovines and constitute nearly 80 per cent of the cases that are attended by the physician. Simple digestive upsets are treated at home by experienced cattle owners by administration of common digestive herbal preparations used traditionally.

Clinical Examination: This should include the enquiry and if possible personal examinations of feed components actually given to animals particularly when there is a herd problem. Crude fibre content should not be less than 15 to 18 per cent. Fodders exposed to rains and humidity usually get lot of black fungus (*Aspergillus. niger*) which can cause acute food toxicity as well as chronic indigestion accompanied with hypocalcemia. Spoilt or sour silage, mouldy feed, grains, containing residues of insecticides used during storage, etc. are the possible problems. In such cases feed sample should be submitted for analysis for toxicity.

Examination of rumen by palpation and auscultation is an important step. Frequency and force of rumen contractions should be noted. Auscultation of reticulum, omasum and abomasum should be practiced in all animals with digestive disturbance. This helps in developing proficiency in detecting abnormality if any. The area of liver should be percussed. Liver can be palpated behind the last rib on right side only when it is enlarged. Examine for jaundice. Consistency, colour and smell of faces should be carefully examined. Undigested portion of fodder is invariably seen when digestion is impaired and liver does not function properly. Examination of faeces for parasitic ova must be carried out in case of chronic or recurrent indigestion and when the animal is not picking up condition or not giving expected milk production.

Research in the recent years has brought about new concepts and the ruminant's Indigestion could be either:

(a) **Alkaline indigestion:** With rumen pH above 7.5.

(b) **Acid indigestion:** With rumen pH below 6.0.

(c) Indigestion *without change* in normal pH.

The normal pH of rumen fluid is between 6.8 to 7.2.

The pH of the ruminal fluid can be examined by pH paper (BDH) with a range of pH 2 to 10.

A small quantity of rumen fluid can be withdrawn by inserting of long needle (4" long 15 -16 gauge needle) attached to a 5 ml. dry syringe. Site is prepared on the left side of abdomen on the lower middle third (*about 6-8 inches below left flank*) by shaving hair and applying strong Tr. Iodine or Alcohol. The needle is inserted in the straight direction at 90° angle through left abdominal wall. A small incision at the site can be given over the skin in case the skin is hard and thick. This will facilitate easy penetration of the needle without use of force. The entire 4" length of needle be penetrated in one stroke and if the site is proper, you can aspirate 1-2 ml. of rumen fluid by making little to and fro movements of the needle. A small quantity of sterile normal saline, or 5 ml. Inj. Terramycin be slowly injected while withdrawing the needle. This will prevent infection (*Fig. 8*).

A drop of rumen fluid should be poured on the pH paper and the colour produced be matched with the colour comparator strip provided with the litmus papers to judge the pH of ruminal fluid.

The rumen fluid can be used for conduction of other tests like protozoan activity, motility, microscopic examination, Cellulose digestion test etc. so as to make proper assessment of microbial digestive rumen function.

(Tr. Iodine swab be applied over the needle punture wound and the procedure of rumen fluid withdrawal is uneventful if animal is properly restrained.)

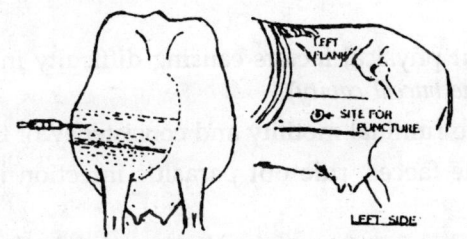

Fig. 8. Aspiration of Rumen Fluid for Examination.

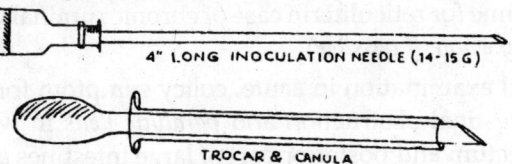

It is observed that the seasonal variation in occurrence of a particular type of indigestion depends upon the type of feeds-particularly the fodders and grasses available in the areas in different seasons. Feeding exclusively dry fodders like kadbi, rice straw, wheat straw etc., in seasons when greens are not available, usually leads to *alkaline indigestion*. Overfeeding greens, silages, grain engorgement and feeding on human food and left over sweets after functions usually lead to *acid indigestion*.

The activity of rumen microflora is governed by pH of rumen contents, availability of substrates such as trace elements like copper and cobalt. A detailed study is necessary in those cases which do not respond in 1 or 2 days. Rumen functions tests are particularly useful (*see under lab. procedure*).

Ruling out traumatic cause or its timely confirmation is very important for the physician. This ability is developed with more and more experience and careful observation of clinical symptoms. Chronic indigestion due to ingestion of indigestible objects like plastic materials is the new emerging problem in urban areas.

Clinical Examination

(i)   Determine whether disorder is primary or secondary (*Rule out fever or any other disease*)

(ii) Enquire about change of feed if any.

17

(iii) Rule out physical factors causing difficulty in prehension (*Examine buccal cavity*).

(iv) Examine ruminal motility and consistency of the contents.

(v) Examine faeces, rule out parasitic infection in a chronic case.

(vi) Look for signs of toxemia, shock and dehydration.

(vii) Examine for reticulitis in case of chronic ruminal indigestion (*X-ray exam. if possible*).

(viii)Rectal examination in acute, colicy symptom for diagnosis of intestinal obstruction and *paralytic ileus* in which cases the rectum and posterior part of large intestines are empty).

General Principles Treatment

(i) ˙ Correction of motility.

(ii) Relieve over distension.

(iii) Reconstitute ruminal flora and correct the pH.

(iv) Relieve pain and spasms.

(v) Replacement of fluids and electrolytes in dehydration and toxaemia.

(vi) Antihistaminics in shock and acute condition.

(vii) Recommend exploratory rumenotomy if no response within 4 -5 days.

Stomatitis (*Inflammation of buccal m.m.*)

Examine for injuries due to foreign bodies, sharp grass spikes. Enquire if any undiluted irritant drug like turpentine or lime (*chuna*) was given. Also enquire if blood vessels of tongue were punctured (as is done as a crude treatment).

Deficiency of Riboflavin, niacin (*B-complex member*) commonly causes ulcerative lesions characterized by salivation in dog.

Make differential diagnosis from specific infectious diseases like F.M.D., Rinderpest, Bov. Malignant Catarrh, Mucosal Disease in cattle and buffaloes. Sheep pox, Blue tongue, Contagious ecthyma etc. in sheep and goats.

18

Collutoria (*Mouth washes*) with any of the following:

(i)   0.1 per cent soln. of Potassium permanganate.

(ii) 2.0 per cent soln. of Alum.

(iii) 0.5 % soln. of "Listerine" or "Dettolin" or Betadine (dilute).

(iv) **Rx.**

Pot Chlorate	1 g
Borax	12 g
Glyerine	60 ml

or

(v)   **Rx**

Tannic acid	30 g
Glycerine	150 g

Mix well and smear on buccal mucosa.

(vi) Turmeric (*haldi*) powder mixed with coconut oil or butter makes a very good antiseptic and soothing application over lesions in buccal cavity for bovines, sheep and goats.

Supportive:

Vit. C (Ascorbic Acid- (*Roche*) Inj. 5-10 ml iv

Vit. B-Complex with Liver extract

(Belamyl; Livadex; Beekom- L; Levoplex;

Bivinal forte; Liverjet; Savameel, Nutriliv etc.)

10 ml im for large animals

0.5 to 2 ml for small animals

Feed gruel with little sweet oil to prevent irritation. Maintenance by iv fluids like Rintose in dysphagic patients

Simple Indigestion and Ruminal Impaction

Ruminants are more susceptible to dysfunction of the forestomach than the other segments of the gastrointestianl tract. Rumen motility, giving microorganisms, anaerobiasis, correct pH of rumen liquor (6.8-7.0), fluidity of ruminal mass and various substrates are essential for normal digestive process. The changes in these functional activities of rumen are reflected by loss of appetite, suspended rumination, atony of rumen and other attended abnormalities.

(i) **Rx**

Mag. Sulph.	150-250 g
Sod. Chlor.	125 g
Pulv. Ginger	30 g
Sod. Bicarb	30 g
Pulv. Nux. vom.	10 g
Aqua	500 ml
Mft. : Haust	**Sig.** : Stat

(ii) **Rx**

Mag. sulph. 250 g with 50 g **Himalayan Battisa** (*Ind. Herbs*) or **Universal Battisa** (*Universal Ayurved*) in a litre of luke warm water as a drench given carefully.

(*The above two prescriptions can also be given in intestinal impaction and constipation. The treatment is more effective after rumen pH is corrected first*).

(iii) **RUMENTON** (*Pfizer*), **"ONFEED"** bolus (*Cadila*), **FLORATONE** (*Concept*) **BIOBOOST** (*Lyka*) **BOOST UP** (*Dosch*) **RUMILAC** (*Indobiocare*) **HIGEST** (*Natural Remedies*), **RUMENTAS** (*Intas*) **RUMEN FS BOLUS** (*Alembic*).

2 boluses dissolved in water once or twice daily for 2-4 days depending upon severity of condition.

Other supportive preparations which support digestion are as under:

(i) **ECOTAS BOLUS** (*Intas*): 2 boli daily for 2 days.

HERRBOSAL (*Respel*): 25 g twice daily for 3 daily.

(ii) **RUMICARE** (*Intercare*) 125 g twice daily with water as a drench.

(iii) **RUCHAMAX** (*Dabur*) : 7.5 g B.D. for 3 days

(iv) **PACHOPLUS** (*Dabur*): Herbal rumentoric bulus.

(v) **GASTRICARE** (*Himalaya Drug*) An ayurvedic preparation. 15 g B.D. or 2 boluses twice a day for 2- 3days.

(vi) **Biobloom powder** (Sarabhai zydus) 15 g/day.

(vii) **Tonokind bolus** (Vet mankind) 1-2 bolus daily.

(viii) **RUMENTO PLUS-15** (*Cattle Rem*) 15 g B.D. for 2-3 days

Stomachics did not affect rumen pH but total volatile acid produciton in treated animals was significantly high. This was attributed to increased rumen propionate production in treated animals as acetate and butyrate production remain unaffected. Total bacterial and protozoa counts were higher in treated animals. Rumen and circulatory histamine concentrations is reduced due to this treatment.

Antihistaminics :

Inj. Avil, Zeet or Chloril Inj. 10 ml (any of the following)

Supportive:

(Any one of the following)

Inj. Tribivet (Intas)

Inj. Belamyl

Inj. Livadex   5-10 ml

Inj. Bivinal - forte

Inj. Livobex (*TTK*) Nutriliv

MAXERON OR PERINORM OR REGLAN (*Metaclopromide monohydrate*) regulates the tone and contraction of stomach and helps in relieving ruminal stasis. Injectable dose @ 60-80 mg (6-8 ml) im dose for 2 days has been found useful in cases of impaction. In some obstinate cases in which anorexia persists without any apparent reason, a course of Inj. Thiamine 5-10 ml im for 2 -3 days has given good results.

Acute Ruminal Acidosis

Acid indigestion is usually the result of stock consuming large quantities of grain or pellets to which they are unaccustomed. Pasture - fed cows not yet adapted to grain may become acutely ill or die after eating only moderate amount of

21

grain, whereas stock accustomed to diets high grain content may consume large amounts of grain with little or no effect.

The severity of the signs of grian poisoning will depend on the quantity of grian eaten and the degree of adaptation of the animal to the grain diet. A range of signs frequently seen in the condition are: Subnomal body temperature, inapperance, salivation, grunting, rumainl stasis, diarrhoea, lameness, prostration, colicy pain, increased pulse and respiration, pressing and dropping of head, renmebucy, coma and death.

Severe diseases can normally be diagnosed by clinical examination; however, field and laboratory tests may be of some additional values. Clinical diagnosis of acidosis depends on measurement of ruminal acidity which usually fall below 6.0. Microscopic examination of rumen fluid for rumen protozoa and bacteria. In positive samples predominance of gram -ve flora over gram +ve one, pH of urine, faces is decreased.

Three basic principals for treatment of rumainl acidosis include correction of ruminal and systemic acidosis and prevent further lactate production, restoration of fluid and electrolyte balance and revival of ruminal and intestinal motility. In an attempt to manage this condition following steps need to be undertaken.

Prevent further access to grain, withdraw water for 12-24 hrs. Give exercise to animals to encourage movement of ingesta and other good quality palatable hay whenever needed.

Neutralisation of acidity by use of magnesium hydroxide, magnesium carbonate 200 gm Sodium or magnesium bicarbonate.

Use of tetracycline 8-10 gm, Chloramphenicol orally can be repeated 12 hourly.

Ringers lactate to correct systemic acidosis, 2.5-5% sodium bicarbonate solution iv (1-2 ml/kg b. wt.). Administer N.S. or Dextrose 20% iv @ 30 ml/kg b. wt. at 6 hourly inverval to check dehydration. Inject calcium gluconate 25% or Calcium borogluconate @ 200-300 ml for 2-3 days to prevent hypocalcaemia and sustain rumainal contractility. Fresh rumen liquor 3-4 litres.

22

Antihistamine (Pheneramine maleate @ 0.2 mg/kg b. wt. intrauminally for 2 days. Thiamine hydrochloride @ 300 mg twice iv Liver extracts can be employed as supportive treatment. Ruminotorics, feeding of straw or hay help restoring ruminal flora.

Alkaline Indigestion

Clinical symptosm in acute cases: Anorexia, mild tympany, salivation, increase in the pulse and respiration rate, semisolid faeces, groaning, kicking at belly, arched back, ataxia, tremors and convulsions.

Chronic cases - Anorexia, lowered milk yield, suspended rumination and passing of scanty pasty raeces. Body temperature normal rumen fluid pH around 8.0.

Treatment - Evaculation of rumen contents by lavage.

5-10% Acetic acid 5-10 ml/kg b. wt. orally. 3-5 litres of 2% vinegar, Hydrochloric acid 0.2%, 1 litre orally, Lactic acid 2% 500 ml orally, Lactic acid 5% 200 ml orally, Antibiotic - streptomycin 6-10 gm/day orally, Intravenous administration of glucose. If tetany, infuse calcium salts.

Ruminal Tympany

Ruminal tympany is of two types : Primary tympany or Frothy bloat and Secondary tympany or Free gas bloat.

Primary Tympany (Forthy Bloat)

Primary bloat is caused due to production of stable foam that traps the normal gases of fermentation in the rumen. Failure to eructate these gases accentuates the condition of tympany. Causes of primary tympany include excessive intake of tympanogenic plants, intake of excessive cereals and absolute lack of fibrous feed in the diet.

Secondary Tympany (Free Gas Bloat)

Physical obstruction to eructation process is the principal cause for secondary bloat. It may develop due to the presence of foreign body in the esophagus, stenosis due to pressure from the outside. Impaired rumen motility in acidosis or hypocalcaemia may also induce free gas bloat.

Clinical symptoms

Obvious distention of abdomen, specially the upper left para-lumbar fossa due to accumulation of gases in the rumen is the most conspicuous feature in bloat. On percussion of the abdomen dull sound is heard in forthy bloat whereas drum like sound is expected from secondary tympany. Ruminal constractions are usually increased in strength and frequency during the early stage but reduced in later stage. Animal becomes inapperent, dull depressed, restless, frequently rises and sits, kicks at belly and sometimes rolls on the ground. Constipation and occassionally diarrhea are evident. Dehydration and associated signs of dyspnoea, tachycardia, drooling of saliva, protrusion of tongue, grinding of teeth and forward stretching of neck follow this. In severe and uncared cases death is the ultimate outcome.

Diagnosis

History of feeding, kinds of feed offered, clinical signs are key to successful diagnosis. Ruminal pH (acidic) measurement may provide some guidelines to diagnosis. Finally the cases of bloat should be differentiated from ruminal acidosis. Vagal, indigestion, diaphragmatic hernia, esophageal obstruction, anthrax, black quarter, lightening stroke and snake bite for its possible associations.

Treatment

As an emergency measure where there is danger of asphyxia, trocarization is advocated. In milder cases gases can be released by administering antifoaming agents. It is often necessary to advice an owner to adopt certain first-aid measures to relieve the patients before the arrival of veterinarians. This includes withdrawl of feed and water, keeping animals in anterior elevated positon. Some medicinal formulations are being extensively used for treating tympany in cattle.

(i) R$_x$

Acid Carbolic (*Phenol*) 4 ml

Oleum Terebinth 30 ml

Oleum Lini' 500 ml

Mft : Haust **Sig.. : Stat**

(ii) R$_x$

Formalin 8 ml

Tr. Ginger 30 ml

Aqua 250 ml

Mft : Haust **Sig. : Stat**

(iii) **Homeopathic** *Nux Vom.* 200 C. or *Ars. alb.* 200 C or Carboveg 200 C may be tried. Give 5 drops of liquid tincture twice a day.

(iv) R$_x$

Milk 500 ml in sweet oil 500 ml

Mix and Shake well.

Give as a drench.

(v) R$_x$

Oil terebinth 30- 60 ml **OR** Formalin 5 to 10 ml

Sweet oil 500 ml. Aqua....500 ml

Mft. :Haust Sig. :Give as drench. Mft :One Dose/ Drench.

(vi) R$_x$

(vii) **TERRAMYCIN** (*Pfizer*) liquid 300 ml in 100 ml sterile water, injected intruminally using a long needle or **ANTIFLAT** 15 to 25 gm with jaggery, B.D.

(viii)**BLOATOSIL** (*Wockhardt*) or **BLOATONIL** (*Balloun*) or **DEBLOAT** (Ethicare) **BLOATON (KTS) BLONIL (Sterling Lab) 50 - 100 ml as a dench.**

(ix) **TYREL** (*Natural Rem.*) Herbal antifrothing and antizymotic for all types of bloat.

(x) Antihistaminics

Anthisan (*M & B*)	
or Avil (*Intervet*)	10 ml
or Phenavil (*J.P.*)	
or Chloril (*TTK*)	
or Zeet (*Alembic*)	10 ml
or Cadistin (*Cadila*)	intramuscular
or Phenargan (*M & B*)	
or Antihistamin(*Intas*)	
or Cural (*Mirind-vet*)	

After recovery from bloat, the animal should be given rumenotorics, Tonakind bolus (Vet mankind), Rumentas bolus (Intas), Rumenton Tablets (Pfizer) 1-2 bolus daily.

Rumicare powder (Intervet) 125 g thrice daily.

Biobloom powder 15 g/day.

Inj. Tribivet (Intas) Inj. Pepcid-C (Concept), Inj. Kayplex - Forte (Kayvet) Inj. Albamyl (Albatross Healthcare) Any one 10 ml iv

Vagus Indigestion

It is a chronic unusual type of indigestion manifested by inco-ordinated contraction of forestomach and abomasum. The etiology has also been controversial. Vagus nerve injury due to traumatic repiculoperitonitis in cattle mainly causes vagus indigestion. Perireticular abscesses near reticulo-omasal orifice can cause the disease. Adhesions between rumen and abomasum may cause the same problem.

Clinical Symptoms

In general, decreased appetite for several days, classical abdominal distension that may be constant or intermittent but tends to be progressive i.e. bloating of the left flank and the right ventral abdominal wall or papple shaped abdomen i.e., pear shaped on the right and apple shaped on the left or 'L' shaped rumen viewed from the rear or palpated per rectum, increased frequency of rumen contraction with decreased intensity, recument free-gas bloat which can be fatal, scanty pasty farry coloured faeces, bradycardia heart rate ≤ 60 beats/min dehydration. Prognosis in most cases is unpredictable.

Diagnosis

Is based on sub-acute or chronic history, typical abdominal distension (L shaped rumen, viewed from rear or through per-rectal examination) as there are no other diseases of cattle, which hyperactivity of rumen.

Through physical examination should be performed. When physical examination fails to reveal the primary lesion, ancillary tests may be helpful to diagnose the same. Most vagal indigestion patients, suprisingly, have metabolic alkalosis (hypochloraemia, hypokalaemia), aciduria and hyponatraemai. There may be increased level of chloride in the ruminal fluid. In valuable animals, a left side exploratory laparotomy and rumenotomy will often be necessary in order to make a diagnosis.

Treatment

There is no specifc treatment. Some medical causes of vagal indigestion require symptomatic therapy for the primary problem. Adequate hydration and correction of acid base or electrolyte deficits should be achieved by iv fluid therapy. Oral administration of mineral oil with adequate fiber may be given daily for 3-5 days for the correction of abomasal impaction of dietary origin. Injection of vitamin B- complex daily through im route may be administered. Valuable pregnant animals near parturition may be maintained on fluid and electrolyte therapy with dexamethasone therapy until near enough to term to induce parturition. Some animals will recover following parturition, but the condition may recur in the next pregnancy. Recovery is slow but progressive in those cases that respond to therapy.

Differential Diagnosis of Traumatic Reticulitis

It is essential to differentiate the case of indigestion as "Traumatic" or "Non-Traumatic" as early as possible i.e., before the foreign body penetrates through the reticulum into the peritoneal cavity. Following points of clinical examination would help in differential diagnosis.

Traumatic		Non-Traumatic
(i)	Circumstantial evidence such as location, possibility of access to foreign bodies due to proximity of industrial or domestic waste-matter piles etc. Stray grazing near such places in crowded urban localities is an important factor	Less common in village conditions where there are no workshops and animals mostly graze in adjoining forest grazing land
(ii)	Animal suffers repeated attacks of indigestion (not always recurrent tympanites) **non responsive** to treatment whenever the foreign body causes injury by getting embedded	Attack of indigestion is usually associated with some known change in feed, over eating or toxic feed material. The condition responds to treatment
(iii)	The type of indigestion usually may not cause alteration in rumen micro-flora or pH, but there is atony of rumen	The condition is usually accompanied with change in rumen micro flora and pH to a certain extent
(iv)	Symptoms of pain at reticular region as evinced by bamboo test, arched back and facial expressions	Signs of pain are not evident by any tests or clinical symptoms or postures
(v)	Mild fever and leucocytosis are observed although intermittently	Usually afebrile and not associated with blood changes
(vi)	Many cases get precipitated during advanced pregnancy due to increased pressure of uterus over rumen-reticulum	Such relationship with stage of gestation is not observed

Passing urine in small quantities and frequently instead of voiding it with normal force, abrupt stopping water consumption and rumination and facial expression of pain are some of the important clinical observations in case of traumatic reticulitis.

Radiological exam. and test with metal detector offer further evidence for confirmatory diagnosis. For such a radiological examination 500 mA X-ray machine is required and this facility is available only at Government Veterinary Polyclinics in most states. A timely diagnosis and decision for exploratory rumenotomy is necessary to save the animal from complications of peritonitis and pericarditis. Even if traumatic foreign body is not recovered on rumenotomy indigestible plastic materials and nonpenetrating materials are invariably removed and evacuation of impacted feed helps in restoration of rumen activity and is beneficial in recovery. Hence decision for exploratory rumenotomy should be taken before animal becomes very weak.

Omasal Impaction

The most commonly reported disease of omasum, chronic omasal impaction is difficult to diagnose. It is usually confirmed at autopsy. Omasal impaction occurs when feed is rough fibrous loppings from fodder trees, draught condition.

Clinical symptoms

Complete anorexia, cessationof defaceation, an empty, rectum, sub acute abdominal pain and disinclination to move or preferance to lie down.

Diagnosis

Swinging papaltion might detect the rebound of an abnormally hard omasum.

Treatment

Treat the primary cause.

Saline purgative, stimulants as for rumen impactions.

Large dose of liquid paraffin.

Tonic powder orally - Nux vomica.

Gentian ammonium carbonate and ginger 8 gms each

Traumatic Pericarditis

Perforation of the pericardial sac by an infected foreign body, occurs commonly in cattle.

Clinical findings include friction sound initially, followed by muffling of the heart sounds, jugular distension with pulsation and decreased pulse pressure.

Diagnosis of TRP often presents difficulties since there are no specific laboratory tests. Radiological investigation is obsolete to field practitioners. The problem of differentiation between piercing and non-piercing metalic objects in reticulum has limited the use of metal detector.

In bovines suffering from TRP, trypsin inhibitor concentration in blood is substantially elevated. A bovine animal exhibiting clinical signs of TRP and having the plasma TI level higher than 8 mg/ml (cut-off value) could be diagnosed positive for TRP.

Trypsin Inhibitor Assay

The trypsin inhibitor (TI) assay was based on the competitive inhibition of proteolysis of gelatin of the x-ray film by known amount of trypsin. The assay is done with plasma from the suspected animal. A serial dilution of 0.5 ml plasma was constituted in normal saline in several test tubes to bring about dilutions of TI present in the test material. 0.1 ml trypsin solution (10mg/ml) was added to each test tube, which were incubated at the ambient temperature for 10 minutes (Fig. 9). 20 µl aliquots from each test tube were applied on a 1.5x10 cm. Unexposed x-ray film strip at a distance of 1.5 cm. The strips were kept at room temperature for 10 minutes and washed in running water. Absence of digestion of the gelatin of the x-ray film indicated the presence of TI. When the gelatin was digested, the blue undersuface of the x-ray film was evident as transparent to the bare eye, which indicated absence of TI in plasma.

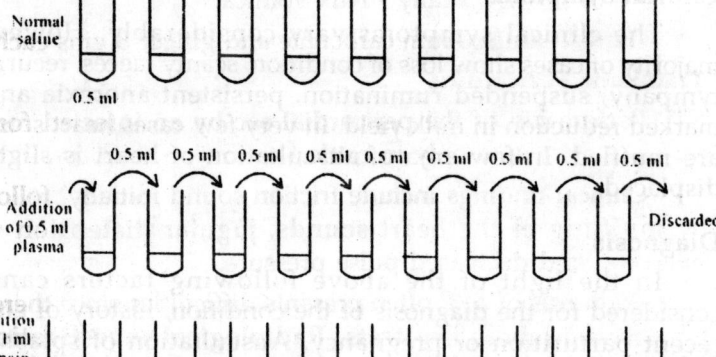

Fig 9. Serial dilution of plasma and addition of Trypsin solution during Trypsin - Inhibition test.

Diaphragmatic Hernia

In recent years diaphragmatic hernia has frequently been reported from all over the country. It is generally an acquired malady characterized by herniation of the abdominal viscera, mostly the reticulum, into the thoracic cavity through a rupture in the diaphragm. Frequency of recorded diaphragmatic hernia is much higher in buffaloes than in cattle. The affection is more common in adult buffaloes, the age varying between 3 to 10 years. Invariably there is a history of recent parturition or the animals are in different stages of pregnancy.

Etiology

Etiological factors of the malady are obscure. Following factors can be considered as the probable cause for diaphragmatic hernia. Heriditary, innate weakness of the diaphragm, traumatic reticulo-peritonitis, trauma, increased abdominal pressure.

Clinical symptoms

The clinical symptoms vary considerably. However, majority of cases show loss of condition, scanty faeces, recurrent tympany, suspended rumination, persistent anorexia and a marked reduction in milk yield. In very few cases heart sounds are muffled. In few area of auscultation of heart is slightly displaced.

Diagnosis

In the light of the above following factors can be considered for the diagnosis of the condition, history of either recent parturition or pregnancy. Auscultation of splashing sounds beyond 6th and 7th ribs. In facilities a plain radiograph will be suggestive of herniation of the reticulum which can then be confirmed by contrast radiography. Lapro-rumenotomy is a sure means of diagnosis of the condition.

Treatment - Surgical

Abomasal Displacement

A condition commonly reported in exotic cattle particularly cows soon after parturition. Immediately following emptying of the uterus on parturition, the rumen gets more space on right side in abdomen and as a result of lying down or changes of position during the bouts of labour pain, the abomasum gets trapped below the rumen and commonly to the left side .

Clinical symptoms

Sudden decrease in appetite which becomes irregular. Faecal volume is reduced and feces are pasty. Secondary ketosis. Ruminal movements present but very weak. An obvious bulge immediately and below right costal area. Rectal examinaiton reveals distended abomasum in the right lower quadrant of the abdomen. In torsion distended tense resilient viscus is palapble. In LDA palpation in the left paralumbar fossa reveal nothing between the body wall and the rumen. Swelling is tympanitic and splashing sounds of its fluid contents may be audible on auscultation. Confirm by aspirating abomasal contents of strong acidic reaction without protozoa by exploratory puncture (Liptak Test) for pH examination, which is usually 2.0. Ruminal fluid will have protozoa and a pH of between 6.0 and 7.0.

Treatment

Rolling and manipulation may be attempted. Cast the cow on back & roll vigorously to the right and give an abrupt stop. This may release the compressed abomasum if the rumen is not very much full. If this is not successful, the condition has to be corrected surgically. In cases of abomasal dilatation Buviopan, injection may be useful.

Abomasal Ulcers

Abomasal ulcers occur in cattle of all ages. The disease is associated with diets high in starch.

Clinical symptoms

Whe examining an animal with abomasal ulceration various clinical pictures are observed based on which ulcers can be classificed as:

Non perforating	Partial anorexia; decreased rumen motility; positive fecal occult blood
Nonperforating with severe blood loss (bleeding)	Partial anorexia; decreased rumen motility, anaemaia, pale m.m.; melena; large blood clots in feces; tachycardia; cool extremities
Perforating with local peritonitis	Total anorexia; low-grade fever; decreased to absent rumen motility; localized abdominal pain
Perforating with diffuse peritonitis	Total anorexia; fever early then hypothermia; ileus of entire GI tract; tachycardia; shock terminally reumbent with grunt on respiration

Diagnosis

The most useful diagnostic test for abomasal ulcer disease is the **Fecal Occult blood test.**

Treatment

Removal of very starchy feed and replacement with good quality hay. Blood transfusions may be necessary in severe blood loss.

Broad spectrum antibiotics are administered with signs of periotonitis.

Use of antacids such as calcium carbonate, magnesium carbonate are recommended.

Peritonitis

Inflammation of peritoneum may be
(i) Acute local
(ii) Acute diffuse
(iii) Chronic with multiple adhesions

A perforating foreign body from reticulum is the most common cause of peritonitis (TRP) in bovines. Whether a foreign body entering the peritoneal cavity will produce acute local or diffuse peritonitis depends on the the type of pathogenic bacteria brought along with it.

A sharp pointed foreign body like a needle may cross the diaphragm and enter thoracic cavity after producing only a local peritonitis which leaves back only a small adhesion.

Other causes of peritonitis
(1) Post operative complication after laprotomy or rumenotomy due to a accidental entry of rumen contents into peritoneal cavity.
(2) Any trauma like punctured wound, resulting from trocarization done without following aseptic precautions.
(3) Rupture of bladder, or perforation of uterus or prolonged and persistant intestinal obstruction in case of paralytic ileus.

Clinical Diagnosis
(i) History of the case is very important.

(Ex. trocarization, laprotomy, retained urine in male bovines, dystokia leading to rupture of uterus, trauma due to accidents etc.)
(ii) **Acute local peitonitis:** Fever, anorexia, signs of pain and tenderness on deep palpation of abdomen. Mild leucocytosis.

(iii) **Acute diffuse peritonitis:** High fever, anorexia, signs of severe pain and tenderness, abdomen tucked up, *facial expressions of the pain distinctly evident, severe leucocytosis and signs of toxaemia.*

(iv) **Chronic peritonitis:** Low grade fever, rapid loss of condition, toxemia, bowel movements very much reduced due to adhesions, persistent indigestion not responding to treatment. Animal becomes unproductive and a liability.

Treatment

Condition better prevented than cured. Use high doses of antibiotics over prolonged period. Long acting tetracycline (*Pfizr or Sarabhai*) with 200 mg/ml concentration be given @ 1 ml per 10 kg b. wt. and repeated on 3rd day. Peritoneal lavage could be attempted. The suggested lavage fluid is 1 to 20 dilution of warmed povidone iodine solution in lactated Ringer's or plain lactated Ringers. The above (3-10 liters) fluid is infused intra peritoneally, allowed to remain for 30 minutes and then drained off such three to four cycles a day are recommended. Initially perform twice a day followed by once daily for 2-3 days more. Treatment is expensive and may be employed in very precious animals. Useful if done in early stage. *No success after adhesioins are formed.*

Enteritis (*Diarrhoea and Dysentery*)

Although a very common and life threatening condition in very young bovines(neonatal calves below 3 to 4 months) diarrhoea is not so common condition in adult bovines. When occurs, it is invariably a sign of parasitic infections (either intestinal worms or liver flukes) or as a result of some feed toxicity or chronic liver disorder or overfeeding. Diarrhoea is a most important and a pathognomonic symptom in certain specific contagious diseases like *Rinderpest , Mucosal Disease Complex, Viral Diarrhoea, Johnes disease, Malignant Catarrhal Fever or Acute Metal Poisonings.* Diarrhoea is the most natural protective response of body to throw out irritant material, toxin etc. It need not be stopped suddenly, unless signs of dehydration are imminent. **Dehydration must be watched and prevented in every case.** Specific case must however be identified and treated.

Diagnosis

The sequential approach to diagnosis of diarrhoea is:

Take history, note change in diet, treatment given and whether diarrhoea is acute or chronic, note appetite, water intake, single or multiple cases.

Perform physical examination. Systemic signs, fever, rumen activity, weight loss, oral lesions. Perform rectal examination.

Examine feces. Gross inspection; note whether blood is present. Microscopic examination for ova and parasites. Culture if animal is febrile.

Take rectal scrapings. Make thin smear on slide for acid fast staining for Johne's disease.

Astrigent Mixtures

(i) **Rx.**

	Adult	Calf
Pulv Creat perp.	30 g	10 g
Pulv Catechu	30 g	15 g
or		
Acid Tannic	15 g	
Kaolin	30 g	15 g
Pulv. Ginger	15 g	5 g
Give in gruel once in 12 hours		

(ii) **Rx.**

Tr. Opi.	30 ml	5 ml
Tr. Zingib	30 ml	10 ml
Tr. Catechu	30 ml	10 ml
Aqua	ad 250 ml	100 ml
Mft: Haust	Sig. once or twice daily	

Any of the following

(iii) **KABJOL** or **DIASTRIN**
powder (*Univ.*)

(iv) **DIASPEL** (Ethicare)   30-50 g   5-10 g

(v) **STOPIT** (Kosmores)   twice daily

(vi) **CATORRHOEA** (*Cattle Rem.*)

(vii) **PESULIN** Bolus -vet (*Cadila*)   3-4 bol. B.D.

In Chronic Diarrhoea (*Rule out Johne's Disease by faecal examination and examination of rectal pinch for acid-fast bacilli* , and parasitic infections by faecal sample examination)

(i) **Rx.**

Ferri Sulph. essci.	4 g
Acid Sulphuric dil.	4 ml
Tr. Zingiberis.	30 ml
Aqua	ad. 200 ml

  Mft: Haust   Sig. Once daily for a week

In chr. incurable diarrhoea with **wasting and debility** homoeopathic drug *Phosphorous* and *Phosphoric acid* or *Croton tiglium* be tried. Tincture of 30 or 200 potency, 5 drops twice a day for 3 to 4 days.

Enteritis: (with primary or secondary bacterial infection)

ANTIMICROBIALS

Inj. **Biotrim** (*Ranbaxy*)	1 ml/ 30 kg b.wt. im
Inj. **Sultrim**	3 ml / 64 kg b.wt.
Inj. **Oriprim** (*Cadila*)	
Inj. **Vesadin** (*Rhon P*)	6 ml / 9 kg b.wt. im or iv

BROAD SPECTRUM ANTIBIOTICS

Inj. Intamox (Intas)   6-10 mg/kg b. wt.

Inj. Conmox (Alved)   2-7 mg / kg b.wt.

Inj. Bacipen (Alembic)

Inj. Mox el *(Alembic)*

Inj. Chlorectin *(Dosch)*   2-4 mg / kg b.wt.

Inj. Neochlor *(Vet-care)*   20-30 mg / kg b.wt.

Inj. Chlorovet *(G.Lucatos)*   4-11 mg/ kg b.wt.

Inj. Enrodine *(Cadila)*

Inj. Floxidin *(Intervet)*   2.5 to 5 mg/ kg b.wt.

Inj. Enrox (Alembic)

Inj. Bayrocin (Pfizer)

Inj. Gyroflox (Indian Immunologicals)

White Scours (*Bacterial Enteritis or* Colibacillosis)

Usually occurs among young calves upto 2 months age. Buffalo-calves highly susceptible. Although a very common bacterial infection caused by **enterotoxigenic** *E. coli.* **Salmonella and Campylobacter and possibly by BVD, Corona and Rota virus** which are ubiquitous in distribution and numerous and antigenically different from each other.

Clinical symptoms

Affected calves reveal dullness, dehydration, enopthalmia, reduced suckle reflex, hypophagia, severe diarrohea with increased frequently, tachycardia, feeble pulse, weakness, convulsions and terminal coma.

Diagnosis

Is based on the isolation of enteropathogens from diarrheic calves. Protozoa and detected by fecal flotation.

Treatment

(i) Any of the astringent mixtures prescribed under 'Enteritis' above as adjunct.

(ii) **Sulpha Drugs** same as prescribed under Enteritis.

    Av. dose; 1-2 boluses (5 g)

Pesulin, Robotran, Cotrimal, Disulf, Oriprim, Wocktrin, Pabadine, Metrofural are the common antibacterials.

Supplement oral therapy with parenteral treatment of 33/1/3% solution of any of the following in severe condition.

Sulphamezathine (ICI), **Vesadin** (*M & B*)

    Dose : 15-20 ml by any route

(iii) Broad Spectrum Antibiotics:

    Same products as prescribed under "Enteritis".

    Doses : 500 mg tablets 1-2 daily 3 days

    soluble powders 15 g B.D. 3 days

(iv) Other Drugs :

VETFUR-TL BOLUS (*Dosch*)	2 boli. B.D. 3 days.
OFZOKIND-01 BOLUS (*Vet Mankind*)	2 bols B.D. 3-5 days.
SULPHADIMIDINE TAB (*Sterling Tab*)	2 tabs. 5 kg. b. wt. daily 3 days.
SORAKAY Vet (*Roussel*) 10-20 ml	TDS 3 days.
SYMOXYL (*Zydus*) Calf bolus (*Amoxycillin*) 750 mg	
KOLIMOX VET POWDER (*Intas*)	5 /100 kg. b. wt. 3-5 days
LORNITAS LIQUID (*Intas*).	5 ml/20 kg. wt. 3-5 days
PESULIN or **ORIPRIM** Bolus (*Cadila*)	
ROBOTRAN BOLUS (*TTK*)	1-2 bolus B.D.
CFLOX-TZ TAB (*Intas*)	1 tab./5-25 kg b.wt. 3-5 days

Fluid Therapy

Ringers lactate is the ideal solution to be used in calf diarrhoea. Caution needs to be taken if there is concomitant hepatic disorders.

Diarrhoeic calves in "shock" state have to be rapidly administrated with required fluids. Veterinarians should periodically monitor the heart rate, respiratory rate and accordingly the flow rate has to be adjusted.

To combat developing acidosis, intravenous infusion of sodium bicarbonate may be adapted, taking care of the cautions and precautions of the therapy.

Oral Fluid Therapy

Whether the etiology of diarrhoea is infectious, nutritional or environmental, oral rehydration has been shown to be effective in calves.

Suggested oral-electrolyte solution for the calves:

NaCl   :   117 g

KCl   :   150 g

NaHCO$_3$:   168 g

K$_2$HPO$_4$:   135 g

Now, add 35 g of this mixture to 250 g of dextrose and 4 litre water.

Management of White Scours

First step in the treatment is to isolate the sick calf and maintain strict hygiene combined with good nursing. Stop Feeding milk.

Feeding with colostrum hastened the recovery from diarrhoea.

Intestinal adsorbents can be given.

Adjunct to antibiotics and antidiarrhoeal

Ecotas bolus (Intas) 2 boli daily for 4 days.

Rumicare (Intervet) ½ sachet once or twice daily.

Boost up Bolus (Dosch) ½ bolus daily for 3 days.

Biobloom powder (Sarabhai zydus) 5 g/day.

Prevention

(i)   Feed colostrum @ 10% of body weight within first 12 hours of birth.

(ii) Apply Tr. Iodine to umbalicus and prevent infection entry.

(iii) Keep floor clean by use of disinfectants.

(iv) Floor should be dry, clean and comfortable.

(v) Utensils of milk and water be cleaned daily.

(vi) Protect from cold winds and rains.

(vii) Avoid overcrowding and isolate sick calf.

(vii) Regular deworming and nutritious diet

Vaccination

Motherhood vaccination of pregnant cows as well as oral vaccination of newborn calves is a common practice for prevention of calf scours in U.S.A.

Scour Guard-3 (K)/C is the vaccine used for healthy pregnant cows and is a liquified preparation containing Bovine Rotavirus, Corona virus,Enteropathogenic strain of *E. coli* (K99)and *Cl. perfringens* type-C antigens which produce antibodies against all and are transferred to the newborn calf via colostrum.

"Calf-Guard " is a oral vaccine used for newborn calves and administered within first 24 hours of birth or as early as possible, and contains Bovine Rota and Corona viruses propogated on cell lines, attenuated and preserved by freeze drying . These vaccines are manufactured by Animal Health Division of Pfizer,New York, U.S.A.

All the above facts emphasise the importance of feeding colostrum to the newborn calf as early as possible after birth to safeguard the life by ensuring the transfer of the maternal immunity against whatsoever pathogens to which the mother cow has had the contact in the surrounding environment so as to offer protection by transferrimg passive antibodies to the newborn calf which it badly needs till it can combat infections himself with his immunocompetent reticuloendothelial system

DIGESTIVE SYSTEM (HORSE)

Approach to Diagnosis

History : The nature and duration of abnormal clinical signs are very important. Any treatment given must be determined. Change in diet should be noted. The breeding history and pregnancy status should also be noted. Enquire about fecal passages last observed, and their consistency. Progression of chemical signs and the response to therapy are most useful.

General examination: Ascertain degree of abdominal distension. Look for evidence of self trauma.

Clinical examination : Record pulse rate and quality, respiratory rate and quality, rectal temperature, mucous membrane moistness and colour, capillary refill time, skin turgor, temperature of the extremities, digital pulses and abdominal borborygmi.

Further a complete rectation be carried out and for this proper restiarnt, as well as tranquilization, if necessary should be practiced. Fever in the rectum should be evaluated for consistency blood or melena, foul odour and mucus. If no feces are present and large amounts of mucus are observed, a prolonged duration of the condition is suggested. In intestinal obstruction, positive anatomic identification of structure is difficult. Absence of borborygmi suggest absence of mobility.

Rule out febrile condition. Examine for distension of abdomen, particularly caecum and colon, palpate to know whether tympany or impaction. Examine faeces. Enquire whether animal is passing stool regularly and rule out obstruction by rectal examination if necessary. For this the animal must be properly restrained by the lifting one of the forelimbs.

Colic

The most important problem faced by horses is colic especially impaction and obstructive. This might be due to frequent change in feed, reduced fibrous content in feed, poor dentition, due to greedy feeding habbit and also due to lack of water which is prime factor in India especially during the dry seasons. The horses usually respond well to the following treatment.

Purgative: Indicated in constipation with moderate colic. Animal dull, off feed, faeces hard and scantly. *No fever.*

(i) **Rx.**

Aloes barb   15 g

Ext. Bellad Sicc.   1 g

Pulv. Gentian   10 g

Oil. Mentha pip.   1 ml

Excipient (*Treacle or wheat flour*) Q.S.

Mft. : Bolus   Sig : Stat

(ii)   Rx

Aloes barb   15 g

Calomel (*Hydrargyri Subchlor*)   2 g

Pulv. Gentian   10 g

Oil. Mentha pip.   1 ml

Excipient : Q. S. **Mft** : Bolus **Sig** : stat

Drench liquid Paraffin in 2 litre

Flatulent Colic

Occurs mostly on succulent green feed. Some secondary
to physical obstruction of large intestine. Severe acute pain.
Visibly distended abdomen. Loud gut sounds present early.
Colic of increasing intensity if distension increases; increased
pulse and respiratory rate, profuse sweating, animal sits on
hauches (*as a sign of gastric distension*). In untreated fatal cases
possiblity of gastric rupture indicated by vomiting and signs of
shock. In case of distension of caecum or colon, there is
distension of right abdomen with resonant percussion. Confirm
caecum and colon involvement by auscultation and rectal
examination. Rule out obstruction and volvulus.

Relieve free gases by passings stomach tube. Attach a funnel
to stomach tube and administer the following :

Rx.

Ol Terebinth   20 ml

Acid carbolic   2 ml

Oil. Lini   300 ml

Mft. Haust   **Sig. Stat**

Analgesics

Inj. Ketop (Alembic) 2-4 mg/kg. b. wt. im or iv

Inj. Esgipyrin (Sarabhai Zydus) 2.2 - 4.4 mg/ kg. b. wt. iv

Inj. Spasmovet (Wockhardt)

Inj. Xylazine 0.1 - 1.0 mg/kg. b. wt. iv or im

43

Antibiotics

Inj. Dicrysticin (Sarabhai Zydus) 2.5 g im

Inj. Duocryst (Kayvet) 4 g im

Inj. Durapent - 48 (Kayvet) 4 g im

Inj. Genster (Sterling Lab) 1-2 mg/ kg. b. wt.

Inj. Metronidazole

Fluid and Electrolyte

Lactated Ringer's Solution

4 - 6 L iv

Promotility Agents

Inj. Perinorn

Inj. Maxeron   0-2.5 mg/kg iv slowly

Inj. Reglan   May be toxic

The response to above therapy should be monitored every hour; for a horse with possible intestinal obstruction; for a horse with probable colonic impaction examinations every 4 hours are adequate; for a chronic colic on examination every day is usual. The following should be assessed:

Behaviour - Severity of pain, frequency and duration of attack, appetite, amount and character of feces and frequency of urination.

Pulse rate - A rate of more than 60/min and a steady rise in heart rate of about 20 beats/min at each hour signal deterioration. A small amplitude, thready pulse characterizes severe shock.

Mucous membrane and CRT: Deep congestion (dark red) or cyanosis (purple) and CRT>2 seconds are indicators of peripheral circulatory failure.

Borborygmi - The disappearnce of intestinal sounds indicates ileus. Ping on ausculation percussion indicates accumulation of gas under some pressure.

Rectal Examination

The empty rectum with mucous signal complete intestinal obstruction. The passage of oil but no feces suggests a partial obstruction.

Feces - Failure to defecate within 12 hours of treatment is a bad sign.

Trocarization

Occasionally is severe cases in which the abdominal distention is impairing respiration, it may be necessary to undertake trocarization which is usually performed through the right paralumbar fossa immedaitely caudal to the last rib. The exact point for trocarization can be located by percussion over the suspected area with finger and auscultaion. The area of loudest ping will indicate the point of insertion of trocar.

Impaction of Colon (*with colic*) confirm by rectal palpation

Rx

Aloes barb	15 g
Aqua ferv (warm water)	Q.S.
Oil Terebinth	60 ml
Chloral Hydras.	30 g
Ol. Lini.	500 ml

Mft: Haust **Sig** : Dissolve Aloes and Chloral Hydras in warm water and shake well with oil of turpentine and linseed oil. Administer as drench slowly.

Spasmodic Colic

Occurs after severe exertion, drinking large quantity of water, lack of nutritious food, excitement and as a reflex effect. Acute restlessness with intermittent bouts of pain. Rolling on the ground, biting, kicking, sweating. *Abdomen not distended.* Rectal exam and feces normal.

Rx.

Chloral Hydras	30 g
Ol. Terebinth	30 ml
Ol. Lini	500 ml
Mft. : Haust	**Sig:** Administer by stomach tube

It is safer to treat by injectable anitspasmodics such as Inj. **Analgin** (*Intervet*) **Spasmovet** (*Wockhardt*), Inj. Xylazine, Inj. Ktop (Alembic), Inj. Esgipyrin (Sarabhai zydus). Drench mineral oil 2 litre orally. A very effective homeopathic remedy for acute

45

and spasmodic colic is Colocynth 30 dose every 15-30 minutes upto 6-8 doses.

Impacted Colic

As the name suggests this is due to a slowing down or stopping of the normal and continous bowel action. This involves a wave motion of the intestinal muscle gradually moving the contents towards the caudal end. The pain is usually mild to moderate and may extend over a few days, with the passage of only a few hard balls of feces.

Treatment

Magnesium or sodium sulfate orally

Mineral oil orally

Obstructive Colic

This may follow impacted colic and indicates a complete stoppage of bowel movement and consequently great pain, which is not relived by treatment.

In the early stages there may be loss of appetite, restlessness and uneasiness. This will soon be followed by mild, moderate to severe bouts of pain, stamping of the hind feet, kicking at the abdomen, looking towards the flank and groaning. As the condition progresses the animal may lie down and then get up again frequently, accompained by rollings and sweating. Additional signs to look out for are the conjunctivae becoming discoloured, the pupils dilated the pulse rate accelerated and increased respiration.

Surgery is the only hope in such a case, but the risk of death due to shock and build up of toxins is great.

In the event of this to counteract shock homoeopathic drug may be tried. Give Aconite 30, 3-4 doses at 10-15 minute interval as soon as symptom appear. Belladona may follow well after a few doses of Aconite. Belladona 30 dose every two hours upto 4-6 doses as necessary.

Chronic Indigestion

Poor appetite, dull appearance, teeth and gums have a dirty brown coating, coat lustreless, faeces pasty with offensive smell,

46

fatigue after exertion. Examine faecal sample to rule out parasitic infections. Record temperature. Examine conjunctivae for anaemia and icterus.

Rx

(i) Tr. Nux. Vom.   10 ml
     Tr. Gentian co.   20 ml
     Acid HCL dil   4 ml
     Aqua   ad 100 ml
     Mft. *Haust*   sig B.D. x 3 days

(ii) Himalaya Battisa (*Ind. Herb*) Any one 30 g B.D. for
                                     6 days.
     or Universal Battisa (*Univ. Ayur*)
     or Digivet (*Charak*)
     or Catone (*Cattle Rem*)

(iii) Liqr. Arsenicalis   30 ml
      Ferri Sulph Excici   20 g
      Tr. Gentian co.   30 ml
      Tr. Zingiberis   30 ml
      Aqua   Q.S.
      Mft : Haust   **Sig.** : Give once daily
                                     mixed with food for 6
                                     days.

Inj, Tribivet (*Intas*)
Inj. Vibejex (*Ranbaxy*)   Any one @ 5 ml im
Inj. Belamyl (*Sarabhai*)   twice a week for 2
Inj. Livadex (*Agrivet-Virbac*)   weeks

(iv) **Liverty** Powder (*Aphali*) or **Valiliv** (*Univ. Ayur*) or
     Tefroli (*TTK*)10 g B.D. for 10 days.

(v) Liv-52 (*Himalaya Drug*) or **Livol** (*Ind. Herbs*) 10 gm.
     powder daily in feed for 10 days.

(vi) **Zigbo** (*Natural Remedies*) bolus 2 once daily or Liquid
     30 ml once daily.

(vii) **Linto** *(Cadila)* Concentrated Liquid 50 ml daily or
     Powder 5 g twice a day.

47

DIGESTIVE SYSTEM (DOG)

Clinical Examination

Diseases of digestive system may affect dogs of any age, sex or bread.

History is very important in differentiating clinical signs associated with different segments of the digestive system, and in planning diagnostic tests. Dysphagia and hyper salivation are the most important clinical signs of the oral cavity disorders. Regurgitation, a common sign of oesophageal disease. Regurgitation should be differentiated from vomiting assocaited with gastric or intestinal disease. The animal should be clinically examined. Abdominal palpation findings of animals with primary gastric disease are usually non-specific. Cranial abdominal pain, distension or mass or the presence of melaena are most consistent with gastric disease. Assess hydration status.

Diagnostic Radiography

Plain and contrast radiographs are valuable when evaluating the stomach.

Endoscopy

Gastroduodenoscopy is useful for diagnosis of gastric disease. It allows direct inspection. Small lesions not detected by radiographs are easily seen with an endoscope.

Simple Indigestion

Appetite reduced and irregular, stools, hard and scanty; dog looks dull, inactive, tongue and teeth have brown coating. *No fever.*

Laxative Mixture (*mistura alba*)

Rx

(i)	Mag. Sulph.	15-25 g
	Mag. Carb levis	4g
	Aqua mentha pip	ad 180 ml
Mft. Mist		**Sig.** 2-4 teaspoonful according to size

(ii) Ext. Cascara sagrada   liq 2-4 ml

(iii) Ol. Ricini(castor oil)   15 ml

(iv) Liquid Paraffin   30 ml

(v)   Milk of Magnesia   (Philips)   30 ml

(vi) Tablets of **Glaxenna , Vaculax** or **Dulcolax** 1-2 tabs.

(Any one of the above may be given for a day or two).

Supoortive: Inj. **B-plex** forte , Inj. **Livadex,** Inj. **Tribivet**

1- 2 ml im alternate day.

Liv- 52 *(Himalaya Drug)* 2 Tab. B.D.

Gastritis

A common condition in dogs. Gastric irritation due to overeating, irritant foodstuffs viral and parasitic infections, drugs and in poisonings. Characterised by vomiting, exacerbated by eating or drinking. Rule out poisoning by enquiry during history taking. Examine the degree of dehydration *(P.C.V. is a good index).* Physical examination usually normal. Diarrhoea may be present.

Consider possibility of Parvo Viral gastroenteritis.

Carry out Endoscopic examination in case Chronic Gastritis with ulceration if it is suspected or to visualize the gastric mucosa.

Treatment

(i)   In persistent vomiting, oral intake of food and water should be withold.

(ii) Dextrose saline is given @ 40-60 ml/kg. b. wt. to prevent dehydration. Lactated Ringers solution is a good alternatvie.

(iii) **Rx**

Gastric Sedatives *(Triple Carb)*

Mag. Carb lev.

Bismuth carb. |

Sod. Bicarb. | 2.0 g each

Mft. Pulv 6 | **Sig .** given 4 hourly

49

(iv) Tablets of **Zyemets , Digene, Gelusil or Almacarb** 1 B.D.

(v) **Polycrol-gel or Digene or Gelusil Liquid or Mucaine gel**   1-2 teaspoonful

In persistent Vomiting

Rx.

Tr. Opii	8 ml
Spt. Chloroform	30 ml
Aqua Mentha pip	ad 180 ml
Mft. Mist	Sig . 2-4 teaspoonful 3 hourly.

(ii) **Inj.Largactil** (*M & B*) 1-2 mg/kg. b.wt.
   Av. Dose : 1-2 ml. of 2.5 % soln.

(iii) **Inj. Siquil** (*Sarabhai*) 0.5- 2 ml
   Tablets of Largactil, Avomen, Stemetil or Siquil.
   @ 25 mg can be given orally twice daily.

(iv) **Inj. Maxeron or Perinorm** 0.25-0.5 mg/kg. b.wt. every 8 hourly.

Hemorrhagic Gastroenteritis (HGE)

Caused by specific canine virus (Paravovirus) is comonly reported. This causes severe vomiting and hemorrhagic diarrohea resulting into rapid dehydration and reduced circulatory blood volume. The packed cell volume gives a good indication of degree of hemo concentration. If PCV is more than 67-70 mm then lactated ringers solution should be given @ 50 ml per lb b. wt. as a slow iv drip till PCV comes down to 40-45 mm. In dysenteric animals where circulating collapse is observed Dextran 40 may be used. When adeuqate electrolytes & glucose are given by injection the oral administration of medicines, food, water etc. should be totally avoided. This prevents vomiting and helps in early recovery. Homoeopathic *Ipicac-30* given at hourly interval has been found very useful in controlling vomiting. Inj. **Stadren, Clauden or Botropase** be given to control intestinal haemorrage. High doses of Vit-C (500mg) given with iv fluids is beneficial. Supportive antibiotic therapy. The vaccine against HGE caused by Parvo virus is available and is incorporated along with Distemper and other vaccines. (*See under Care & Management of pet dog*).

Enteritis (Diarrhoea/Dysentery)

Caused by sudden diet change, incorrect diet, scavenging, in poisonings, due to bacterial, viral, protozoal, and most commonly in intestinal parasitic infestations and toxicities. History and clinical examination will usually indicate whether a dog has a systemic illness and any abnormal findings on abdominal palpation can be confirmed by radiography.

Treatment

Assess dehydration and calculate fluid deficit and maintenance requirement iv Lactated Ringers solution most useful. Oral rehydration fluids if animal is drinking not vomiting.

Withold food for 12-36 hrs depending on severity.

Intestinal Astringent with Antiseptic (*for adult dog*)

Rx.	
Salol	0.5 g
Bismuth Carb.	0.5 g
Tr. Opii camphorata	0.5 ml
Aqua Mentha pip.	ad 10 ml
Mft: Mist	Sig : B.D.

If enteritis with toxaemia, acute haemorhagic diarrhoea.

Give any one of the following:

(i)	Tab. DEPENDAL-M	1 tab. T.D.S. x 3 days.
(ii)	Tab. FUROXONE	1 tab. T.D.S. x 3 days.
(iii)	Caps. IMOSEC—F	1 cap. B.D.
(iv)	Suspn. GRIPTOL	5 ml B.D.
(v)	SPEKTOLE-M Liq (*Inventa Lab*)	5 ml T.D.S.
(vi)	SOFRAKAY-VET (*Roussel*)	5 ml T.D.S. orally

(vii) **NORMET** suspn.	1 Tsp. B.D. for adults.
(viii)**Tab. CIPTAS-L** (*Intas)*	½ to 1 tab. B.D.
(ix) **FUMEDIL** tabs.,	1 T.D.S.
(x) **DYSFUR -M**	Tabs or syrup 6 hourly.
(xi) **LOMOTIL**	2 tabs 6 hourly.
(xii) **Tab. FURADENTIN**	1 ab. T.D.S.

SPOROLAC VIZYCAL, RINIFOL, daily for 6 days is useful in non-specific diarrhoea, and restores intestinal microflora.

Parasitic Enteritis

Is most common and caused by *Toxocara* in young puppies and *Ancylostoma caninum* a common blood sucking hookworm in all age group dogs. Tapeworms *Dipylidium caninum* and *Echinococcus granulosus* has zoonotic potential. Pup may get the infection of Toxocara in utero from its mother if she was heavily infected with worms. These worms cause diarrhoea, with presence of blood, vomition and rapid exhaustion due to anaemia and dehydration. Pups should be dewormed with Piparazine at weekly interval from 15th day till the age of 3 months. Periodical deworming with broad spectrum anthelminitcs such as Mebendazole, Pyrental pamoate, qrazipuentel keeps the worms away. Females should be dewormed preferably before breeding so that pups are born healthy and free of worms.

Diseases of Liver

Liver has tremendous functional reserves and hence signs of liver disease are not clinically recognised early. Clinical signs are seen when nearly 80 per cent of liver is damaged.

Since the liver has so many functions, there are many possible signs of liver disease depending upon which functions are failing to meet the animals need.

Diagnosis of liver disease is not so easy as the clinical manifestations of hepatic disease are often non-specific. While evaluating a patient with suspected liver disase it should be borne in mind that liver disease may be acute or chronic primary or secondary. However, with the aid of clinical history, thorough physical examination and appropriate laboratory tests, the clinican can reach to a presumptive diagnosis.

Clinical Examination

Normally not palpable. Enlarged liver is palpable behind the right costal arch.

Signs of Liver Disorder

(i)   Lethargy, depression. Enlargement in the size with or without pain
(ii) Chronic indigestion, anorexia, constipation and diarrhoea
(iii) Dullness, clay coloured faeces, nervous signs
(iv) Icterus (*Jaundice*)
(v)   Odema, ascites, weight loss
(vi) Abdominal pain

Liver Function test

A wide range of tests are available to decide whether the liver is involved in the disease or not. These tests detect liver disease based on assessment of functional potentials of the organ.

Liver Function Tests Routinenly Used

1. Arginase
2. Alanine aminotransferase (ALT/GPT)
3. Aspartate aminotransferase (AST/GOT)
4. Glutamate dehydrogenase (GLDH)
5. Gammaglutamyl transferse (GGT)
6. Isocitrate dehydrogenase (ICDH)
7. Lactate dehydrogenase (LDH)
8. Sorbitol deydrogenase (SDH)
9. Blood ammonia concentration

Complementary Diagnostic Procedures

1. Radiography
2. Ultrasonography
3. Liver Biospy

Principles of Treatment

(i) Identification of cause and specific therapy (*Example* Liver fluke disease, Leptospirosis & poisonings).

(ii) Feeding easily digestible carbohydrates, sugars and fat free and protein rich diet.

(iii) Dextrose by iv route whenever necessary.

(iv) Good protein supply containing amino acid methionine.

(v) Liver tonics (Liver extracts) and lipotropic factors such as choline.

(vi) Supplementation of vitamins A, B, C, E and K.

(vii) Antibiotics if associated with fever for prevention secondary bacerial invasion because host resistance is reduced.

Treatment

For specific treatment **Refer under specific diseases**. (Fascioliasis, ICH, Leptospirosis and under Poisonings).

(i) Inj. Liver Extract and B-Complex: 5-10 ml as per body wt.

(ii) Dextrose 25% soln. 500-1000 ml for large animals and 50 ml for dogs.

(a) 25 % Dextrose soln. or
   Rintose(*Wockhardt*)

(b) **Liv-52 , Livety, Valiliv,
   Zigbo** powder
   orally as a supportive therapy.

(iii) **Livadex** (*Virbac*)

Belamyl (*Sarabhai*)	(Any one prep.) 1-2
Bivinal forte (*Alembic*)	ml i m for small
Liviplex (*KTS*)	animals and 5-10 ml
Savaplex (S/F forte (*J.P.*)	for large animals
Nutriliv Inj. (*Vetcare*)	

(iv) For Glucose therapy in small animals either 5% dextrose 200-400 ml (as per size of animal) given as a drip or alternatively 25-50 ml of 20% dextrose soln. (available or 25ml. ampule) can be given by slow iv.

(v) Liv-52 drops or **GASTRICARE** (*Himalaya Drugs*) tablets used for dogs and cats.

(vi) **Digeplex** (*TCF*) or **Provitex** (*ICF*), **Vetril** (*Vestas*), **Dexorange** (*Franco India*) or **Livofornai** (*Inventa*) or **Hepatoglobin** (*Raptakos*), **Myprotein, Appatase** (*PCI*) and **Ferrohepatine, Sorbiline** one teaspoon B.D. along with food. This helps in improving appetite by restoring liver function.

(vii) Antibiotics with corticosteroids in diffuse liver disease to control secondary bacterial infection and to prevent fibrosis. Use judiciously and in required doses.

Animal should be given complete rest. Progress be monitored by periodical liver function tests.

Total protein level should be watched carefully and liver soup be given in the diet for small animals as a food supplement.

Chapter 3

Respiratory System

Respiratory disease remains the most economically important disease complex in cattle today. Bovine respiratory disease continues to be the major challenge to the livestock industry.Respiratory infections are more common in young animals in their early life. Incliment weather; feed and water deprivation, exposure to rains and low resistance due to malnutrition, worm infection, crowding and modern intensive management systems etc. are the predisposing factors. Mostly bacterial infections are common. Occasionally viral pneumonia may be encountered. In adult animals respiratory diseases are seen associated with specific diseases like Pasterurellosis, CBPP. Aspiration pneumonia resulting due to faulty drenching is often fatal. Rate of mortality in pulmonary involvement is very high.

Clinical Exam : Careful auscultation is the important method in clinical practice necessary to determine whether the involvement is restricted to URT or has extended to bronchi and lungs. Whether both lungs are involved and how much portion of lungs is affected should be ascertained. Blood exam, particularly leucocyte picture gives valuable indications. Radioligical examination, Bronchoscopy, and aspiration and microbial examination of pleural fluid, form important diagnostic measures in modern medicine in small animals

X-ray Examination : Radiological examination of the chest is most important because many localized and even some widespread infiltrative lesions may produce no abnormal signs. Serial x-rays form an integral part of the estimation of progress in many diseases.

Bronchoscopy : By means of a bronchoscope the main bronchi and their branches can be directly inspected , small portions of tissues can be removed for biopsy, and therapeutic procedures carried out. With the aid of modern flexible bronchoscope very small bronchi can be visualized and the washings for cytological examination from separate lung segments.

Pleural Aspiration : Pleural effusions may be drained by inserting a wide bore needle into the filled pleural space through 6th or 7th intercostal space below the fluid level. Aspiration may be therapeutic to relieve the respiratory embarrassment due to large effusions or diagnostic. To remove fluid for examination the aspirated sample of fluid will reveal it's gross and microscopic features, and thus, assist in the diagnosis.

Cardinal Symptoms: Nasal discharge, cough, alteration in the rate and character of respiration, adventitious sounds on auscultation. Fever depending upon extent of involvement. Rule out specific diseases like H.S. CBPP, CCPP, Distemper etc. In these specific diseases the animal has high fever, dull, has total anorexia, profound depression, soft cough, abnormal abdominal respiration with stiff movements. In upper respiratory tract involvement, the signs are restricted to only nasal discharge and moderate cough. Febrile reaction is also very mild.

General Principles of Treatment

(1) Provide good ventilation and oxygen through fresh air, at the same time avoid direct exposure to wind drafts. *Avoid dry dusty feed,* Give antiseptic inhalations.

(2) Examine for physical obstruction of respiratory passage.

(3) Antibitics- to control primary and secondary bacterial infections.

(4) Respiratory stimulants in case of depressed respiratory centre (*irregular arrythmic breathing with coma*).

57

(5) Expectorants

(A)	Cough painful & Exhausting with tenacious exudate	*Sedative expectorants* Ex : Potassium and Ammonium salts
(B)	Chronic bronchial irritation with soft cough	*Stimulant expectorants* Ex. : Turpentine, Creosote, Eucalyptus
(C)	Spasmodic, exhausting and dry cough	*Anodyne expectorants* Ex., Codeine, Morphine, Belladona

(6) Administer medicines in the form of electurie, boluses or tablets, avoid drenching.

(7) Antihistaminics as bronchodilators, in dyspnoea due to spasm of bronchi and in conditions of allergic origin.

Upper Respiratory Tract (URT) Infections (Rhinitis, Laryngitis, Tracheitis)

Upper respiratory tract infections are most common in young animal and pet animals. Nasal discharge and cough are present in lower respiratory tract involvement also but in URT reaction is mild and general systemic reactions and toxemia are absent. Respiratory distress is mild and only due to blocking of nasal passage with exudate. URT Infections can extend to bronchi and lungs if neglected. Hence attention is necessary.

Antiseptic Inhalations

Eucalypus oil, Ol. Turpentine, Tr. Benzoin co. or Creolin	Add about 30 ml. of any of these in a bucketful of hot water nearing boiling point

Hold the head of animal above bucket. Cover with clean towel and allow the animal to inhale vapours. For young pups **Vicks Vaporub** or **Rubex** can be employed for inhalations. For URT infections associated with fever, severe cough, severe systemic reactions and in pneumonia use any of the following drugs for prevention and control of bacterial infections. Blood examination-particularly leucocyte picture is a useful investigation which helps to know about severity as well as about prognosis.

The selection of proper antibiotic regimen for the treatment of BRD is an important part of the treatment programme. Selection of an effective antimicrobial depends on identification of the pathogen most likely responsible for the disease.

Sulpha Drugs (*quite effective in respiratory infections*)	Dose Rate
Sulphamezathine (*ICI*) 5 g tbs. and 33.33% soln. as injection	1 g /7.5 kg b.wt.
DIADIN (*Pfizer*) 5 g tabs.	Av. First day dose: 30 g
BAIFIDINE (*BAIF*) 33.33% sol Inj.	for adult cattle and horses
SULPHA BOLUS (*Sarabhai*) 5 g tab.	
VESADIN (*M & B*) 33.33% soln.	Half the above dose
VETYDINE (*TCF*) 33.33%.	on second and third day

ORIPRIM-Vet (*Cadila*) 2 g bol. & Inj.	
BIOTRRIM Inj. (*Ranbaxy*) 10 ml vial.	These are long
ROBOTRAN (*TTK*) bolus and Powder	acting sulpha
COTRIMAL (*Alembic*) bolus.	drugs doses are
ANTRIMA (*Rhone P.*) Bolus & Powder	half of above

ANTRIMA (*M & B*) **BACTRIM** (*Roche*) **SEPTRAN** (*Welcome*) and **WOCKTRIN** (*Wockhardt*) also contain long acting sulpha drugs in tablet form.

For dogs and cats sulpha drugs in use for human treatment such as **Elkosin, Oriprim-DS, Maliprim, Bactrim, Ciplin-DS** etc., can be used in dogs but their use be avoided in dogs maintained on non vegetarian diet.

ANTIBIOTICS- (*Narrow spectrum*) PRONAPEN (*Pfizer*) Procaine penicillin 4, 20 and 40 Lakh I.U. vials. CRYS-4 (*Sarabhai*) 20 Lakh I.U. vials. PROCAINE PENICILLIN (*Alembic & H.A.L.*) OMNACILLIN (*Hoechst*) 4 and 20 lakh I.U. with omnadin	**Dose Rate:** 20-40 lakh, I.U. for large animals and 4-8 lakh I.U. for small animals daily for 3-6 days

Long acting Penicillin e.g., **Pendirue** (*Wyeth*) or **Penicillin** in oil (*Sarabhai*), **Longacillin - VET** (*HAL*) Durapen - 48 (Kay vet) are absorbed slowly over a period of 3-4 days and when given in adequate dose, are convenient as it avoids frequent visits.

COMBIOTIC (*Pfizer*) 20 Lakh I.U. and 2.5 g	**Doses**
BISTRTRIPEN (*Alembic*)	Same as Penicillin
VETOPEN (*HAL*)	
DICRYSTICIN (*Sarabhia*)	
DUOCRYST 5.4 gm (Kayvet)	

Strepto-Penicillin preparations

with omnadin as specific antigen.

(4: 0.5) vials for dogs also available.

MUNOMYCIN (*Agrivet*) 20 lakh I.U. and 2.5 g with specific bacterial antigens.

Broad Spectrum Antibiotics

(i) **TERRAMYCIN** (*Pfizer*) oxytetracycline

Injectable sol. 50 mg / ml conc.

10, 30 and 100 ml vials for im or iv use.

TERRAMYCIN -LA (*Pfizer*)

200 mg / ml conc.

Terramycin 500 mg bolus, and soluble powder for oral use.

(ii) **OXYSTECLIN** (*Sarabhia*)

Injectable soln. 50 mg/ml conc. 30 and 50 ml vials for im or iv route, & **OXYVE-LA** (*Sarabhai*) 200 mg /ml conc.

(iii) **STECLIN** intramuscular (*Sarabhai*) Tetracycline Hydrochlor 500 mg Steclin granules and boluses.

(iv) **OXYVET**(*KTS*) and **OCTICIM** (*IDPL*)

(v) **WOLICYCLINE** (*Wockhardt*) Inj. and **WOLICYCINE-DS** 100 mg/ml.

(vi) **HOSTTACYCLINE-**(*Hoechst*) Tetracycline Hydrochlor water soluble powder 100 mg

(vii) **ALCYCLIN** (*Alembic*) Tetracycline Hydrochlor 500 mg bolus

Inj. Enrox (Alembic)

Inj. Floxidin (Intervet)

Inj. Bayrocin (PFizer)

Inj. Gyroflox Indian Immunologicals

Inj. Flobac (Intas)

Inj. Suin Intas (Intas)

Inj. Flobae SA/Inj. Fortuis

2.5 mg - 5 mg/kg. b.wt. im or iv

30ml/400 kg b. wt. single injection by i.m. route.

Inj. Meriflox (Vetoquinol) 15 ml vial

1.5 mg/kg b. wt. Twice daily

5 mg/kg b. wt. iv once daily

Inj. Cflox (Intas), 0 ml/80 kg b. wt. daily

50 ml vial im or iv

Inj. Cflox (Intas) 10ml/80 kg b. wt. daily im or iv

Inj. Cflox powder (Intas), 15ml 300 kg b. wt. daily 15 ml and 50 ml vials

Inj. Tylin (Obcow)

4-10 mg/kg b. wt. im or sc

(viii) **AMPICILLIN** : is a synthetic broad spectrum antibiotic effective against bacteria resistant to pencillin. **Dose rate** : 2-7 mg/kg b. wt.

Prop-Preparations

Inj. **Polbactum** (*Polchem*)

3 g and 4.5 g

Inj **Campicillin- vet** (*Cadila*)

for im vials of 250, 500 and 1000 mg

Inj. **Vetampin** (*Wockhardt*)

Dynacil-vet (*HAL*)

Rosecillin Inj. Vet. (*Ranbaxy*)   500/1000/2500 mg

Bacipen (*Alembic*)   500/ 1000/2000 mg

Ampicillin + Cloxacillin

Inj. AC-Vet Forte (Intas)

　　　　3 g vial

Inj. AC-Vet (Intas)

　　　　2 g vial

Inj. AC-Vet Max (Intas)

　　　　4.5 g vial

Inj. Binocin (Concept)

　　　　500 g vial

Amoxicillin + Cloxacillin

Inj. Moxikind (Vet Munkind)

　　　　2.5 g and 4 g vial

Inj. Conmox (Concept)

　　　　2 g and 4 g vial

Inj. Intamox (Intas)

　　　　3.5 g and 4.5 g vials

Inj. Moxel -D (Alembic) 4 g vial

Inj. Doxmox Forte (Dosch)
　　　　3 g vial
Inj. Inimox Forte (Intas)　　　　7 mg / kg b. wt. im or iv
　　　　3 g vial

Amoxycillin + Sulbactam

Second and Thrid Generation Cephalosporins

Inj. Intacef (Intas)
    1, 2, 3, 4, gm vial
Inj. Intacef Tazo (Intas)
Inj. Moxcef (Alembic)
    2 g vial
Inj. Moxcef (Alembic)
    2 g vial
Inj. Wocef-XP (Vetoquinol)   5-10 mg/kg. b. wt.
    3 g vial
Inj. Seftivet (Indian Immunologicals)
Inj. Polcef (Polchem)
    3 and 4.5 g vial
Inj. Safevet (Dosch)
    3 g vial

Inj. Bovicef (Indian Immunologicals)
    300 mg and 1000 mg vial
Inj. Xnel (Pfizer)   1-2 mg/kg b. wt.
    1 g vial

Alternatives for gram - negative pathogens

Inj. Primicin Vet (HAL)
Inj. Gentavet (PCI)   2-4 mg/kg b.wt.
Inj. Genster (Sterling Lab)

In bacterial pneumonia of any cause, inadequate duration of therapy can lead to treatment failure. The response should be monitored examining especially respiratory rate and temperature. The temperature should be monitored carefully at the cessation of antibiotic therapy. Rest is must during treatment of pneumonia and return to work (in case of bullocks) should be gradual.

COUGH ELECTURIES (*Horse and Cattle*)

(i) **Rx**

Amm. Carb	4 g	Amm. Chloride - 8 g	
Pot. Iodine	5 g	Pot. Chlorate 8 g	
Pulv. Camphor	2 g	Pulv. Anisi - 30 g	
Pulv. Glycerrhizae	30 g	Tracle	Q.S.
Treacle	Q.S.	Mft. : Elect Sig. : B.D.	
Mft. : Elect		Sig. : B.D.	

Pulmonary Emphasema

Is seen mostly in working bullocks in summer, when they are fed only dry and dusty fodder. Due to overdistension and exaggerated respiratory efforts break the alveoli and air escape into sub cutaneous tissues. Secondary infection may occur. Animal looks swollen from all sides with crepitation on palpation. Antibiotics, antihistamine and complete rest advocated. Sometimes a disease of cattle characterized by sudden onset of acute respiratory distress, shortly after a change of forage from dry grass to lush green pasture is encountered. Monensin sodium (**RUMENSIN-60** *Elanco- USA*) @ 200 mg twice daily intra ruminally for 5-7 days has been found effective along with other treatments.

Anodyne Electury (*H & C*) for dry exhausting cough and pulmonary Emphasema

Rx Ext. Belladona sicc	1 g
Pot. Iodide	4 g
Codeine phosphate	0.5 g
Pulv. Glycerrhiza	30 g
Treacle	Q.S.
Mft. : Elect	Sig. : B.D.

CAFLON or **KOFLIX** (*Ind Herbs*) or **CATCOUGH** (*Cattle Remedies*) 25	30 g of any one B.D. as electury

Cough Mixture for Dog and Cat

(i) **Rx**

Pot. Iod.	0.5 g
Tr. Camphor Co.	2.0 ml
Tr. Scilla	2.0 ml
Spt. Amm. Arom.	3.0 ml
Syrup Vasaka	5.0 ml
Aqua	**ad** 20.0 ml
Mft. Haust	**Sig.** 2 teaspoon B.D.

(ii) **Rx**

Syrup Codeine Phosph.	2 ml
Tr. Ipicac.	1 ml
Syrup Tolu or Vasaka.	5 ml
Aqua chlor.	15 ml
Mft. Haust	**Sig.** 2 teaspoon B.D.

Cough syrups like **PHENSDYL** (*Rhone P*), **COREX** (*Pfizer*), **GLYCODINE** (*Alembic*), **BENADRYL** (*P.D.*) 1 - 2 TSF. T.D.S. T -TONE Tablets (Alarsin) 2 B.D. for 7 days.

Analgesics & antipyretics in the form of tablets of *Novalgin, Analgin, Veganin, Crocin, Anacin, Aspro, Coldarin, Coricidin, Nalgis, Nise, Dart,* and decongestant like **Sudafed Actifed** syrup can be prescribed when indicated.

Antihistamine Preparations

Indicated for relieving respiratory distress, bronchial spasm, pulmonary emphysema and in chronic bronchitis.

(i) **ANTHISAN** (*Rhone P.*)   5% sol. 10-20 ml im

  Dog : 2.5% sol 1-5 ml im

  Cat : Vallergan (*M & B*) 1% 1 ml, im

(ii) **PHENARGAN** (Rhone P.)   5% 15-20 ml, im

  Dog and Cat : 0.5 - 1 ml

(iii) **PHENAVEEL** (J.P.) 10 ml, im...... Dog - 0.5 ml

(iv) **AVIL** (*Hoechst*) 10 ml, im.... Dog- 0.5 ml

(v) **CHLORIL** (TTK) 2 - 5 ml, im

(vi) Inj. KAYPHEN (Kay vet) 5—10 m/im Dog 0.5 -1 ml, im

(vii) Inj. ZEET (Alembic) 5—10 ml im Dog 0.5-1 ml, im

(vii) Inj. ANTISTAMIN (Intas) 5—10 ml im Dog 0.5-1 ml, im

For dog and cats, human medicinal preparations like tablets of **Incidal, Trexyl, Cortasmyl, Polaramine, Celestamine, Avil** etc. are very useful antihistamine preparations.

EPISTAXIS (*Bleeding from Nose*)

Is fairly common in all animals and sometimes a very severe problem particularly in large animals. Although it is common in hot summer it may occur at other time also. The capillaries of the nasal mucosa rupture and start bleeding profusely. It is usually a surface bleeding and exact cause may not be known. External injuries, inhalation of irritant vapours, ganulomatous lesions (*nasal granuloma*) or some tumors are the possible causes. Nasal cavity should be examined carefully. See whether bleeding is unilateral or bilateral. Continuous shaking of head, sneezing and movements make the case very difficult to deal particularly in large and ferocious animals. It is sometimes associated nasal Schistosomiasis but granulomatous lesions are observed if nasal cavity is examined and it is basically a chronic condition and examination of smears of the nasal mucosa gives the correct diagnosis.

Treatment- Keep the animals as quiet as possible if necessary by use of tranquilizer like **Siquil, Diazapam or Xylazine.** Apply cold water or ice packs over head and swab of **Stadren drops** or **Botroclot-forte** with **Cadisper-C** 1 T.D.S. useful in small animals.

Inj. **STADREN, CLAUDEN, COAGULEN** or **BOTROPASE** or **ETHASYL, STADREN-V and** with **VIT-K** may be tried in appropriate doses. Head should be held high and ice water be used for slow but continuous irrigation over the head.

Sometimes the epistaxis occurs recurrently in some animals. Following homoeopathic medicines have been found very effective in controlling the epistaxis, and should be tried.

(1) **Hamamelis** (*bleeding with bad odour*)

(2) **Melilotus** (*profuse bleeding*)

(3) **Milefolium** (*blood bright red*)

Tinctures of 200 potency be administered 5 drops orally at one hourly interval and then the interval be increased as the case shows progress. The above 3 medicines can be used simultaneously in case selection of one becomes difficult.

Pulmonary Oedema (moist rales with severe dyspnoea

Confirm by x-ray in small animals)

Oxygen supplementation

Fluid therapy

Plasma or Dextran-40

Frusemide can be tried

Respiratory Stimulants

Indicated in respiratory failure, coma, overdose of anaesthetic, anaphylactic shock etc.

(i) **Oxygen** Cardon dioxide mixture for inhalation along with artificial respiration. (O_2 95% : CO_2 5%)

(ii) **Caffeine citrate :** H & C 1-4 m Dog : 50- 250 mg

(iii) **Nikethamide** (*Coramine*) H & C : 10-25 ml **Dog :** 1 -3 ml

(iv) **Amphetamine** H & C : 200 mg sc **Dog :** 1 - 4 mg /kg

(v) **Cardiazol** (*Laptazol*) Injectable as well as syrup and tablets Dose : H & C 200 - 400 mg Dog : 100 mg

(vi) **Adrenaline** Inj. 1 : 1000

H & C 2 - 4 ml iv **Dog :** 0.1 - 0.3 ml, iv

"2 - 8 ml sc 0.1 - 0.5 ml, sc

(*Do not use in respiratory failure due to the chloroform and Chloral hydrate anaesthesia*).

(vii) Amm. Carb. and Pulv. Camphor as electury.

(viii) Cortisones, *Prednisolone, Dexona, Vetalog, Betamethasone or Decadron in case of respiratory failure due to anaphylactic shock*)

(ix) Artificial respiration should always be tried in small animals.

(x) Camphor in oil (1 in 20) 10 - 20 ml, sc for large animals is the good old treatment.

Chapter 4
Urinary System

Diseases of urinary bladder and urethra are common in farm animals and dogs. Pyelonephritis caused by *Corynebacterium renale* usually occurs as an ascending infection. Nephritis due to *Leptospira* is common in old dogs. Cases of chronic renal failure are commonly detected by canine practitioners.

Attention should be paid to the following points : Quantity, frequency, colour and transparency of urine and the naked eye characteristics of the urinary deposit.

Quantity : The normal quantity of urine passed daily varies widely depending upon the fluid intake. Normally much larger quantity of urine is voided during night hours. A pathological increase (polyurea) occurs in diabetes mellitus and isipidus in dogs, elimination of oedema fluid following administration of diuretics and may be evident in renal failure. Abnormal reduction of urine (oliguria and anuria) may be due to water depletion, in diarrhoea, vomiting,fever or acute diffuse disease of kidney. Complete cessation is uncommon and is a sign of urethral obstruction in bovines and cystic or renal calculi in dogs.

Colour and transparacy : Hematuria and heamoglobinurea need to be differentiated to diagnose the origin of the pigment. Heamoglobinurea gives a coffee or tea colour (a sign of babesiosis if associated with fever). Presence of frank blood is to be confirmed by centrifuging the fresh sample of urine. The source could be from kidney to urethra. Administration of certain drugs also are responsible for urine discoloration e.g., Yellow colour due to tetracycline and B-Complex, Red colour (due to phenothiazine). A urine sample in a test tube may look turbid due to presence of pus, leucocytes, bacteria and phosphates.

Clinical Examination

In case of large animal the clinical symptoms of urinary tract diseases are not easily identified. Examination of urine is therefore more useful aid. In case the urine contains high conc. of abnormal constituents such as pus and bacteria, the palpation of kidneys per rectum for enlargement may be useful. Kidneys are located below the lumber vertebrae on the roof of posterior area of abdominal cavity and can be palpated by fairly anterior exploration. Similarly enlarged ureters can also be palpated by experienced vet. Palpation of bladder per rectum is very useful in male bovines which occasionally suffer from urethral obstruction causing retention of urine. Palpation of urethra may be useful locating the urethral calculus causing obstruction.

In case of females, history of recent parturition with retained placenta, dystocia and uterine infections can easily lead to ascending infection to urinary tract through urethral opening which lies on the floor of vagina. In case of canines urinary tract infections are fairly common.

Leptospirosis cause chronic insterstitial nephritis, particularly in older age group patients. Recurrent fever, pain on lumbar region by palpation, oedema are quite evident in case of infections.

Water intake and urine secretion should be carefully considered. Pain while passing urine should be observed. Haemoglobinuria and myoglobinuria have extra renal causes.

Other Investigations

In small animals urinary system can be examined by intravenous pyelography (*IVP*) wherein a Iodine containing radio opaque dye **UROMIRA** (*Pharmed*) or **CONRAY** is injected by iv route and X-ray films of kidneys, ureters and bladder taken at various intervals and can visualize anatomy of entire urinary tract and the outflow of urine. This examination is useful in detection of pyelonephritis, renal failure and urinary obstructions, cystic claculi, tumors, constriction of ureters etc.

Cystography and Urethroscopy

The interior of the bladder and urethra may be inspected through a cystoscope and urethroscope respectively. The main value of these investigations is in the diagnosis of tumors of the epithelium of bladder and in assessment of disease of the prostate particularly in canines.

Renal Biopsy

This is a rare investigation performed and the specimen is obtained by passing a special needle inserted in the lumbar region. This requires considerable skill and involves risk to the patient.

Clinical symptoms

(i) Pain and dysuria.

(ii) Presence of abnormal constituents in urine particularly albumin, casts, blood, pus cells, crystals and bacteria.

(iii) Oedema and uraemia in terminal stages. (*Estimation of Serum Urea and Creatinine is very useful index*).

Principles of Treatment

(i) Control of infection by judicious selection of antibiotics, preferably after conduction of culture and sensitivity test. Estimation of serum urea and creatinine is beneficial particularly in dogs and gives idea about extent of uremia.

(ii) Continued treatment over a prolonged period (10 - 15 days) at high dose because urinary infections are difficult to eradicate completely. Antibiotics such as **Ampicillin, Nitrofurans and Norfloxacin** are used for a prolonged period. Injectable preparations containing Trimethoprim and sulpha combinations (**Biotrim or Oriprim**) im or iv are quite effective in urinary tract infections in ruminants. **Pyridium** (*Phenazopyidine - Warner*) and **Norbid** (*Alembic*) are the two new antibiotics specially recommended for urinary tract infections, pain and urethral swelling. These should be tried after sensitivity test and for adequate number of days till symptoms disappear.

(iii) Control side effects of drugs, prevent crystaluria and formation of calculi, particularly while treating canine patients. Adequate water intake- if necessary by intravenous Dextrose%, maintenance of alkalinity of urine by administration of Alkasol or Cital syrup is very necessary.

Diuretics

Are not of much use in disease of urinary system and must be employed with caution. These are employed to help excretion of toxic and waste products of metabolism.

Diuretics for Horses and Cattle

(i) **Rx**.

Rx. Phenacetin	4 g
Treacle	Q.S.
Mft. Elect	**Sig**. B.D.

(ii) **Rx**.

Sod. Salicyl	30 g
Pot. nitras	8 g
Spt. Aether Nitr	60 ml
Aqua	Q.S.
Mft. Haust	**Sig**. B.D.

Diuretics for dogs

Rx	
Sod. Salicylas	0.5 g
Pot. Acetas	0.5 g
Spt. Amm. Arom	1 - 2 ml
Syrup	5 ml
Aqua	ad 15 ml
Mft. Haust	**Sig**. T.D.S.

Tablets of APC (4 - 6) or Inj. **Paracetamol** can be used as antipyretic and diuretic.

For ASCITES (*In small animals*)

Inj. **Lasix** (*Hoechst*) 1to 2 mg/ kg b. wt. im

Inj. **Neptal** (*Rhone P*) 1 ml, im

Urinary Antispetics

Indicated in cystitis, urolithiasis, urethritis, post operative in urethrotomy. These are better given along with antibiotic therapy.

Horse & Cattle

Rx

Hexamine	4 g
Sod. Acid phos	30 g
Teacle	Q.S.

Mft. : Haust   **Sig.** : Stat

CYSTONE (*Himalaya Drug*) Powder

H & C : 2 - 3 g T.D.S. for 10 - 15 days

CRYSTONE (Alarsin) tablets

BANGSHIL (*Alarsin*) tablets.

Dogs : 2 tablets T.D.S. x 10 - 15 days

continue at half dose rate for a month

Urinary Incontinence

Involuntary and uncontrolled urination is occasionally seen in canines. This could be due to severe infection, irritation, or due to spinal injury (Loss of neuromuscular control and sphincter weakness).

Treatment: Treat infections after selecting appropriate antibiotic after culture sensitivity test. Give urinary sedatives, course of Vit. B1, B6, B12 injection. In Sphincter mechanism incompetence Testosterone propionate 0.5-1 mg/kg b. wt. 2-3 week im. Oestradiol benzoate 1 mg daily for 3 days then reduce to 1 mg every third day. Homeopathic remedies *Causticum* & *Kreosate* may be tried.

Hematuria (Nepheritis, Cystitis & Urethritis) Confirm by microscopic exam. of urine. Differentiate form haemoglobinuria and myoglobinuria. (by presence of RBCs).

Treat infections first. Give urinary sedatives, Inj. **Stadren, Clauden, R. C. Chrome, Vit-C** in high doses. Homoeopathic drugs *Hammalelis or Cantharis* may be tried.

URINARY SEDATIVES : (In Cystitis & Urethritis)

Horse & Cattle
Rx

Tr. Hyocyamas	30 ml
Sod. Bicarb	30 ml
Aqua	125 ml
Mft .Haust	**Sig** . B.D.

For dogs
Rx

Tr Hyocyamas	0.5 - 1 ml
Sod. Bicarb	1 - 2 ml
Aqua Chloroform	4 - 5 ml
Syrup	5 ml
Mft . Haust	**Sig** . B.D.

Urinary tract infections are moe common in females due to shorter length of urethra and concurrent uterine infections during or after parturition which facilitates entry of infections through urethral opening at the floor of vagina. Treatment of urinary tract infection mainly comprises of judicious use of antimicorbial therapy for sufficient duration. Parenteral Sulphadrugs (Combination of Sulphamethaxazole and Trimethoprim) given in adequate dose are quite effective and in bovines there is no risk of crystaluria. For canines use of **Norfloxacin, Furadantin** or **Ampicillin** is preferable.

Chapter 5

Cardiovascular System

The functional cardiac and cardiovascular diseases are comparatively less common or may be less frequently identified in bovines by the general practitioner. Equines particularly race horses and bullocks used for heavy draft work, do suffer from condition like cardiac dilatation and other decompensatory changes. In canines various types of cardiac and cardiovascular disorders including the congenital abnormalities have been diagnosed with the help of electrocardiography and angiography. Lack of psychological stressors, abundant exercise etc., are some of the reasons why functional and organic cardiovascular diseasea are comparatively less common in domestic animals as compared to human beings. Traumatic pericarditis and myocarditis are economically important conditions in bovines. Probably more investigational approach in near future may be useful in this area.

Symptoms of Cardiac Involvement

(i) Poor exercise tolerance and dysponoea at rest. Arching of back with abduction of elbows (as a sign of chest pain).

(ii) Arrhythmia (Bradycadia and Tachycardia).

(iii) Cardiac murmurs on auscultation.

(iv) Muffled heart beats and splashing sounds indicating pericarditis with effusion or hydropericardium.

(v) Oedema of brisket and extremities, prominent jugular pulsation.

Traumatic Pericarditis

Traumatic pericarditis and myocarditis are the common conditions observed in bovines when the foreign body crosses the reticulum-peritoneum-diaphragm and reaches the heart.

There is usually suppuration and effusion. The pericardial sac contains exudate in significant quantity.

Diagnosis

A definite history of chronic, repeated attacks of indigestion and recurrent attacks of tympanites or impaction with atony of rumen.

Symptoms of chest pain *Expression of pain clearly evident on face.* Arched back, extended neck, abducted elbows and unwillingness to walk, oedema of brisket and prominent jugular vein. A pericardial friction sound is detectable on auscultation of the cardiac area in the first stage. The second stage of effuson is manifested by muffling of heart sounds if gas is present in the pericardial sac each cardiac cycle may be accompanied by splashing sound. Tinking and spalshing sounds are audible when heart beats are increased due to exertion. Animal sits or stands cautiously, voids urine in small quantities with signs of pain while arching of back.

Treatment

Medicinal treatment is of no avail. Pericardial lavage and attempts to remove foreign body may be attempted by experienced surgeon but chances of saving animal are very meagre. Long acting antibiotics in high doses may be employed.

Early diagnosis and rumenotomy could save progress of foreign body.

Special Investigations

Thoracic radiography is essential in the proper assessment of the cardiovascular system and so are considered as part of routine examination. Standard dorso-ventral and right lateral views of thorax give much information.

Electrocardiography and angiocardiography are the investigations to diagnose organic and functional cardio vascular problems in canines. Use of ultrasound evaluation has become useful technique to obtain images of cardiac structures like valves and atrio ventricular flow of blood.

Angiocardiography consists of injecting a contrast material into the chambers of heart,the great veins (aorta and pulmonary artery) or the coronary arteries while serial films are exposed.

Cardiac Arrest (*Acute Heart Failure***)**

Causes

 (i) Sudden and unexpected cardiac arrest during operation involving manipulation of mesentary.

 (ii) Obstruction of respiratory tract resulting in asphyxia and reflex vegal inhibition.

 (iii) Rapid and excess adminstration of anaesthetic or rapid iv administration of hypertonic solution.

 (iv) Existing heart disease and shock.

Symptoms of Cardiac Arrest

 (i) Dark blood indicating cyanosis.

 (ii) Increased rate and shallow respiration.

 (iii) Irregular pulse.

 (iv) Absence of bleeding, dilatation of pupil and coldness of skin.

What to do?

Irreversible brain damage occurs within three minutes of cardiac arrest. Hence **act immediately**.

 (1) Note presence or absence of heart sounds.

 (2) Stop administration of the anaesthetic or iv solutions and administer **Sorbitrate** tablets.

 (3) In case of small animals raise the hind quarters and lower the head.

 (4) Provide pulmonary ventilation by oxygen.

 (5) Artificial respiration and external cardiac massage possible in small animals.

 (6) Inject Epinephrine or Adrenaline 1 : 1000 soln. 1 ml intracardially.

 (7) Open chest massage possible in dogs and cats.

Peripheral Circularory Failure

Causes

(i) Failures of venous return or peripheral vasodilation as in shock.

(ii) Hypocalcemia (*Milk fever*)

(iii) Reduction of circulatory blood volume (CBV) as in excessive haemorrhage and dehydration.

Symptoms

Profound depression, fall in temperature to sub. normal, increased intensity but heart rate feeble. Imperceptible pulse. Skin cold and bloching of mucus membranes. Respiration increased in rate but shallow, coma, clonic convulsions.

Treatment

Clearly identify whether due to vasodilatation or reduced CBV.

Inj. Adrenaline (1 : 1000 soln) 2 - 4 ml, iv for combating vasodilation.

In case of haemorrhage and dehydration restore CBV by blood transfusion. Dextrans like Dextravan 40, 70, 110, 150 as plasma extenders of different molecular weight are available for varying degrees of dehydration. Do not use adrenalin if CBV is reduced as it will cause vasoconstriction and blood flow will be further restricted.

Dexamethasone and prednisolone in high doses

Cardiac stimulants are of no value in peripheral circulatory failure because of the absence of cardiac efficiency.

Heart Tonics

For improving functional capacity of heart muscle. Weakness of myocardium occurs in chronic anaemia, vitamin E and Cu deficiency, certain poisonings, effect of FMD virus and in B.Q. cannot sustain excessive exercise. Slight exercise causes excessive increase in heart rate. Dilatation of heart occurs as a compensatory effect (increase in area of cardiac dullness). Arrhythmia, auricular fibrillation and systolic murmur.

Heart Tonics (*In Congestive Heart Failure*)

Horse & Cattle

Rx

Tr. Digitalis	8 ml
Tr. Nux Vom	16 ml
Tr. Zingiberis	30 ml
Aqua	ad 125 ml
Mft . Haust	**Sig**. once daily for 8 days

Digitalis is still the most accepted drug for correcting functional heart diseases.

Inj. Lanoxin (Burroughs Wellcome) contain Digoxin 0.5 mg/2ml

Horse : Initial iv loading dose of 1-1.5 mg/100kg

Followed by a maintenance dose of 0.5-0.7 mg/100 kg every 24 hours.

Cattle : Initial iv loading dose of 2.2 mg/100 kg

Followed by 0.34 mg/100 kg every 4 hrs.

Dog : Emergency digitalisation - 0.05 mg/kg bwt P.O.

Rapid digitalisation - Loading dose of 0.05-0.20 mg/kg b. wt. to be given orally in divided doses over 48 hrs. Slow digitalisation - 0.02 mg/kg b.wt. daily in divided doses for a period of one week.

Horse & Cattle

Rx

Tr. Scilla	15 ml
Tr. Digilalis	10 ml
Mft. Haust	**Sig**. once daily for 8 days.

Dog :

Rx

Tr. Scilla	0.5 ml
Spt. Amm. Arom	1.5 ml.

Syrup	10. 0 ml.
Aqua	ad 20.0 ml.
Mft . Haust	**Sig . B.D. for a week**

Haematinics (*In iron deficiency anaemias*)

Indicated in anaemias. Confirm by haemoglobin estimation and watch the improvement by periodical estimation.

Horse & Cattle

Rx

Ferri Sulph Exsci	5 g
Copper Sulph.	0.2 g
Cobalt Sulph.	0.2 g
Treacle	Q.S.
Mft . Elect	**Sig. one daily for 10 days.**

Tab. Cofecu

Inj. Ferritas

Inj. Imferon with B12 -H and C 10 ml im every 10th day. **Dog** : 3 ml im every 10th day. Sometimes anaphylactic reactions are reported with iron dextran which may prove fatal.

LIVOFORINA (*Inventa*) Liquid - 30 ml daily can be given to horses orally as haematinic and liver tonic.

For Dogs :

Rx.

Ferr. et. Amm. Citr	5 g
Syrup	20 ml
Aqua	ad 125 ml
Mft . Mist	**Sig . One teaspoonful BD.P.C.**

FERRADOL, or **TONOFERRON** or **MINOLAD** (*TCF*) or **LIVOFORINA** (*Inventa*), or **SHARKOFERROL** (*Alembic*) **DEXORANGE** etc. 1 teaspoonful B.D. with food.

Fesovit Capsules Rediplex tabs 1 B.D.P.C.

Advice Liver soup in the diet.

(Several other haematinic preparations are available in market)

Blood Transfusion

Very useful and can save animal in emergencies of haemorrhage and shock as well as in extensive haemolytic anemias (*Theileriosis, Anaplasmosis*) when hemoglobin level goes down below 4 g%. Blood transfusion is also useful in conferring passive immunity.

Cross-Matching: Cross matching not essential for first transfusion in cattle. In dogs blood should be tested for A-group if time permits. (*A - negative recipient whereas A positive recipient can receive blood from donor*).

Donor's RBC should be tested in recipient's serum in test tube. No haemolysis should occur in 30 minutes. Recipient's RBC and also be likewise tested in donor's serum, but the first test is more important. Cross matching must be done if the recipient is being given more than one transfusion.

Procedure

Collect blood in a sterile autoclaved saline bottle containing 3.85% soln. of sodium citrate @ 10 ml for each 100 ml blood to be collected. ACD bottles or blood bags used for human blood collection could be used. Blood is to be collected from jugular vein using a wide bore needle or a cannula.

Rate of bleeding for transfusions : @7 ml/kg b. wt. Av 2-4 liters in cattle, for Dogs. : 5 ml. /kg Av. : 100 ml.

Keep the bottle rotating while blood is received on the inner wall of bottle to prevent frothing. Blood can be stored in refrigerator at 4^0C for a week. It can be stored for nearly 21 days for use in emergencies. There is no bad effect except some haemolysis.

Transfusion should be done after bringing blood to body temperature, by iv route.

In some cases the recipient shows restlessness and shivering. Reaction can be controlled by antihistamines. Exceptionally, reaction occurs 10-14 days after transfusion but the reaction is mild and controllable.

Animal Blood Bank is established in Maharasthra Animal and Fisheries Science University (MAFSU), at Mumbai and Madras Veterinary University (TANUAS) the protocol for blood and blood component therapy has been standardised.

Chapter 6

Nervous System

Symptoms of Nervous System Disorders

(i) Change in temperament

(ii) Excitation (*Violent movements, fury*) or

(b) Depression (*Drowsy appearance, head pressing, unconsciousness*)

(ii) Involuntary movements (*convulsions, tremors*)

(iii) Abnormal postures and gait (*Circling, inco-ordination*)

(iv) Paralysis (*sensory or motor*)

(v) Loss of control on anal sphincters , bladder, atony of bowels due to vagal injury

Types of CNS Syndromes

(a) *Increased Intracranial pressure:* Animal is dull, drowsy, head lowered and head pressing, moving in circles etc.. While removing CSF from post occipital site the CSF comes out in the form of a jet.

(b) *Cerebral Syndrome :* Impaired vision, stiff gait, nodding of head, reduced reflexes.

(c) *Cerebellar Syndrome:* Animal balances itself with legs wide apart, incoordinatin of gait, reluctance to walk, paralysis of varying degree, tremor.

(d) *Base of Brain Syndrome :* Pressure paralysis may occur most probably due to trauma *(sudden occurrence)*, gradual development *(growing tumor, abscess or protrusion of intervertebral disc)*. There may be partial or complete loss of sensation and motor function of the area which receives nerve supply from specific branches.

Clinical Examination

The veterinary physician has to depend on the objective symptoms only. Observation by the owner as well as by the physician can bring out symptoms about the change in behaviour, restlessness, mode of walking, dashing against objects due to blindness etc. In country like India, possibility of rabies must always be thought of while dealing with a case of any type of CNS involvement because the reliable history of dog bite (for bites in case of cattle going in forest areas for grazing) is not always reliable and rabies is widely prevalent.

Protective gloves must be used while examination of buccal cavity of all animals-specifically in dog patients. Specific diseases such as **"Surra", Listeriosis, botulism, poisonings "metabolic disorders"** *(nervous form of ketosis, myoglobinuria, acute hypocalcemia, hypomagnesimia with tremors should be ruled out).*

Testing Sensory and Motor Functions

Sensory Functions: Assess Corneal reflex, panniculus reflex (prick method), pain, temperature.

Motor Functions : Assess bulk of muscles, tone of muscles, strength of muscles, reflexes, coordination of movement, gait and involuntary movements.

Special Investigations

The following special methods of investigations are in common use:

Examination of Cerebrospinal Fluid (CSF)

This forms a special examination and is valuable in certain conditions.

Sites For CSF Collection

(1) *Post Occipital* : Animal has to be sedated and restrained appropriately. *This site is convenient in case of dogs.* Head is bent forward & downward as much as possible, with proper restraint. Site is prepared by shaving and disinfected. A sharp beveled pointed 10 -15 cm long needle with 1.5 mm bore diameter is used for cattle. The needle

is inserted in the midline, behind the poll below the occipital in the foramena magnum. Injury to nerve tissue and infection should be avoided. If the site is correctly approached clean CSF appears through the needle with moderate force (like a jet in case if intracranial pressure is increased). The CSF should be aspirated with dry sterile syringe and collected in a vail. For dogs use 3" long 20 gauze needle. Needle size in dogs shall depend on the age and size of animal. In all cases use brand new needle and a carefully sterilised one (preferably disposable and sterile).

(2) *Lumber Site* : This site is more convenient in cattle and CSF can be collected while animal is restrained in standing position. If the animal cannot be stable, it may be casted down and controlled. The site is in the midline between two tuber coxae, in the hollow between the spinous process of last lumbar vertebra and the sacrum. Needle is inserted first vertically and then slightly oblique with gradual forward and backward adjustment, the CSF appears as a clear drop of fluid which should be aspirated by syringe.

CSF is examined for protein contents (*Pandy's test*), cell count, glucose, smear exam for bacteria, tryps and if necessary other investigations may be carried out depending upon the case.

The Electroencephalogram (EEG)

Electrodes applied to the patient's scalp pick up small changes of electrical potential, which after amplification are recorded on the paper. The EEG is of particular value in the investigation of epilepsy and in localization of cerebral tumors and other expanding intracranial lesions.

Myelography

This is a method of demonstrating the subarechnoid space in the spinal canal. A lumbar or cisternal puncture is performed and a spinal radiopaque medium is injected in the subarechnoid space . This is a very useful method for accurate localization of tumors in the spinal canal.

Computerised Axial Tomography (C T scanning)

The CT scanning provides tomographic sections of the brain of very high resolution, without the need of contrast procedures. A crystallographic X-ray detection device is used instead of conventional X-ray film and a photographic picture is produced by computerized imaging techniques . The method gradually reduces the need for encephalography and angiography

Principles of Treatment

(1) Specific treatment in specific diseases. (i.e.,Trypanosomiasis, Listeriosis, Nervous form of Ketosis and other metabolic disorders).

(2) Antibiotics for control of infections. However, blood brain barrier makes the situation difficult.

(3) Intracranial pressure of fluid can be relieved by iv Inj. of hypertonic solutions or diuretics.

(4) C.N.S. depressants.

(5) C.NS. stimulants.

CNS Depressants (Cattle and Horses)

Indicated in nervous excitement, epilepsy, hysteria, tetanic convulsions and seizures for example in strychnine poisoning etc.

Rx.

(i) Chloral Hydras	30 g
Aqua	125 ml
Oil Lini	500 ml
Mft : Haust	Sig : Stat

Rx

(ii) Amm. Bromide	
Sod. or Pot. Bromide	4 g
Treacle	Q.S.
Mft : Haust	Sig : as required

(iii) Chloral hydras 30 gm in 200 ml distilled water can be given by slow iv route.,

(iv) Inj. **Largactil** (*Rhone P.*) 1 mg/kg b. wt.

6 -10 ml. of 5% sol. im for cattle

(*Produces irratic results in equines hence not used*)

(v) Inj. **Siquil** (*Sarabhai*) 5 mg/100 lb b. wt. ml im or iv

(vi) Inj. **Anazepam** (*J.P.*) 4 - ml/100 kg b. wt. im

For Dogs :

Inj. Largactil (*Rhone P.*) 25% soln.

1- 2 ml im or iv or tablets 25 mg B.D.

Inj. **Diazepem** (*Anazepam or Calmpose*) 0.025 mg/kg b. wt.

Inj. **Siqul** (*Sarabhai*)   20 - 40 mg sc or iv

Siledin (*Alarsin*) tablets   2 T.D.S.

Gardenal (*Rhone P.*) 1−2 mg/ kg b. wt. p.o.

(*Dose to be adjusted in individual cases*)

"**Duodil**"or"**Muraxyl**"tablets as antipyretic and tranquilizer.

Tranquilizers used in human medicine can be suitably employed for dog. Ex. : **Dilentin caps, Sedonol, Equanill, Valium** *or Calmpose tablets, Intravel sodium (Rhone P.)* can be administrated by slow iv injection for profound sedation @ 25-30 mg per kg body weight (0.5 gm. in 20 ml distilled water for an average adult dog weighing 20 kg).

Epilepsy in dogs (*Convulsions & Seizures*)

Is fairly common and the tiology is not precisely known. Frequency and duration of epileptic fits varies. The diseases of CNS should be ruled out and treated. Treatment is required to be given over a long duration. Anticnvulsants (barbiturates and allied compounds) are widely used. Doses are to be regulated in individual cases.

Ex. **Dialentin Caps** (P.D.) 100 mg

Epileptin (*IDPL*) 100 mg Caps

Epilex (*Reckits*) 200 mg Caps

Epsolin (*Cadile*) 100 mg tabs

Mysoline (*ICI*) 250 mg tab.

85

Phenytoin (*Samarth*) 50 mg tab.

Any of these compounds may be used after computing doses as per individual case.

Ignatia 30 is the homeopathic drug which is worth evaluating in the condition.

Nervine Stimulants & Tonics

Indicated in various types of paraplegias, weakness, depression, atony of bowels due to autonomic dysfunction, after anaesthesia and in certain CNS depressant toxicities.

Rx

Caffein Citrate H and **C** : 2-4 mg, sc

Dog : 50 - 250 mg

Amphetamine H and **C** : 100 - 300 mg

Dog : 1-4 mg/kg b. wt.

Leptazol (*very useful to counteract effects of barbiturates*)

H and **C** : 0.5 -1 g **Dog** : 50 - 100 mg

Nikethadine (*Coramine - Ciba*) better for counteracting chloral hydrate and morphine.

H and **C** : 10 - 25 ml **Dog** : 1 - 3 ml

Strychinine Hydrochloride (*Spinalcord stimulant*)

H and **C** : 15 - 60 mg **Dog** : 0.3 - 10.0 mg

(Dog is highly susceptible)

Liqr. strychnine Hydrochlor

4 - 8 ml for horse and cattle to be given orally or i.m.

Rx

Tr. Nux Vom	15 ml
Liqr. Arsenicalis (*Fowler's soln.*)	30 ml
Aqua	Q.S.
Mft . Haust	**Sig.** once daily for 7 days.

Inj. **Tonophosphan** (*Hoechst*) or Inj. **Hivit** (*Ranbaxy*) or Inj. **Cobaphos** (*Agrivet-Glaxo*) **H** and **C. 10-20 ml sc or iv**

Dog. : 1 -3 ml being a phosphours compound, is useful in stimulating motor activity.

Calcium preparations e.g., **Calboral** (Rhone P.) or **Calmex** (*Ranbaxy*) are commonly employed as nervine stimulants.

Inj. **Thiacal** (*Wockhardt*) a calcium preparation with thimine is also useful in large animals.

Calcium (*Sandoz*) 5 - 10 ml for dogs.

Vit B_1 B_6 B_{12} (*Glaxo*) **Vibejec** (*Ranbaxy*) or **Triradisol-H**, **Neuroxin-12** (*Cadila*), **Tribivet** (*Intas*) or **Neurobion** Injections commonly employed in dogs. **Aristoneuron** capsules 1 B.D. for 10 days are also recommended for dogs.

Chapter 7

Musculoskeletal System

The locomotor system includes the muscles, tendons, bones and the joints.

Bones : For examing the long bones of the limbs, look for any alteration in shape, or outline, for localized swelligs in the bone, for signs of fracture and for evidence of undue pain. Alteration in the shape of bones occurs in rickets. Localized swellings may occur in infections, cysts and tumors.

Joints: These must be examined while inspection and palpation for the range of movements, for enlargements or irregularity for redness, pain and heat and also note whether the overlying skin is moist or dry. In case of enlargement determine whether it is due to effusion in the joint space and if tenderness is identified try to localize the accurate point.

Gait: Make the animal walk away from you, turn around and walk towards you. Note if the alteration is due to local lesions or of a neurological origin.

Synovial Fluid Examination

In inflammatory lesion and trauma the synovial fluid may get accumulated and make the joint painful on palpation. If the condition becomes chronic, the synovial fluid needs to be examined for inflammatory cell count, turbidity and presence of bacterial infection.

The common conditions are myositis; sprain of muscles and tendons, rheumatic muscular pain, stiffness of gait and lameness. *Rule out fractures.*

Local applications with Liniment Ammonia in Cattle and Horse. **Relaxyl** or **Iodex, Sloan's Liniment,** or **Rumalaya** cream, **Diathermy** for dogs and small animals.

Rx. Inj. **Analgin, Savalgin** (J.P.) **Ronalgin** (*Ranvaxy*), **Valginate** (*TTK*)

H & C : 10 - 20 ml im **Dog** : 0 .5 - 1.0 ml Inj. **Esgipyrin** (*Sarabhai*), as analgesic and antirheumatic or antiinflammatory, **Proxyvet** -DS (*Wockhardt*) **Inj Melonex**(*Intas*) is a new product to reduce fever, pain and inflammation.

Rx Sod. Salicylas	30 g
Pot. Iodide	2 - 3 g
Treacle	Q.S.
Mft. Elect	**Sig.** B.D. for 4 - 6 days

Inj. Sod. Salicylas with Sod. Iodide 20 ml iv for large animals once or twice a week.

Rx R. COMPOUND (*Alarsin*)

H & C : 10 tablets. T.D.S. x 15 days

Dog : 2 tablets T.D.S. 15 days

RUMALAYA (*Himalaya Drug*)

H & C : 8 - 15 Days

Dog : 1 tab. T.D.S. for 15 days

Homoeopathic Remedy : **Rhus tox** 200 x tincture 5 drops B.D. for 3 days. In Sprains and contusions : **Armica 200 x** tincture as above.

Arthritis

In addition to above treatment, the following may be tried. Infra - red fomentation useful.

Rhus tox - 200, twice day daily as homeopathic remedy be tried.

Inj. Maxxtol (Intas) C4B 4 mg/kg b. wt. im or iv single dose or 2 mg/kg b. wt. to be repeated a after 48 hrs.

Inj. Phenybutazone

H & C : 9 - 12 ml im or 1- 2 day.

Dog : 2 - 3 ml. im

Tabs Triaction, Esgipyrin, Suganril, Oxy-P, Ibugesic, Flamar-P, Emflam-200, 400 or Dolonex, 1.B.D. should be tried for 3-4 days in case of dogs and small animals. Several products with similar composition are available.

Inj. **Prednisolone** (*Hoechst*), **Decadron** (*MSD*), **Vetalog** (*Sarabhai*), or **Dexona** (*Cadila*) - 1-2 ml into the joint capsule.

Strict aseptic precautions are necessary.

Radial Paralysis

Paralysis of forelimb (one or both) and inability to bear weight occurs in cattle when casted down for a long time or due to falling down of animal, the radial nerve gets pressed and resultant paralysis occurs.

The condition usually responds to massage with liniment ammonia, fomentation and injections of **Tonophosphan, Inj. Tribivet,** and **Neurobion.** Some cases take a very long time to recover and create a very awkward situation for the veterinarian if radial paralysis occurs due to casting of animal.

After ruling out fractures, dislocation and tendon rupture the condition can be treated by perineural injections of Vit B1 or a mild irritant such as Inj. **Terramycin** at various sites along the course of radial nerve on the inner aspect of arm. This usually causes rapid recovery and animal gets up within a few hours.

Muscle Relaxants

Indicated for relieving the tetanic spasms of skeletal muscles and in combination with general anaesthesia.

(1) **TUBARINE** (*BW*) (*Tubocuraine Chloride*)

(i) Miscible Inj 15 mg in 1-5 ml suitable for combination with thiopentone sodium at the rate of 1 mg per 0.5 ml of 5% solution.

(ii) Stabilized inj. 50 mg / 5ml

Dose : To be computed in individual cases as per b. wt. initial dose 10 - 15 mg iv

(2) **MIDARIN** (B.W) (*Succinyl choline chloride*)

For transient action can be mixed with thiopentone sodium or by slow drip for prolonged action.

Dose - 30 - 100 mg iv to be computed in individual case under observation.

(3) **FLAXEDIL** (*Rhone.P*) (*Gallamine triethiodide*)

For iv use Dog : 1 mg/kg b. wt.

Chapter 8

Diseases of Skin

S kin and hair coat are the protective coverings of body. Smoothness and shining of body coat is an indication of good health and nutrition. Occurrence of skin diseases and ectoparasites is an indication of unhygienic management and negligence on the part of owner. It also indicate malnutrition and deficiencies. The disease of skin could be either due to parasitic infections (*mites, fungi or bacteria*) or due to nutritional deficiency of some kind or due to allergic reaction. Chronic skin diseases are also indicative of reduced vitality and resistance. Depigmentation or hyper pigmentation can occur due to hormonal imbalances.

For the examination of the skin one should seek the presence of any eruption. It must be remembered that every cutaneous eruption consisting of a primary lesion, to which a secondary lesion may or may not be superadded.

Primary lesions: Macules, papules, vesicles,pustules, weals, burrows, plaques, and scales.

Secondary lesions: These are either produced mechanically or are as a result of changes which take place in primary lesions in the course of it's growth or decline. The commonest of the secondary lesions of mechanical production are excoriations due to scratching and fissures.

The following are the secondary lesions produced by changes in those which are primary : Infiltration, richenifaction, dyschromia, ulceration, scar formation.

Proceed now to palpation of the skin and note the following points : whether it is smooth or rough, thin or thick, dry or moist? The elasticity of skin should be assessed.

The condition of the subcutaneous tissue should also be assessed, presence of oedema, subcutaneous emphysema should be looked for.

Microscopic examination of skin scrapings could be a good beginning point and *must* always be done to establish the causative factor. In chronic lesions complicated with bacterial infection, the culture and sensitivity test proves useful.

The distribution of skin lesions is of a great diagnostic importance. The lesions may be discrete, circumscribed, patchy or diffuse. Identify the causal agent by examination of scrapings if necessary. Note whether accompanied with pruritus (*itching*) or pain. Rule out allergic eruptions (*Urticaria*). Note whether primary or secondary.

General Principles of Treatment

(i) Isolate the animal (If infectious cause suspected).

(ii) Clip the hair and remove debris so that topical applications would come in contact with lesions.

(iii) Prevent secondary bacterial infections.

(iv) Control itching and extensive injuries caused thereby, by administration of sedatives and ointments containing anaesthetics.

(v) Prevent dehydration from extensive lesions by electrolyte and fluid therapy and anti-histaminics.

(vi) Ensure diet rich in protein-particularly sulphur containing amino acids.

Dermatitis with Bacterial Invasion

(*Pustular dermatitis & Pyoderma*)

Apply one of the following ointments after thorough cleaning and drying of the lesions.

(i) **TERRAMYCIN** ointment (*Pfizer*)

(ii) **SAVLON** (*ICI*) antiseptic cream

(iii) **CAMBISON** ointment (*Hoechst*)

(iv) **HIMAX** ointment (*Indian Herbs*)

(v) **Antiseptic cream** (*Rhone P.*)

(vi) **VEGECORT** ointment (*Himalaya Drugs*)

(vii) **VETCREAM** and **VELTON**

(viii)**FURACIN** (*SKF*)

(ixi) **SOFRAMCYIN** - Vet cream (*Roussel*)

(x)   **PIVIPOL** (*Kosmorex*) liquid.

(xi) **BETADINE** (*Natural Rem*) cream.

(xiii)**HEALMAX** ointment (*Sunrise*)

(xiv)**CHARMIL** (*Dabur*)

Parenteral antibiotics in combination with local application would speed-up recovery. In obstinate cases culture and antibiotic sensitivity test of exudate should be done.

Inj. **MUNOMYCIN** (*Glaxo*), **OMNAMYCIN** (*Intervet*)

For **Allergic Dermatitis**

(**Urticarial eruptions with itching and rash**).

Inj. **SIOLAN** (Milk with Iodine)

PHENARGAN Cream (*Rhone. P*)

ANTIHSAN Cream (*Rhone. P*)

BECLOMAC-N ointment (*Liva*)

BECALTE - C or **N** (*Cipla*)

Supplemented by parenteral antihistamine therapy.

For controlling intense pruritus (itching).

Xylocain ointment or **GESICAIN** ointment.

VEGECORT ointment (*Himalaya Drugs*).

Inj. **Largactil** (*Rhone P.*) or **Siquil** (*Sarabhai*) for controlling irritation and injuries.

Eczema

Eczema is of allergic origin. Exact etiology is not known. It may be dry or moist. Cause may be dietetic in origin. Feeding excess carbohydrates is a common cause in dogs. Some foods, meat, beef, milk etc. are sometimes responsible. Try a change in food.

For Eczematous Lesions

Rx.

Acid Salicylic 2 g	Inj. Placentrex (*Albert David*)
Acid Tannic 2 g	2 ml im once week may be tried.
Spirit 30 ml	
Mft . Lotion	**Sig.** for external application.

VEGECORT ointment or **HIMAX** ointment (*Ind. Herbs*) **Caladryl** lotion (*PD*) may be also be tried. Ointments containg corticosterioids and antibiotics are largely used in pet dogs. (*Beclate-N, Kenalog-S etc*). Efforts be made to improve nutrition and correct deficiencies including that of selenium.

Dermatomycosis

Circular, raised, asbestos like lesions common in calves. Caused by *Tricophyton* and *Microsporum spp. of fungi*. The typical circular lesions may not always be seen in dogs. There is loss of hair. Confirm by exam. of scrapings or with the help of Wood's illumination lamp.

Rx

Acid Salicylic	2 g
Acid Carbolic	2 g
Vaseline	30 g

Mft . Ointment (*Do not use in dogs*)

Strong **Tr. Iodine** applied after scraping the lesion thoroughly is also effective.

Any of the following antifungal preparations should be used for topical use :

MULTIFUNGIN oint. (*Boehringer*)

DERMOQUINOL cream (*East India*)

MYCOSTATIN oint. (*Sarabhai*)

FARIDERM lotion (*Walter Bush*)

SPECTRAZOLE cream (*Ranbaxy*)

TINADERM soln. (*Fulford*)

ZOLE lotion (*Guffic*)

Internally any of the following preparations containing Griseofulvin could be given :

GRISOVIN (*Gllindia*)

IDIFULVIN (*IDPL*)   3 tabs. O.D. x 10 days for **calves**
MCORAL (*Plasma*)   1 tab O.D x 6 weeks for **dogs**
                          (Depending on body weight)

Copper sulphate- unslaked lime spray in case of herd problem in bovines. Agricultural Bordeaux mixture.

Scabies

A most common skin disease of all domestic animals.

Caused by mites of *Sarcoptes* and *Psoroptes sp.* Infection can be transmitted to man.

Symptoms

Clinically intense pruritus even to the extent of causing bleeding, erythematous lesions, loss of hair and secondary bacterial infections. Confirm by exam. of skin scraping.

Treatment

Isolate the animal. Clean the lesions by use of soap water after clipping the hair.

(i)   **Golden Lotion** (See under Lotions)

       For external application twice daily. This is a good old and very effective treatment.

(ii)   **ASCABIOL** Lotion (Rhone P) to be applied with brush at 2 - 3days internal. Do not use in cat.

(iii) **GAMASCAB** lotion (Nulife)

(iv)   **TETMOSOL** lotion (Nulife)

(v)   **SCABIEZMA** lotion.

(vii) Inj. **SCABIEZMA H** and **C** : 4 - 5 ml, sc twice weekly Dogs: 1 - 2 ml, sc twice weekly.

(vii) Inj. **IVOMEC** (Ivermectin- MSD) found very effective 200 microgm/kg b. wt. or 1 ml 50 kg b. wt. sc once weekly till the resolution of lesions.

(ix)   Homeopathic "*Sulphur*" 6X to be given orally for 6-8 days.

(x) Herbal preparations : Ointments prepared from extracts of garlic, neem leaves or seetaphal leaves in the medium of vaseline or coconut oil have been proved useful.

Supportive : Use Antihistamines. (See page 54).

Demodicosis

Caused by *Demodex spp.* which are deep burrowing mites. Infection difficult to cure. Lesions are in the form of raised nodules, usually commence on face but may spread all over body. Secondary bacterial infection causes formation of pustules. When pressed, release pus which contain mites. Severe itching is absent. Seen in dogs usually at young age as well as in calves.

Treatment

(i) **AMITRAZ** (*MITABAN-UpJohn*) 19.9% Emulsifiable conc Use 0.025 aqueous emulsion in lukewarm water for external use. Apply once in 2 weeks using a sponge.

(ii) **NEGUVAN** (*Bayer*) for external application 2 % aqueous sol. once a week Inj. 500 mg kgb wt subcut. only once.

(iii) Inj. **IVOMEC** (*MSD-USA*) Ivermectin-1 percent w/v Inj. 400 microram/kg once a week has been found highly effective. Combination with Levamisol is found effective in calves and dogs as an immunomodulator.

(iv) A combination of Inj. **Neguvan** and local application of 1% **ASUNTAL** (*Bayer*) once a week is highly effective.

(v) **SCABPER** cream (*Nulife*) local applicatopn once a week can be tried.

(vi) **GAMASCAB** lotion (*Nulife*). local application once a week can be tried.

Local applications are effective in case of local lesions but in case of diffuse lesions a parenteral treatment coupled with immunomodulators, vitamin supplementation and improved nutrition will be preferred.

Flea - Dermatitis

Is a common condition in dogs and cats. May become a severe problem in long haired breeds. The fleas cause continuous irritation due to introduction of salivary secretions during bite. It also causes allergy (*flea-bite hypersensitivity*) characterised by itching and erythema. Animal becomes restless and irritable. The flea faeces contain blood and make the coat dirty.

Treatment

Regular grooming and brushing. Use shampoo like **CANIFUR** (*Cadila*) **SII** (*Serum Instt*), **SOFTAS** (*Intas*) or any other similar product be used for bath once a week regularly. Spraying with **BUTOX-VET** is very effective 1- 2 ml per litre in water once in a fortnight.

"**ASUNTAL-50**" (*Bayer*) 1/4 to half teaspoon powder mixed with about 5 litre water is used for application over the body after bath. Do not wipe out this water and allow it to dry.

This keeps the fleas and lice away. It is not recommended in case of multiple bite injuries because the drug may get absorbed through aboded skin. Protect mouth parts and eyes while application and take other precautions to avoid toxicity.

Tick-flea repellent collors are also available but have limited effect in heavy infestations and are more useful for prevention of reinfestation.

In case of hypersensitivity, antihistaminic preparations (oral or injectable) and local application of corticosteroid ointment may be used.

Photosensitization

Is a type of dermatitis which occurs commonly in case of cattle and the lesions are observed over *unpigmented* parts of skin which are directly exposed to sunlight. Certain toxic plants such as *Lantana camara* - a strongly smelling plant with small bunch type flowers- commonly called as *Ghaneri, phenothiazine* compounds and other unknown factors are responsible. The concentration of *phylloerythrin* increases in the body and causes oedema, inflammation, erythema of skin and ultimately causes extensive sloughing of skin.

There are several other plants, weeds, fungi and chemicals which can cause photosensitization. There is liberation of histamine which causes oedema of subcutaneous tissue.

Treatment

Protect animals from sun light. Antihistaminics (*See page 54*), Antibiotics to check bacterial infections and liver tonics to counter hepatotoxic effects. Purgatives be given. This helps in preventing further absorption and excretion of the toxic material.

Zinc sulphate is administered in appropriate doses for accelerating healing of lesions.

Chapter 9

Metabolic Disorders

M ost important in *high yielding dairy* cows and buffaloes and occur within a few weeks after parturition. Poor nutrition during pregnancy, sudden stress of heavy lactation, nutritional and hormonal imbalance are some of the precipitating causes. These are becoming important emerging problems with increase in the number of high yielding animals due to cross breeding program.

Rule out other parturient disease such as *Mastitis, Metritis and other systemic disorders* likely to cause sudden illness.

These are better known as *"Production diseases"* or *"Homeostatis disorders"* due to the fact that there are intrinsic faults with either mobilization, conversion and maintenance of essential nutrients and minerals in the body and as such are directly related with milk production.

Milk Fever (*Parturient Paresis*)

Clinical Symptoms

Usually occurs within a week of parturition. More commonly within first two days. There is a sudden drop in blood calcium levels, sudden drop in milk yield, shivering, muscular weakness, inability to stand, subnormal temperature (*body surface and extremities cold*) pupils dilated, salivation, sternal recumbency (*animal sits with resting its head on flank a typical posture*) anal sphincter relaxed, dyspnoea. Heart rate feeble but accelerated.

Diagnosis is based on the history of recent parturition and high yield of colostrum.

Treatment

Any of the following parenteral Calcium preparations:

Rx.
Ionik (Obcow)
Inj. Qualidrops (Pfizer)
Inj. **Calborol** (Rhone P.)   **Dose** : 300-
Calcium Magnesium Borogluconate (*Sarabhai*) 450 ml by
Calcium Borogluconate 20% soln. (*Ethicare or* slow iv route
Agrivet)
Cal - B - Vet (*TCF*)
Pfizer milk fever formula
Calmax (*Ranbaxy*)   **Dose** : 300 -
Thiacal (*Wockhardt*)   450 ml by
Calcicat (*Cattle Rem*)   slow iv route
Intacal M (*Intas*)
Polcal (*Polchem*)

Warm the bottle to body temperature. The full dose (450 ml) should be administered slowly in 20 minutes. Careful auscultation of heart is very essential during infusion. Exceptionally two bottles are required for complete recovery or may also require a combination of magnesium, glucose and phosphorus in the treatment.

If milk fever is complicated with hypoglycemia and hypomagnesemia then. **MIFEX** (*Rhone P.*) or **CALMEX-M** (*Ranbaxy*) **PFIZER** Milk Fever Formula **MAGICAL** (*Cadila*), **CALCIMAG** (*Cattle Rem*).

Treatment gives a magic relief and the recovery confirms the diagnosis.

SANCAL-Vet (*Sandoz*) - 15-20 ml im daily for 3 days is very useful. This should be given along with above calcium therapy or afterwards to avoid relapse.

Supportive

Hyporid (Intas) 180 g orally once daily or 90 g twice daily. Feeding should be initiated immediately after iv calcium injection and to be continued for 3 days.

Inj. **Tonophosphan** (*Hoechst*) 10 - 20 ml 10 - 20 ml by iv, im or sc route.

Ostocalcium with B$_{12}$ Syrup (Glaxo) or **ASCAL** Syrup (*Alembic*) or **CAL-D-RUBRA** (*Cadila*) **VETKAL** (*Sarabhai*)

100 ml orally twice a day.

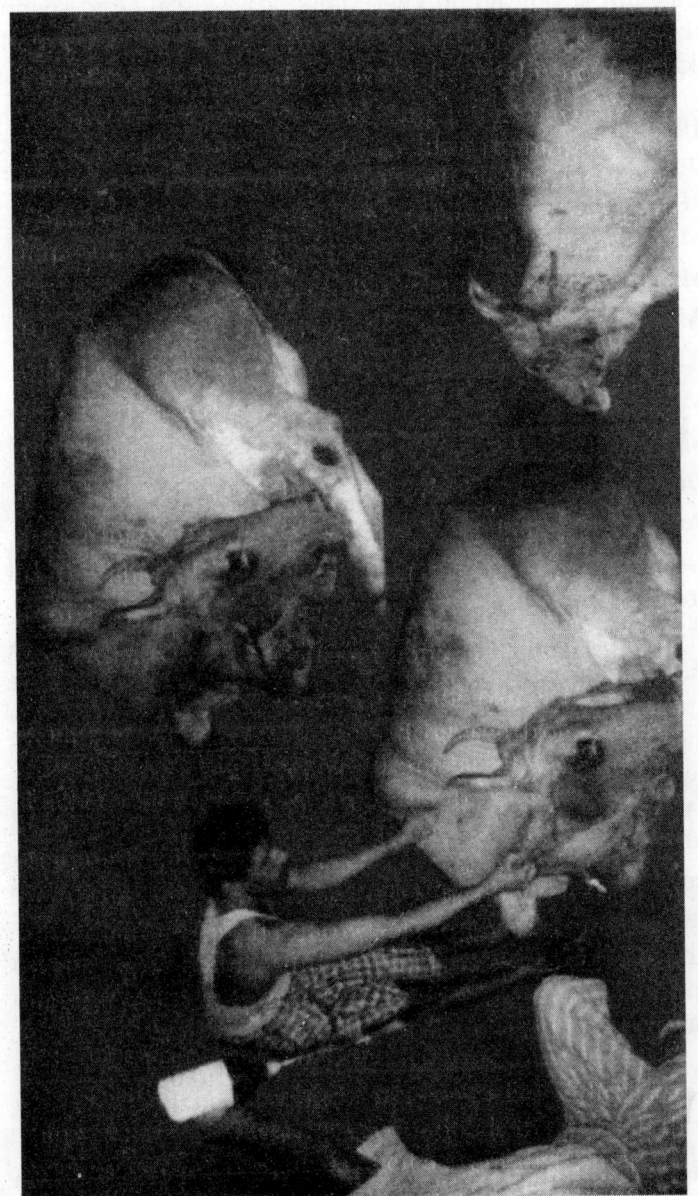

Fig. 10. A cow suffering with a typical symptom of milk fever showing sternal recumbancy and response to treatment.

Calcium strong liquid (Vet Mankind), Doscal Goid suspn (Dosch), Polcal (Polchem), Calshakti Platnia (Intas), Merical (Wockhardt).

Prevention

Inj. Vit. D_3 Arachitol 10 million iu as a single dose one week prior to parturition.

MILKMIN (*Sarabhai*)   or 1 kg in 100 kg feed

Minal Forte (*Alembic*)   or 28 g daily in feed.

Alvite - M (*Alembic*) C and B - 25g/day

Alvite -M Chelated (*Alembic*) C and B - 30 g daily

Minfa (*Intas*) C and B - 30 g/day

Minfa Gold (*Intas*) C and B - 25-30 g/day

Dosmin Forte (*Dosch*) C and B - 25 g/day

Polmin Forte (*Pol Chem*) C and B - 25 g/day

Goumix (Indian Immunologicals) area specific mineral mixture 50-200 g daily.

Hypocalcaemia may coexist along with hypophosphataemia or hypomagnesaemia. Getting incomplete response to injectible calcium therapy and recurrence usually indicates such co-existence. Presence of tremors, hyperaesthesia and nervous signs are the usual signs of co-existing hypomagnesemia. Dullness, inactivity and stupor are suggestive of co-existing hypophosphatemia.

Recurrence of hypocalcemia may call for estimation of paratharmone activity.

The photographs of a cow suffering from hypocalcemia are typical of usual case of milk fever for which a veterinarian is usually called in panic (Fig. 9).

A bottle of Mifex or Calboraol must always be kept at hand because the veterinarian may have to attend the emergency at any odd hour when medical shops may not be open.

Slow administration of warm solution of Calcium borogluconate in the ear vein is pereferable as it enables the vet. to watch the animal and auscultate the heart when the animal is at ease. The animal usually responds quickly and shivering, return of consciousness, attempting to balance the neck and head, passing big volume of urine and faeces are the signs of recovery.

Incomplete milking for first 2 - 3 days and giving feed rich in phosphorous content before calving are some preventive measures which may be resorted to.

Subclinical Hypocalcemia

Apart from clinical cases of hypocalcemia or *"Milk fever"* which are encountered as typical cases within 48 - 72 hours after parturition, it is likely that there are large number of animal which are having low levels of blood calcium but not so low as to manifest clinical symptoms of milk fever. The normal range of serum, calcium level is between 8 to 12mg/100 ml. Clinical symptoms of tremors, recumbancy and subnormal temperature are observed when the serum Ca. level drops below 5 mg/100 ml. However, when a survey of recently calved animals was conducted and particularly those animals in which the serum calcium levels ranged between 6 to 8 mg/100ml. This indicates either poor mobilization of depot calcium due to weak hormonal response or due to poor dietary absorption (*high alkalinity of diet as one of the factors*). Internal parasitic infestation is also responsible to a certain extent. Fungal toxicity due to *Aspergillus niger* (Black fungus) through mouldy feed exposed to rains causes increased oxalic acid content and results in hypocalcaemia and toxicity.

Its therefore desirable to estimate Ca levels whenever possible. For this purpose a rapid field test (*semiquantitative*) based on the amount of Sodium EDTA required to prevent clotting of a sample of blood is worthy of trial.

It is therefore necessary to correct the diet by proper supplements and ensure proper calcium homoeostasis for getting best and steady milk production.

"Downer Cow" Syndrome

Is a condition wherein the predominant symptom is the inability of a cow to get up. Usually occurs after parturition but exceptionally may occur in pregnant animals. Metabolic disturbances, injuries to musculoskeletal system, infections, toxaemias and such other possibilities are various etiological factors.

Affected animal is quite alert, appetite usually normal, attempts to get up unsuccessful. Animal if made to stand forcibly cannot bear weight either on forelegs or on hind legs. Sort of numbness and flaccid atrophy of hip and thigh muscles.

Treatment

First rule out fractures and sprain by careful examination, examine for sensory and motor reflexes, metritis and mastitis, malpositions and fixing of foetus in advance gestation by rectal examination.

Prognosis is favourable in this syndrome if due to metabolic disorders.

Inj. **Tonophosphan** or **Cobaphos** or **Alphos-40** iv and **Mifex** or **Mifical** 200 ml. by slow iv once daily for 3-4 days.

Inj. **Berin, Vibjex, Triradisol-H, Tribivet** or **Neurobion** 10 ml. for 3 - 4 days.

Potassium acetate10% sol. 100 ml slow iv daily for 8 days together with **DIANABOL** *(Ciba)* 100 mg im daily for 3 days. Supporting the animal with slings, massage with liniment camphor, infra red fomentation, diathermy, prevention of bed sores and intensive supportive therapy and patient might respond in variable periods.

Ketosis (Acetonaemia or Hypoglycaemia)

Primary Ketosis occurs usually within 6-8 weeks after parturition commonly during peak yield. This is due to impaired carbohydrate metabolism. Blood glocose level falls down considerably with simultaneous rise in blood ketones. Synthesis of glucose is less as compared to fast drain in milk. In sheep the condition occurs during late pregnancy and is called as *pregnancy toxaemia* of ewes.

Sometimes occur concurrently with hypocalcemia. Sudden drop in milk yield. Signs of nervous excitement and mania, no recumbency. Temperature, pulse, respiration, within normal range. **Rapid wasting and loss of subcutaneous fat**

(*Gluconeogenesis*). Sweet smell to breath and urine. Selective appetite (*feeding on hay but refusal of conc. mixture*). Confirmation by exam. of urine by *Rothera's test*. Also by estimation of blood glucose.

Treatment

Dextrose sol. 25- 50%. (*Ethicare or KTS*) or **Glucine** (*Abhi*) or Inj. **RINTOSE** (*Wockhardt*).

Av. Dose : 500 - 1000 ml by iv route is the specific replacement therapy. In emergency sterile solution of *Dextrose monohydrate* - good grade, in dist, water can be administered.

It has been observed that concurrent administration of insulin 0.5 units/ kg b. wt. sc improves utilization of glucose.

Any of the following corticosteroids could be combined with glucose therapy:

Inj. **Prednisolone** (*Intervet*) 10 ml, im Inj. **Dexona** or Inj. **Vetalog** (*Sarabhai*) or **Betnesol** (*Glaxo*) 2-5 ml/ im. This stimulates gluconeogenesis but utilisation of glucose for milk production is suppressed. And there is complete suppression of milk production.

Rx

Chloral Hydrate	30 g
Aqua	125 ml
Oil Lini.	250 ml.
Mft . Haust	**Sig** once daily for 3 days

This controls nervous symptoms and improves digestion of cellulose.

Supportive

Inj. **Liver Extract with B-Complex** (*any prep.*)

5 -10 ml, im alternate daily, 3 days.

Advise feeding of crushed maize 2 kg & 250 g of molasses per day as a readily available source of carbohydrates. Treatment of pregnancy toxemia in sheep is same but the doses will be proportionately less as per body wt.

Prevention : Khurak (Alembic) 150-300 g/animal/day

Fatomax (Intas) 100 g/animal/day

Lactogain (Polchem) 100 g/day/animal

Hypomagnesaemia

In cows (*lactation or Grass Tetany*) is said to be due to grazing exclusively on lush green pasture grown on heavily fertilized soil. May occur at any stage of lactation. Symptoms of hyperexcitability, convulsion, muscle tremors and tachycardia (*heart rate 100- 120 per min*).

Confirmation

By estimation of magnesium in serum and by ruling out other diseases which show CNS disturbances. Exam. of CSF Mg. levels is useful.

In young calves this is called "whole milk tetany" and occurs in calves fed exclusively on milk. Symptoms of hyperesthesia, convulsions and tachycardia. The calf may die suddenly after bellowing. Concurrent hypocalcaemia is commonly recorded.

Treatment

MIFEX (*Rhone P.*) or **CALMAG** (*Ethicare*) or **MIFICAL** (*Cadila*) or **CABCODEX** (*BAIF*)

Dose : 200 - 300 ml for adult

50 - 100 ml for young given by slow iv route

Magnesium sulphate sterile 20 % solution.

Dose : 100 - 200 ml **subcutaneously** for adult.

Feeding of magnesium oxide @ 100 - 200 g daily for one week.

Azoturia (*Paralytic Myoglobinuria*)

(Monday morning Sickness of horses)

A diseases of horses, occurring during beginning of exercise after a period of rest. More common in welfed horses.

Symptoms

Sudden stiffness of muscles, inability to walk, profuse

sweating, muscles painful, respiration rapid.

Treatment

Stop further exercise and give complete rest. *Give treatment on the spot.*

Chloral hydrate 30 gm as a drench or

Inj. **Largactil** (*Rhone P.*) 5% sol. 4 - 6 ml iv

Thiamine Hydrochloride (*Inj. Berin*) 500 mg, im Antihistaminics (*see p. 54*) 10 - 20 ml im

Vit E. injectable (Ecare-se) and iv saline.

Inj. Sodabicarb 2.5 % 25- 50 ml, iv

Hypophosphataemia (Post - Parturient Hemoglobinuria)

This is a condition commonly recorded in certain areas when soils are deficient in phosphorus. Sporadic cases occur in animals usually in post parturient stage. More commonly seen in buffaloes. A well known disease in Haryana, Punjab and in Marathwada region of Maharasthra.

Symptoms

Usually afebrile, the rectal temperature normal or slightly elevated. The important symptom is haemoglobinuria. Animal continues to give normal milk yield for 24 hours after appearance of haemoglobinuria, weakness, depression, anaemia and dehydration develops rapidly. Dyspnoea, jaundice and tachycardia in late stage.

Diagnosis

Rule out Babesiosis by blood smear examination,and associated symptoms of high fever and tick infestation. Confirmation by estimation of serum inorganic phosphorus level which fall from 4.7 to less than 2 mg/dl. Rule out haematuria. Diagnosis not very difficult where incidence is common.

Treatment

Dissolve 60 g of Sodium acid phosphate (NaH_2PO_4) in 300 ml of distilled water and give slow iv is the specific therapy. Continue by subcut route at 12 hours interval consecutively for

3 times. Oral administration of bone meal 100 gm. twice daily in feed is recommended. Continue treatment with Inj. **Cobaphos** or **Tonophosphan, Alphos-40** (*Alved*) Inj. **Fertophos** (*Glaxo-SKF*), Novizac (*Intas*) for 2 -3 days.

Herd Health Management

Metabolic Profile Test

Study of the nutritional status and energy requirements of a dairy herd can be conducted by Metabolic Profile Test. This test comprises of estimation of blood glucose, calcium, phosphorus, magnesium, iron, cobalt, copper and other trace elements, serum proteins and other haematological values of the **high, medium** and **low producing** animals in a herd for three different seasons. This type of study gives a clear cut picture as to whether the nutritional requirements are adequately met with or not. Comparison of the several herds can be done and with the necessary corrections in the feeding. The incidence of metabolic disorders can be prevented to a greatest extent.

A **mini profile test** comprise of estimating blood glucose, serum urea nitrogen and albumin in cows between 4 - 10 weeks after calving. This gives idea as to whether energy and protein intakes are adequate. Sampling is done at 4 - 6 weeks interval. This test is useful to detect gross inadequacies of nutrition in any herd.

Chapter 10

Diseases Due to Deficiency of Vitamins

Vitamins are vital substances necessary for growth and normal body functions. Their importance is felt when they are deficient in the body. Preformed Vitamins or their precursors are present in feeds and fodders.

Estimation of vitamin in body fluids and tissues is complicated and expensive procedure. Disappearance of clinical symptoms after suitable supplementation provide a better clue to diagnosis of deficiency in the field. The deficiency diseases are therefore better called as "Responsive Diseases".

Vitamins are classified as under:

(1) Fat Soluble Vitamins (Vit A, D, E and K)

These are usually stored in the Liver.

(2) Water Soluble Vitamins (Vit B. complex group and Vit. C) These are not stored in the body (except B_{12}) and most of them are synthesised by microflora in rumen and intestines.

Vitamin A Deficiency (*Hypovitaminosis-A*)

Hypovitaminosis -A occurs as a primary disease of dietary deficiency of Vit A or its precursor Carotene, if continued for prolonged period of time so as to produce visible signs of deficiency.

The alcoholic form of Vit. A present in carotene does not pass through placental barrier but the ester form present in fish liver oil passes through placental barrier and increases level in the foetal liver. Feeding greens in advance pregnancy therefore does not increase levels of Vit. A in foetus but significantly increases Vit. A content of colostrum which acts as a source of Vit. A for new born calf.

Secondary Vit. A. A deficiency may occur in chronic diseases of liver or intestines and during high atmospheric temperature in summer.

Pathogenesis

Vit. A is essential for regeneration of visual purple necessary for dim light vision. Deficiency results in night blindness. Vit. A is necessary for normal growth of bones and maintenance of normal epithelial tissue. Exfoliated epithelial cells of urinary tract form a nidus for formation of urinary calculi. Vit. A deficiency affects the reproductive functions and reduces conception rates. Deficiency also increases susceptibility to infections and hence the vitamin is called as "anti infective" or "anti stress". Intestinal worms proliferate if the animal is deficient in Vit. A.

Clinical symptoms

Night blindness is the earliest sign. Cornea becomes thick and cloudy in dogs and calves. Reproductive problems, infertility, stunted growth, abortions and retained placenta are common.

Treatment - Immediate treatment with Vit. A at 10 to 20 times the daily requirements usually @ 440 i.u./ kg b. wt. is preferable by parenteral injections.

Daily dietary requirements are as under:

- Growing calves & sheep : 30 - 40 iu kg b. wt.
- Pregnant and milking cows & sheep - 70-80 iu /kg b. wt.
- Dogs - 500 iu per 100 g diet (*dry basis*).

Some proprietary preparations containing Vit. A.

(1) Inj.**Prepalin** forte (*Glaxo*) 3 lac IU/ per ml

(2) Inj. **Vitacept** (Concept) (Vit ADE) 10 ml, im

(3) Inj. **AQUASOL**

Feed Suppliments

(4) **VITABLEND -AD 3** (*Glaxo*)

(5) **VIMEROL** (*Roche*)

110

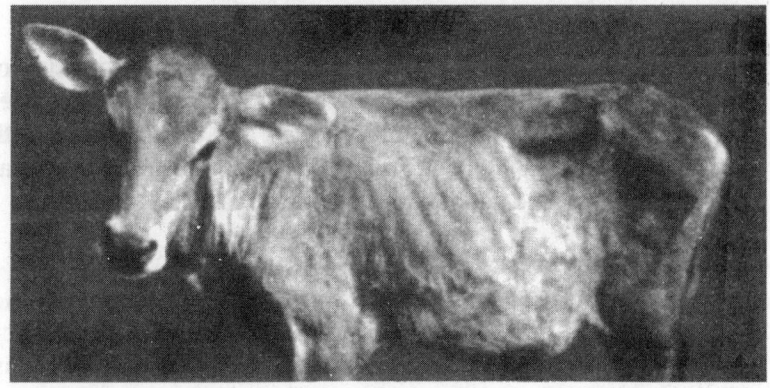

Fig. 11. A calf suffering with deficiency of Vitamin A.

Vitamin supplement for oral administration useful for calves and dogs.

(6) **AROVIT** tablets for dogs and cats.

Feeding of green grasses, yellow maize and fish liver oil are the common feed supplements.

Vitamin— D Deficiency (*Hypovitaminosis - D*)

Vit. D exerts a profound action in regulating calcium, absorption and metabolism together with hormones calcitanin and *paratharmone* and as such is very important for all growing animals, pups and dairy animals in which regulation of calcium and phosphorous is important Vit. D is also known as an *"antirachitic factor"* because of its role in prevention of rickets in small animals.

Source— Vit. D is formed due to ultraviolet solar radiation in the skin of animals and in the plants and sun dried hay. Dietary sources are fish liver oils, egg yolk, milk butter and sun-dried hay.

Etiology

Keeping animals indoors in areas where sunlight is inadequate may cause deficiency, particularly in pet animals. Pregnant ewes and post parturient cows whose requirements of ionised calcium are increased and are particularly vulnerable for Vitamin D deficiency.

111

Pathogensis

Vit. D is essential for absorption and utilization of calcium and phosphorus. In rickets, the normal ossification of bones does not take place and they become soft and cartilaginous with the result that the skeletal structure becomes misshaped. Similar disease known as osteomalacia occurs in adult animals.

Clinical Symptoms

Normally due to plentiful availability of sunlight and consumption of sun dried hay gross symptoms of deficiency are not usually seen in farm animals in India. It may occur in pigs, sheep with heavy coat and pups. Rickets is common disease in young pet dogs due to defective mineralisation of growing bones.

Parturient paresis (*Milk Fever*) - occurs in high yielding cows, soon after parturition due to sudden and excessive loss of calcium through colostrum and milk and reduced mobilization of calcium bones due to slow release of paratharmone by quiescent parathyroid gland. Similar parturient hypocalcemia occurs in bitches and is known as "Eclampsia".

Treatment and Control

Adequate calcium and phosphorus should be provided along with administration of Vit. D3 given to a cow or a buffalo a week before expected day of parturition is one of the possible ways to prevent attack of hypocalcemia (*milk fever*) Inj. **Arachitol** (Vit. D3) 6 lakh i.u. /ml can be administered for this purpose.

Vitamin - E Deficiency (*Hypovitaminosis -E*)

Vit. E is a fat soluble vitamin and structurally occurs as a mixture of alpha, beta, gamma and delta tocopherols out of which alpha tocopherol is most potent and main biological functions in association with selenium and prevents necrosis of liver and muscular dystrophy in animals.Vit. E also enhances the reproductive efficiency in farm animals.

Etiology

Deficiency of Vit. E and selenium collectively cause nutritional muscle dystrophy and other syndromes.

112

Clinical symptoms

Nutritional muscular dystrophy in lambs and calves is characterised by stiffness, weakness, trembling and inability to stand. Muscles become hard, rubbery and swollen. Animal die suddenly. Plasma SGOT and Ceatinine Phosphokinase (CPK) activity are much increased as a laboratory finding and provide diagnosis for confirmation.

Treatment

Combination of selenumn with Vit.E is preferred. Injectable and oral supplements are available for treatment. Germinated wheat contains high conc. of Vit. E and should be included in the feed.

Vitamin - K Deficiency (*Hypovitaminosis -K*)

Is a fat soluble vitamin synthesised from green leafy vegetables which are the natural source of Vit. K-1 necessary for formation of prothrombin and other clotting factors.

Deficiency causes decrease in prothrombin leading to prolonged clotting time and uncontrolled haemorrhages. Warfarin and sweet clover poisonings are the examples of Vit. K deficiency.

Injectable preparation like **KAPLIN** (*Glaxo*) avaiiable. Other causes of haemorrhage be ruled out.

Vitamin B-Complex Deficiency

Members of Vit. B-complex group are water soluble, thermolabile and are synthesised in the rumen and large intestines by microbes in all animals. These vitamins are not stored in the body and occasional deficiency may occur.

Thiamine Deficiency

Thiamine is synthesised in rumen but can be destroyed by enzyme "thiaminase" produced by certain bacteria and fungi during acidosis. Thiamine has important activity in the metabolism of carbohydrats, fats and proteins.

Clinical Symptoms

Nervous signs, tremors and anorexia are common, which respond to treatment when other causes are ruled out.

113

Treatment

Multidose vial Thiamine Hydrochloride @ 100 mg/ml.

Riboflavin, Panthothenic acid, Nictotinic acid, Pyridoxine, Folic acid, Biotin, Choline, Cyanocobalamine-Vit B12 deficiencies are collectively considered as Vit B.- Complex deficiencies. Some of these vitamins are responsible for maintenance of neural functions, enzymes systems and erythropoiosis (Vit B12) . These are usually available in a combined "B-complex" form as injective preparations or for oral administration as capsules or syrups. These preparations are commonly employed in digestive disturbances, neurological disorder, paraplegia and anaemia as a supportive therapy.

Chapter 11

Post Parturient Diseases (Cattle & Buffalo)

Post parturient metabolic disorders are dealt with separately elsewhere.

Examine uterus per rectum, enquire and look for any purulent uterine discharge and examine mammary gland in every case of illness with history of recent parturition.

Retention of Placenta

Normally placenta is expelled within 6-8 hrs. after parturition.

Cleansing Dose *(to be given after parturition)*

Mag. sulph.	250 g
Ext. Ergot liq.	10 ml
Tr. Zingiberis	60 ml
Aqua	500 ml
Mft. Haust	**Sig**. Stat

UTEROTONE (*Cattle Rem*) 100 ml B.D.or any other as under

HORMOTONE (*Charak*) Liquid 2-3 days.

UTROTONE (*Obcow*) 100 g in luke warm water

METRATONE LIQUID (Polchem) 100 ml BD

EXAPAR (*Dabur*) @ 100 - 200 ml daily for 2 days

Inj. **METHARGIN** or Tablets as per advise

INVOLON (*Natural Rem*)

Above drugs help in expulsion of placenta, clears up lochial discharge and useful in metritis. If the placenta is not expelled

115

inspite of above treatment the placenta should be manually removed with the help of experienced Vet.

Observe strict aspetic precautions. Smear **TEGERON** cream or **SAVLON** on the hand and remove placenta as completely as possible by gentle manoeuring (*rule out possibility of Brucellosis by history and protect yourself while handling*).

Antibiotic Therapy Following Removal of Placenta

(*For prevention of metritis*)

(*The recent hypothesis is that placenta need not be removed manually due to the possibility of injuries and trauma likely during it's removal, and so, uterine infection be properly controlled by intrauterine and parenteral antibiotics*)

Place any of the following pessaries (2 to 4) daily as deep as possible in the uterus at least for 3 days. **FUREA** (SKF) or **FUZONE** (*H. Jules*) or **NUFROZONE** (*KTS*), **OR CLENAX** are the types of intrauterine boluses which contain Nitrofuran and urea which helps in liquifying the organic debris of placenta and help in its expulsion. This treatment is a satisfactory measure to prevent infection.

In case the placenta is retained over a period of 48 hrs and putrefaction has set in, the animal shows signs of fever, uterine colic and toxaemia. In such case placenta should be removed manually taking all aseptic precautions and making use of protective hand gloves. Excessive and rough handling of endometrium or pulling the placenta by force should be avoided. Rectal palpation of uterus and reverse massage of uterus per rectum using gentle pressure by a well lubricated hand helps in èvacuation of uterus of its contents.

In case of moderate to heavy infection of uterus oxytetracyclines should be administered both intrauterine as well as by parenteral route. **Terramycin** (*Pfizer*), **Steclin** (*Sarabhai*) or **Alcycline** (*Alembic*) 500 mg boluses (3 to 4 at a times) be placed in the uterus and oxytetracycline should also be given by parenteral route @ 10 mg/kg body wt im or iv. The entire treatment be continued for the period of 3 to 4 days and if required even longer. Long acting tetracycline at adequate dose are convenient for use. The recent pharmacokinetic studies have indicated that intramuscular administration of oxytetracycline produces varying effective levels of the drug in the uterus and the entire genital tract infections are taken care. **Terramycin** liquid 30 ml or **METROGYL** (*Rhone. P.*) can be used for intrauterine infusion using an insemination pipette, if the os-uterus does not permit insertion of boluses. If possible bacteriological and antibiotic sensitivity test on uterine swab be performed to select appropriate antibiotic. **LIXEN-U** (Glaxo SKF), **BETADINE** (*Wockhardt*) solution 20 ml properly diluted, infused intrauterine for 3 days may be tried. These are non-irritant Iodine preparations.

Inj. **Methargin** (*Ciba*) or **Nexbolic** 2 -15 ml im or iv route and **Hormotone** (*Charak*) 100 ml orally are recommended for rapid involution of uterus. Tablets **Myron** (*Alarsin*) or **Lucol** and **Septilin (Himalaya)** -20 tablets each, B.D. x 10 - 15 days.

Pyometra

Incompletely removed placenta, incomplete treatment, prolapse of vagina, uterus and negligence leads to this condition. Infection such as *Vibriosis*, *Trichomoniasis*, *Brucellosis* are also responsible. Animal looks sick, has fever, drop in milk, purulent foul smelling uterine discharge observed particularly when animal sits down. Examine uterus per rectum for confirmation. Animal has fever and toxemia.

Treatment

Usually os-uterus does not permit insertion of large sized pessaries if treatment is delayed. Hence, first the uterus should be evacuated and discharge removed by gentle uterine massage per rectum. Administration of Inj. **Posterior pituitary** extract or **Methargin** for 2 - 3 days helps in this.

Intrauterine Antibiotic Therapy

Eumetran (*Eu Medica*) bolus containing sulpha drugs, **Streptopenicillin (Combiotic, Dicrysticin or Bistripen)** intra uterine by use of insemination pipette as well as parenterally. Tablets of sulphadiazene or Tetracycline can also be administered for 2 -5 days.

OR

Oxytetracycline intrauterine and any of the tetracycline parenterally as a combined therapy is very useful.

In case there is no response to treatment it is necessary to get culture and sensitivity test (A.S.T.) of the uterine discharge so that the most effective antibiotic can be selected. *In every case complete cure of the condition must be ensured* otherwise chronic and low grade endometrial infection can lead to repeated breeding problems which in turn will affect the production and economics of the herd. **Gentamycin** has been reported to be highly effective on the basis of the AST in the treatment of uterine infection & pyometra Inj. **Genster** (Sterling) 2 mg/kg im for 3 days and intrauterine for 3 days was found very effective in cows as well as buffaloes.

Non antibiotic intrauterine treatment with **Pivipol** (*Ar. Ex*) or **Betadine** (*Wockhardt*) may be tried for 3-4 days. Inj. **Metranidazole** (*Rhone P.*) 50 ml I/U.

Supportive Therapy

Tablets **Myron** (*Alarsin*) or **Lucol** and **Septillin** (Himalaya)	10 B.D. orally for 10 days
Hormotone (*Charak*)	@ 100 ml daily for 3 days be given orally
Endotrin (*Cadila*) liquid	100 ml twice daily for expulsion of placenta and as a cleansing dose

Parenteral calcium - **Calboral** or **Thiacal** 100 - 150 ml. daily for 3 days combined with **Tonophosphan** (*Hoechst*) 10 ml. tones up the uterine muscle and early involution, recovery and restoration of milk yield.

Prolapse of Vagina and Uterus

Usually occurs in cases of retained placenta due to severe irritation and excessive straining. In some cases the oestrogen content of some grasses and silages are thought to be responsible. In some cases exact cause cannot be identified.

Management

Shift the animal on a clean ground with hind quarters resting on the raised level,and place the prolapsed mass on a soft clean cloth. Irrigate with cold water containing 1% **Savlon** (*ICI*) or 0.1% potassium permanganate. Examine for injuries and tears. Control bleeding by topical application of adrenaline, smear local anaesthetic ointment (*Xylocain*) and reduce the prolapsed uterus by gentle manoeuvring. If the prolapsed mass is covered by a clean soft cloth and gentle squeezing of cloth is done, the prolapsed mass gets reduced in size and repositioning becomes easy. Use the pressure of palm of hand or fist and never push by fingers as it may cause injuries.

Inj. posterior pituitary extract 5 ml intra mural will cause uterine shrinkage and reduction will be easier (*in case the bladder is distended, removal of urine by a catheter facilitates the repositioning of uterus*).

To prevent reccurrence of prolapse administer—

Chloral hydras	50 - 60 g
Aqua	200 ml
Oil Lini	500 ml
Mft. Haust	**Sig. stat**

or Inj. **Largactil** (*Rhone P.*) 5% sol. 10 ml, im

or Inj. **Siquil** (*Sarabhai*) 1 - 2 ml im

or Inj. of **Novocain** (*Hoechst*) 10 ml epidurally.

Apply *rope-truss* after reducing the prolapse and treat for 3 days as a case of metritis. In obstinate prolapse with tenesmus, insuflation of air in the peritoneal cavity is done (*after reducing prolapse*) via paralumbar fossa till both fossae get distended. This method has a *risk of infection*.

Homeopathic *Podophyllum* tincture of 200 x potency @ 10 drops orally given alternately at hourly interval may be tried. This has given excellent results.

Aconite dose every 15-30 minutes upto four doses if excessive bleeding and injuries due to manipulations (Shock). After repoitioning of uterus caulophyllum 30 TDS x 5-7 days.

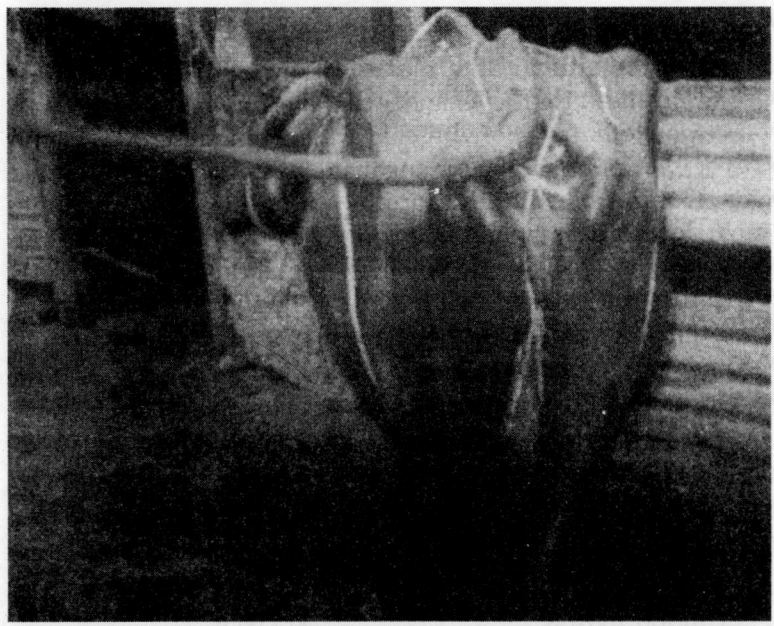

Fig. 12. Rope jacket applied to prevent prolapse of uterus/vagina after its reduction inside.

Antihistaminic (*See page 54*) to prevent, shock due to excessive manipulation. Supportive treatment with Mifex or **Mifical** (*Cadila*) 100 - 150 ml, iv for 2 -3 days has been found very useful.

Mastitis

Inflammation of mammary gland (udder) is the most important disease of dairy animals and probably the most neglected in the field where the vets are required to treat so many clinical cases wherein the gland becomes very hard, loses milk producing capacity of the delicate gland cells (*acini*) and we get the purulent blood mixed secretion instead of milk. In such a case there is hardly anything that can be done to restore normal functioning and milk producing capacity of the udder. The glandular tissue of udder is lost forever and the animal remains uneconomical and a liability for the owner causing considerable loss to the industry.

It is therefore very necessary to protect this vulnerable organ by following certain essential preventive practices described in this book elsewhere.

Detection of Subclinical Mastitis— It is very essential to detect the infection of udder in the early stage so that prompt treatment can be initiated before any permanent damage occurs to the udder. This is called detecting the disease in subclinical stage i.e., before the clinical symptoms such as swelling, alteration in quality of milk are seen by the owner. The Veterinary science has developed some tests to detect early infection. These are called as *"Indirect Tests"*. There are many such tests but the following ones are comparatively superior because there is positive correlation between these indirect test and isolation of pathogenic bacterial infection as proved by cultural isolation techniques.

1) Modified California Mastitis Test (*MCMT*)
2) Electrical Conductivity Test (*ECT*)
3) Modified White Side Test (*MWST*)
4) Modified Aulendorfer Mastitis Probe Test (*MAMP*)

The pathogenic organism responsible for mastitis are mostly *Staphylococci, Streptococci, E. Coli, Klebsiella & Corynebacteria.* It is always better to conduct Antibiotic Sensitivity Test (*AST*) before you start the treatment, which should be continued till a negative bacterial isolation report is obtained.

Although mastitis can occur at any stage of lactation it is most common during early post partum period. Excessive engorgement of udder and oedema occurring in high yielders during last fortnight of gestation should be guarded.

Udder Oedema

Excessive oedema can be relieved by administration of diuretics. Prepartum milking may be done if necessary. *Never use corticosteriods in advance pregnancy as it may cause premature calving.*

Acute Mastitis

Usually caused by *Staphylococci* and *Streptococci*. Gland is hard, swollen, hot and painful. Be watchful for indication of

121

gangrene (*coldness & bluish discoloration*). Milk is examined for the presence of flakes, clots or any discolouration and consistency. There is intense systemic reaction i.e., fever and toxemia.

Treatment

Never delay or neglect treatment of mastitis

(i) Isolate the animal and milk off healthy quarters first before handling the affected ones.

(ii) Remove secretion from affected quarter as much as possible; if necessary by use of a sterile milk-siphon in case the gland is very painful and in obliteration of teat canal. (*Utmost sterile precautions must be taken while using teat siphon*)

(iii) Cultural exam. of milk and antibiotic sensitivity test should be done whenever possible.

Parenteral treatment is advisable when there is systemic reaction and to assist in treating infection of mammary gland. Higher doses are needed, the preferred once being tetracyctines (Inj. Terramycin, Oxysteclin, Inj. Wolicyclin, Oxysure) and Tylosin (Inj. Tylin). They are also used when the udder is swollen so that the diffusion is difficult. 5/4 day course is better than 3/2 day treatment. Good diffusers are erythromycin, tylosin, chloramphenicol (Inj. Chlorectin, Inj. Chlorovet, Chloroamphenicol succinate) and Trimethoprim (Inj. Biotrim, Inj. Sultrim, Inj. Oriprim). Medium diffusers are penicillins (Inj. Fortified procaine penicillin, Inj. Durapen 48, Inj. Albapam), tetracyclines and cephalosprins (Inj. Bovice, Inj. Xnel - 1 to 2 mg/kg b. wt. im, Inj. Wocef, M- Ceft, Inj. Intacef, Inj. Intacef Tazo, Inj. Ceftrivet 5 mg- 10 mg/ kg b. wt. im or iv). Poor diffusers are neomycin, polymixin and streptomycin.

(iv) Udder Infusion - Antibiotics in ointment of aqueous base are infused into the udder after emptying the udder and under hygienic conditions. Infuse any of the following intramammary preparations, *at least for 3 consecutive days after* thorough stripping of milk.

1) **PENDISTRIN & PENDISTRIN -SH.** *(Sarabhai)*
2) **VETCLOX- PLUS** *(Sarabhai)*
3) **FLOCLOX** (Ranbaxy) intramammary
4) **MASTIWOK** *(Wockhardt)* Intramammary
5) **FLOCLOX** *(Ranbaxy)* Intramamamry
6) **CHLORECTIN** (Dosch)
7) **CLAXAMPICILLIN /CAMPIDEX** *(Codila)*
8) **MAMMITEL** *(Intas)* Intramammary

Milk from the antibiotic treated animals should not be used for human consumption for *at least 72 hours* after last infusion. Parental antibiotic therapy should be combined and the same antibiotic as used for intramammary therapy should be employed.

Inj. **"TIAMUTIN"** 10% *(Sandoz)* is recently introduced product.

New antibiotic combinations are constantly introduced in the market wherein superior and new generation antibiotics are used. This is always necessary due to the resistance acquired by the invading bacteria to use of existing antibiotics. Veterinary physician has therefore to remain vigilant at all times.

Antibiotic sensitivity tests on milk samples are very useful as a guide to select best and effective antibiotic.

Inj. Levamisol **LEVAMOL-75** @ 1 ml/7.5 kg for 2-3 days is found useful supportive therapy.

Mammodium (Intas) 50 g daily for 4 days by mixing in jaggery as an electuary orally as an adjunct to antibiotic therapy.

Conventional mastitis treatment and control methods are based on chemical disinfectant and treatment of the affected quartes using antibiotics. Most commercially available drug formulations for udder infusions comprise antibiotics to check infections and anti- inflammatory to reduce congestion. However, antibiotic therapy does not work always and often seems to have very little effect on course of mastitis. Therefore some alternatives of antimicrobial mastitis therapy should be explored to provide holistic approach to disease management.

Glycerine with **Acriflavin** 1 : 10,000, 20 ml per affected quarter for 3 days, is the old treatment and may be employed in absence of antibiotics, **PIVIPOL** (Kosmorex) or **BETADINE** (*Wockhardt*) are the non irritant iodine containing preparations 10 - 20 ml of dilute soln. per quarter may be tried for 3 days.

Homoeopathic *Phytolacca* is also found useful. particularly in subclinical mastitis with blood tinge in milk 4 - 5 drops of tincture be given twice daily orally.

MASTILEP (*Dabur*) is recommended as a topical herbal gel for external application to maintain hygienic milk production and prevention of infection.

WISPREC (*Natural Rem*) is a multispectrum cream to combat skin infections of udder and also as anti inflammatory application to reduce pain and swelling of udder.

Non antibiotic therapy with **Trisodium citrate** @ 30 mg/kg bwt (about 3 gm) in 250 ml water orally of 5 days plus single injection of **Levamisol** 10 ml im (**Lemasol -75** -(*Rambaxy*) as immunomodulator was found effective. This treatment reduces the pH of milk to some extent and thereby does not favour bacterial growth. This treatment may be tried in combination with antibiotics as an additional supportive measure.

Chronic Mastitis

Mostly results due to incomplete treatment, antibiotic resistant bacterial strain and insanitory conditions and gross neglect.

There is little or no local reaction i.e., swelling or pain. Milk may show visible alterations only if examined carefully. Part of gland is fibrosed and this fibrosis extends with reduction in milk yield in each succeeding lactation. The incidence of staphylococcal infections is increasing.

Cultural examination of milk and antibiotic sensitivity test should be done wherever possible.

Line of treatment is the same as in acute mastitis (*prolonged course necessary*). Treatment to control systemic reaction is not usually necessary.

In case of masitis with mild glandular inflammatory reaction, with presence of blood-tinge in milk, the treatment with Homeopathic drug *"Phytolacca"* 200 x tincture, 5 drops, B.D. for 6 days has been found effective.

Prophylaxis

1) Klengard (Intas) for heat dipping. Just after milking 1 tablet/litre of water.

2) Do not neglect any injuries of udder or teat.

3) If a cow suffers from metritis, the infectious purulent discharge running down may produce udder infection. (*metritis-mastitis syndrome*). Hence utmost cleanliness is necessary.

4) Treat preparturient udder oedema by diuretics. Try Homeopathic drugs like **Aconite, Belladonna** 200 C, 3 to 4 times a day.

5) Feed balance diet with moderate protein and supplementation of **Selenium** and **Vit E.** necessary for building defence mechanism.

6) Take a note of slightest swelling of udder and qualitative change in milk.

7) Periodical testing of all animals with CMT be carried out with the indirect test using CMT reagent. This test detects subclinical cases of mastitis and enables you to treat the animal before the gland is damaged. This test is not reliable in recently calved animals and at drying off stage (*for test reagent see under reagents*).

8) Wash the udder with any of the following solutions before milking. One per cent soln. of bleaching powder or **CHLOROSOL or PIVIPOL** (*Kosmorex*), **SAVLON** (*Johnson & Johnson*) or **BETADINE** (*Wockhardt*) or **KOHRSOLIN-TH** (Virbacc-*Glaxo*) soln.

9) Never pass any objects such as wire or siphon with a view to remove teat obstruction.

10) Milk the affected animal at the end.

11) Undertake dry cow therapy (infusing intramammary drug on the last day of drying off) with a suitable intramammary antibiotic preparation.

Agalactia and Hypogalactia

Reduction in the expected milk yield from a cow or buffalo is the most common problem a Veterinary practitioner encounters.

First it must be clarified that milk yield is governed by multiple factors. The problem should be approached in a systematic way as under :

1) If an animal has freshly calved, rule out common post parturient diseases. (*History of retained placenta, metritis and other generalized illness and parasitic diseases.*)

2) Examine the udder and rule out mastitis, fibrosis of the gland and teat abnormalities. Treat these abnormalities first.

3) Enquire if there is letting down problem due to death of sucking calf.

4) Enquire about feed and ensure that feeding is at adequate level and that essential nutrients are fed. Discourage frequent change of feed. Enquire also if the animal was well-fed during advance pregnancy . Feeding of 1 to 2 kg ground maize to high yielders provides the necessary carbohydrates in the easily digestible form.

5) Ensure that adequate minerals and salt etc. are being fed to the animal.

6) Examine for metabolic disorders by urine and blood examinations and from history and clinical symptoms.

Recommendations

1) Feeding the Mineral Mixture (*Any of the following*)

   AVLOMIN (*ICI*) for cattle 30 g for daily in feed.

   SUPER MINDIF (*Boots*) 20 g in feed.

   ALMIN and a **ALVITE-M** (*Alembic*) 25 g daily.

   PRIVIMIN Forte (*Rhone P.*) 2 - 4 boluses.

   MILKMIN (*Sarabhai*) 1 kg in 100 kg feed.

   GWALA (*Sarabhai*) mineral mixture with amino acids 1 @ 1 kg / 100 kg feed.

(2) **LEPTADEN** (*Alarsin*) tablet 10 B.D. x 10 days. corrects letting down problem and improves milk production.

(3) **"MY"**formula A combination of Ostovet Liquid + Vimeral. (*Virback*)

(4) **MORALAC** tablets (*Universal Ayurved*) 10 B.D. for 10 days.

(5) **LACTOVET** (*Charak*) 25 - 30 g B.D. for 6 days.

(6) **VETILK** (*Aphali*) feed supplemnt @ 50 g daily.

(7) **PAYAPRO** (*Dabur*) - herbal galctogogue @ 1 - bolus daily for 8 -10 days.

(8) **CAL-D-RUBRA** (*Cadila*) or **ASCAL** (*Alembic*) liquid orally @ 100 ml daily for one week.

(9) **Fartomax** (Intas), Lactogain (Polchem), Khurak (embic), 100 g/day.

(10) **DUGH-DAN** (*Cattle Rem*) 4 tabs twice a day x 10 day.

(11) **LYVIM** (*Cadila*) for improvement of milk fat

Maintenance of Optimum Breeding Efficiency

The economics of livestock industry and success of breed improvement programs depend entirely on the optimum breeding efficiency of livestock.

Breeding Bulls & Stallions

For maintenance of optimum sexual performance and improvement of libido and semen quality)

(1) **FORTAGE** (*Alsarin*) tablets10 B.D. for 15 days followed by10 once daily for 1 month

(2) **SPEMEN** (Himalaya Drug) powder 12 gm. daily for 40 days.

(3) **TENTEX** forte (*Himalaya Drug*) 10 tab. B.D.

(4) **GERIFORTE** (*Himalaya Drug*) 10 tab. B.D.

(5) Inj. **TONOPHOSPHAN** (*Hoechst*) or **HIVIT** (*Ranbaxy*)

(6) **PALLRYWYN** FORTE (*Charak*) 25 gm. granules daily for 1 month.

(7) **VITACEPT** (*Concept*) Vit. ADE Inj. 10 ml. im weekly.

Breedable cows and Buffaloes

Infertility

There could be several causes of infertility such as lack of development of gonads and reproductive organ diseases and dysfunctions of ovaries, malformations and hormonal deficiencies etc. The detailed examination of the animal by an experienced Gynaecologist opinion should always be sought for in such problem cases.

The following treatments are worth a trial. *The pregnancy diagnosis must be done prior to commencement of treatment.*

Anoestrus

(Some of the remedies are as under and be tried in consultation with Gynaecologist)

(1) **PRAJANA** (*Indian Herbs*) capsules

Cows & Buff : 3 capsules. (Repeat after 24 hrs. if no signs oestrus are observed).

(2) **ALOES** compound (*Alarsin*)
10 tablets B.D. 10-15 days.

(3) **COCU- Plus** or **COFFCU** tablets 1 B.D. x 15 days.

(4) Inj. **TONOPHOSPHAN** (*Hoechst*) or **HIVIT** (*Ranbaxy*) 10 ml, im twice a week.

(5) **JANOVA** (*Dabur*) capsules - claimed to be useful in the anoestrus condition.

(6) **SAJANI** (*Sarabhai*) Non- hormonal herbal capsules for inducing oestrus.

(7) **Hitali** - capsule one for 2 days with **Metrali** powder I teaspoon for 7 days. **Heat quick** - 25 g as a single dose.

(8) **Mineral Mixture** (*see under Agalactia* and *Hypogtalactia*) and Vitamin supplements **VITABLEND AD$_3$** (Virbacc & *Glaxo*) 5 g daily in feed forfortnight or **SUPPLIVITE -M** (*Sarabhai*) 1 kg in 400 kg feed.

(9) Per rectal ovarian and uterine massage.

(10) Hormonal therapy like **Folligon, Receptal - Gn RH analogue** for better conception rate and follicular cysts in consultation with Gynaecologist.

(11) Tamponing of the Os-uterus with Lugol's Iodine using speculum and swab holder.

(12) **FERTIVET** (*Ar-Ex*) @ 300 mg. for 5 days orally

(13) **BOVISYNCHRON** (*VEB - Jena Pharma Bernburg Germany*) 1 ml. twice daily for a fortnight given orally. This is a synthetic progesterone derivative and induces ovulatory oestrus.

(14) **SECRODYL** Inj. (*Glaxo*) One ampoule daily for 4 consecutive days (induce ovulation within 4 to 14 days with good percentage of conception)

(15) **E-CARE -Se**(*Vet Care*)

   Inj. @ 1 ml / 25 - 50 kg body wt im

(16) **Iliren** (*Intervet*) PGF$_2$ x analogue : a master key to open anoestrus lock.

(17) **Buco Fert** (Natural Remedies) 2 boli once daily orall for 3 consecutive days. If no weak sign of heat within 10 days repeat the aforesaid dose. Bucomin -E (Natural Remedies) Administer 1 caplet orally with gur or flour for 10 consecutive days.

(18) **Prostanglandin** injections (**Prostodin** 1 ml Astra I DL) or **Prostavet-C** (Verbac) 2 ml or **Prosolvin** (*Intervet*) 2 ml. can be administered. Usually about 60 percent animal attain oestrus within 25 days and about 40% of them. require second injection. Can be treated after 11-12 days in non responsive animals.

Repeat Breeding

Cows which come in oestus regularly but do not conceive pose a problem at many times. Such cows need a thorough exam by Gynaeecologist. Intrauterine injection one hour before and after inemination / service, insemination in late oestrus after 24 hrs to 36 hrs etc. are some of the remedies. Low grade chronic endometritis is the most common cause. The cultural exam. and antibiotic sensitivity test (AST) helps in selection of appropriate antibiotic. Recent reports indicate that intrauterine Inj. of Chloramphenicol followed by *Lugol's Iodine* on the next day has given good results in 80% of repeat breeders which conceived in subsequent oestrus and carried full term pregnancy.Oestrus period lasts sometimes for more than 30 hours particularly in crossbred and exotic cows. In such cases 2-3 inseminations at 12 hourly interval may be useful.

NBT - 800 (*Ranbaxy*) Flouroquinolone group therapeutic agent 1 tab.dissolved in 15 ml distilled water and infused intrauterine for 3 days during oestrus may be tried.

The repeat breeders are found to be having low serum levels of **iron** and **inorganic phosphorus** is revealed in some pilot studies. Hence corrections by suitable treatment should be tried.

Hormonal induction of Lactation

This method is adopted in problem cases of breeding failure and in sterile cows/heirfers which are otherwise in sound health. This involves a course of hormone injections and one of the schedules is as under :

Inj. Stilbesterol @ 7 mg / 100 kg.
and Inj. Progesterone @ 20 mg /100 m/kg.
(*both at separate site*) daily for 12 days.
Rest for one day.
Inj. Prednisolone @ 20 mg daily for 3 days.
Inj. Reserpine @ 3 mg daily for 3 days.

The total period of treatment is for 19 days and medicines may cost about Rs. 400/.This causes development of mammary gland and milk secretion starts by about 15 to 20 days. Results depend upon the endocrine constitution of animal.

This is likely to stimulate the normal ovarian function and regular oestrus cycle.

Although this is practiced in some parts of India and elsewhere, there are lot of controversial opinions about this practice.

The important objections are :
(i) This is against the law of Nature.
(ii) Other side effects of this procedure are not fully investigated.

(iii) The duration and quantity of hormones secreted in milk is not fully investigated. *Since these hormones if present in milk are not destroyed by heating,* the consumption of such milk may not be totally safe and might involve complications in those who consume the milk continuously over a long period. Milk from such animals must be discarded at least 3 weeks after completion of the course i.e., the last injection. **Recently the use of stiblbesterol has been totally banned and as such this method of hormonal induction of lactation seems to be not possible.**

Caution

Research is in progress and till this time more information on above points is not published by research workers therefore **the method should not be practiced on large scale.** The expert consultation of Gynaecologist must necessarily be sought in every case.

Chapter **12**

Preventive Medicine

General Principles of Dealing with Infectious Diseases.

(i) Isolate the sick animal.

(ii) Laboratory confirmation by sending suitable material.

(iii) Safe disposal of carcass by burial.

(iv) Prophylactic vaccination (wherever available.)

(v) Report to the superior officers of the department.

(vi) Responsibility to safeguard public health if a zoontic infection.

Correct diagnosis and early action is the greatest responsibility because correct and timely prophylaxis depends on this.

COMMON BACTERIAL DISEASES

Actionobacillosis (*Wooden tongue*)

Disease of bovines caused by *Actinobcillus lignieresi*. Acute inflammatory. swelling of soft tissues of head (*Lymph glands and tongue*) followed by indurations and abscess formation of lymph glands.

For confirmation send pus smears.

Treatment :

Biniodide of Mercury   0.2 gm. in water as
Pot Iodide   10 gm. a drench for 7 days.

Potassium Iodide 2 gm. in 20 ml. dist. water iv repeated 2 -3 times at 3days interval.

Streptopenicillin in high dose (*Duocryst-sp, Dicrysticin, Bistripen*) daily for 6 - 8 days is highly effective. Long acting

132

tetracycline (Terramycin-LA, Oxyvet-LA) in recommended dose may also be tried.

Prophylaxis - No vaccine available. The veterinarian and dresser/ attendants should take precautions because the infection is transmissible to human.

Actinomycosis (*Lympy jaw*)

Caused by *Actinomyces bovis*. Affects bony tissue of jaw. Granulomatous, immobile, lumpy hard swelling of jaw bone with multiple intercommunicating abscesses. Physical inteference with prehension. Yellow gritty pus.

Confirmation : By sending pus smears.

Treatment & Prophylaxis : As for *Actionobacillosis*.

Anthrax

Peracute septicemic disease of animals caused by *Bacillus anthrasis*, common in cattle . *Commmunicable to man.*

Clinical Symptoms — Hyperpyrexia, bleeding from natural orifices, sudden death.

Confirmation : Exam. of blood smears. Tarry black blood. Spleen enlarged 8 - 10 times and black. Send either blood or piece or ear neatly packed, for laboratory confirmation (*Ascoli's precipitation test and Guinea pig inoculation test.*)

Treatment : Crystalline Pencillin (PRONAPEN or CRYS - 4) 40 - 80 Lakh i.u. iv and procaine penicilin 40 lakh im. Hyperimmune anti Anthrax serum 100 -200 ml, iv is specific. Repeat crystalline penicillin at 3 hourly interval.

TERRAMYCIN (*Pfizer*) or OXYSTECLIN (*Sarabhai*) in high doses iv could also be used.

Prophylaxis — Anthrax spore vaccine 1 ml, sc

Spore vaccine to be *handled with great caution* and used only where repeated outbreaks are confirmed.

Immunity : One year. Annual revaccination in enzootic areas. *Do not open carcass if Anthrax is suspected.* Deep burial of carcass and disinfection of cattle shed.

133

Black Quarter (*B.Q.*)

Aetiology : Acute infection of young bovines usually below 2 years age, sheep and goats, caused by *Claustridium Chauvoei*.

Clinical Symptoms — Sudden onset, high fever, lameness accompanied with inflammatory swelling of thigh musculature, crepitating sound on palpation of swelling. Severe toxaemia.

Confirmation : Exam. of smears of exudate from crepitant swelling. Also send a piece of affected muscle in 10 % formalin.

Treatment — Same as prescribed for **anthrax.** Incise swelling and drain off the exudates. Inj. Anthisan. Continue antibiotics for 4 - 6 days. B.Q. antiserum in large doses if available.

Prophylaxis — Alum precipitated vaccine 5 ml, sc Immunity for 5 months. Annual revaccination before monsoon is recommended in enzootic areas. Combined **H.S./B.Q.** vaccine commercially available in small dose packings.

Botulism

Fatal motor paralysis of cattle, sheep and birds due to toxins of *Clostredium. botulinum* which proliferates in the decaying animal matter. History of access to decaying carcass on pastures. Deficiency of proteins and phosphorus are predisposing factors.

Clinical Symptoms — Progressive muscle weakness and paralysis *commencing in hind quarters.*

Confirmation — By demonstrating specific toxins in the ingesta on autopsy.

Treatment — Specific or polyvalent anti-toxic serum useful in early stages. Purgatives for removal of toxins from gut.

Prophylaxis - By vaccination with type specific precipitated toxoid in enzootic areas.

Brucellosis

Contagious abortion of cows and buffaloes caused by *Brucella abortus.* **Communicable to human** through milk and contamination with discharge. Abortion occurring usually only once during 6 - 9 months of gestation. Subsequent calving full term and normal, but incidence of retained placenta is common. Typical herd history of abortion storm and breeding problems in subsequent years.

Confirmation : Cultural exam. of placenta, fetal stomach contents (*send on dry ice*);bacteriological exam. (agglutination test) to be conducted 21 days after abortion / parturition. **Agglutination tiltre** of 1 : 40 and above on two samples taken at an interval of 30days (*paired samples*) is considered as a positive test.

Rapid whole blood plate test with coloured antigen gives a qualitative diagnosis and a good field test. A test can also be done on milk (*ABR or Milk Ring Test*) of individual animal or on a pooled milk sample from milk can. For this test also a special coloured antigen is used.

Treatment— **Streptomycin** and **chloramphenicol** are effective but prolonged treatment with high dose is necessary. **Oxytetracycline** 10 g given *intraperitonially* as a single dose, repeated after 30 days has been reported to effect cure by some workers. The treatment seems to be useful in reactors with *low antibody titre* (1 : 80 and below) which *could be* due to some nonspecific cause. In frankly positive cases the titre are always very high. Complete eradication of infection from body is not certain. Segregate the positive reactors, rear their calves in isolation. Test and segregation is the method of control.

Prophylaxis

Calfhood vaccination with "**Cotton-19**" strain vaccine at 4-8 months age in the herd in which the incidence is more than 25%. :**Dose** : 5 ml, sc. *Handle vaccine with care, Vaccinator may get infection due to careless handling because it is a live vaccine.*

Colibacillosis

(*See under digestive system - Enteritis*)

Contagnious Bovine Pleuropneumonia - CBPP

A specific infectious disease of bovines caused by *Mycoplasma mycoides* with localization in lungs and pleura. Typical sings of pneumonia with pleurisy. Auscultation findings are diagnostic.

135

Confirmation

Send serum for complement fixation test. Marbled appearance of lungs with thick interlobular septa is a diagnostic p.m. finding.

Treatment

Tylosin tartarte (Inj. Tylin) 4-10 mg/kg b.wt. im injections once daily is specific. **Terramycin** or **Oxysteclin** in high dose and Inj. Enorox, Floxidin, Inj. Enrodac, Inj. Quintas 2.5 to 5 mg/kg b. wt. is specific.

Prophylaxis

Tail-tip vaccination with natural lymph or culture. Not in common use due to necrosis and possibility of spread.

Contagious Caprine Pleueumonia - CCPP

A specific disease of goats and sheep. Clinical picture and treatment same as in CBPP. Large number of unprotected goats die in some areas every year.

Clinical Symptoms— High fever, respiratory distress, nasal discharge and rapidly developing fatal pneumonia.

Treatment—:Tetracycline in high dose iv in early stage. Enrofloxouin is specific.

Prophylaxis

Live- vaccine available at I.V.R.I. and gives good result. Dose : .2 ml at the *ear tip*. **Immunity** : 6 months.

Enterotoxaemia (*Pulpy kidney*)

Acute toxaemia of ruminants particularly sheep, caused by *Clostridium perfringens Type D*. Organisms inhabits the intestines and liberate toxins, lambs (3 - 10 weeks age) suffer more commonly, but, may also occur in adults and goats calves. Disease is per acute in lambs causing death in 2-12 hrs. Adult sheep show staggering, respirator, distress, bloat, convulsions, muscle tremors and diarrhoea.

Confirmation

Collect intestinal contents (*from posterior portion*) in a sterile container preserve with few drops of chloroform and send on ice. Also send smears of the same contents.

Prophylaxis

Annual vaccination. Dose 2.5 ml sc of Multicomponent clostridial vaccine - **IVRI** or vaccine from **IVBP** Pune. Given booster dose after 21 days. Once animal has been properly vaccinated, an annual booster vaccination is recommended.

Glanders

Infectious disease of equines - **communicable to human.** Usually chronic. Caused by *Burkholderia mallei*. Acute septicemic form rare.

Clinical symptons

In chronic form there is chronic cough, respiratory distress, epistaxix, ulcers on nasal septum with discharge of yellow oily pus, enlarged sub-maxillary lymph glands. Cutaneous form shows sub-cutaneous nodules along lymphatic, which soon burst and ulcerate, discharging pus which resembles honey (*farcy*).

Confirmation

Send preserved serum for C.F. test and pus smears. Perform Mallein Intrademopalpabral (IDP) test. *Inject 0.1 ml concentrated mallein intradermally into lower eyelid.*

Read after 24 and 48 hrs. Marked swelling of eye lid, oedema and sever purulent conjuctivites are the signs of positive reaction. CFT is an internationally recognised test. Other laboratory methods include PCR, MLST.

Treatment

Report to higher authority. The animal has to be destroyed under the provisions of *Glander and farcy, Act, 1899.*

Legal Implications

This act got the Governer-General's assent on the 20th of March, 1899 and is applicable to horses, assess and mules. Under this Act, diseased means affected with Glanders or Farcy or any other dangerous epidemic disease among horses, which the Governer-General in council may by notification in the Gazette of India, specify in this behalf "either generally or in respect of any local area". When this act has been so applied to a local area, the Local Government may by notification in the local official Gazette, appoint Inspectors under this act and to exercise and perform, within the whole of the local area, or such portions thereof as it may prescribe, the powers conferred and the duties imposed by this act on such officers.

Within such limits as aforesaid the inspector may seize any horse which he has reason to believe to be diseased and also within such limits he can enter and search any field, building or other place for the purpose of ascertaining whether there is therein any horse which is diseased. The inspector shall cause such veterinary practitioner as the local government may appoint in this behalf. Provided that when the Inspector is also a veterinary practitioner as appointed, he may make the examination himself. If the veterinary practitioner certifies in writing that the horse is diseased with Glanders, the inspector shall cause the same to be immediately destroyed.

The owner or any person incharge of a diseased horse shall give immediate information of the horse being diseased to the Inspector or to such authority as the Local Government may appoint in this behalf.

Whoever refuses or neglects to comply any notice issued by the inspector under this law, shall be punishable with imprisonment for a term, which may extend to one month or with fine, or both. No suit, prosceution, or other legal proceeding shall lie against any person for anything, which is in good faith, donor intended to be done under this act.

Haemorrhagic Septicaemia (H.S.)

Acute septicaemic disease of cattle, buffaloes, sheep and goats caused by *Pasteurella multocida*. Outbreaks usually occur in early monsoon and during stress conditions.

Clinical Symptoms

The disease mainly occurs in per-acute, acute and sub-acute form. The main symptoms shown are high fever, nasal discharge, dyspnoea, lachrymation, rapid pulse, anorexia, drop in the milk yield, oedema under the jaw/neck. Prostration and death.

In some cattle, buffaloes and sheep there is nervous involvement. In some there may be haemorrhagic diarrhoea.

Confirmation

Blood smear and smear from oedematous fluid. Leishman's staining can show typical bipolars organisms. Send blood and oedematous fluid in sterile pippet (*sealed*) on ice for rabbit inoculation.

Treatment

Effective if given in early stages :

Sulfa drugs : (*Give any of the following*)

VESADIN (*Rhone P.*)	100 - 200 ml (33 1/3 % sol)
DIADIN (*Pfizer*)	as initial dose for adults
SULPHADIMIDINE (*Ind. Immunol*)	Half dose by iv and half sc
DIMDIN (*Kosmorex*)	Repeat half dose after 24 hrs

For chronic pastureliosis Inj. **Trimethoprim Sulpha** (*BAIF*) or **Biotrim** iv (Ranbaxy)-15-30 ml by slow iv. In all forms of disease **Terramycin** (*Pfizer*) or **Oxystectlin** (*Sarabhai*) 40- 60 ml iv are also effective. Maintain prolonged levels by giving **Terramycin-LA** or **Oxysteclin-LA** 20 - 30 ml im.

Inj. **Anthisan** (*RhoneP*) 10 ml sc and (or any other antihistamine).

Prophylaxis

Alum precipitated H.S. vaccine 5 ml sc (*Immunity : 6 months*) Oil adjuvant vaccine 2.5 to 3 ml im (*Immunity : 1 year*). This may produce severe shock the reaction after vaccination in some animals. The reactions can be controlled by prompt use of antihistaminic inj. (*for different types of vaccine see chart No. VI*)

Infectious Footrot (*Cattle and Sheep*)

A disease caused by *Spheophorus necrophorus* and lesions usually get complicated with other bacteria. Severe lameness occurring suddenly in one of the limbs with swelling of coronet and fever. Fissure formation at interdigital space with suppuration.

Confirmation

By pus smear examination. Rule out other causes, trauma and F.M.D.

139

Treatment

Paenteral treatment with sulpha drugs (*See under Resp diseases*) combined with local application of the same drug. Locally a gauze soaked in 5% copper-sulphate soln. or Velton liquid or Dressing all gives good result. Inj. **Metraniazole** (*Rhone P.*) may be tried.

John's Disease (J.D.)

A specific infectious chronic enteritis affecting cattle usually of 2 - 6 years age group. Sheep and goats are also affected. Caused by *Mycobacterium paratuberculosis*. Chronic emaciation in spite of normal appetite. Chronic recurrent diarrhoea which does not respond to treatment. Intestinal mucosa thickend and corrugated. Absorption of nutrients does not occur.

Confirmation

Scrapings from rectal m.m.. for acid-fast bacilli in epithelial cell. Serum for C.F. test. Allergic test. Johnin test (Single intradermal test using 0.2 ml. Johnin in the skin of neck. Appreciable oedematous swelling at 48 hrs. indicates positive reaction. Double intradermal testing with Avian tuberculin is also conducted.

Fecal Microscopic Examination: Collect Faecal samples directly from rectum. One gram faecal sample is triturated with pestle and inortar in NSS. Centrifuge triturated mixture at 2000 rpm for 10 minutes. Prepare smears from supernatant of these samples and stain with hiezl-Neelson method of acid fost staining.

Treatment

Infection is very resistant to treat. **Streptomycin** @ 25 mg/ kg b. wt. given a prolonged period effects only a transient recovery, hence not economical and usually not advocated Inj. **Streptomycin** 5 gm vial is now available.

Control : By segregation. No vaccine available.

Leptospirosis

Caused by any of the several species of *Leptospira infection transmissible to human*. Rodents are carriers, infection through contamination of food and water by urine as well as through skin penetration. Organisms localise in kidneys and liver.

Clinical Symptoms

Jaundice, intermittent fever, abortions.

A common disease of old dogs, producing the interstitial nephritis.

Confirmation

By microscopic exam. of sediment of urine, (*dark ground illumination or fontana's silver impregnation staining*) serum agglutination test. Send kidney and liver pieces in 10% formaline for histopathology.

Treatment

Penicillin and Tetracycline are highly effective when given continuously for 7-10 days. Long acting antibiotics in recommended dose are preferable.

Prophylaxis

Vaccine for large animals available but not used in India. A combined vaccine DH PPI +L is available for dogs.

Listeriosis (Circling Disease)

An infectious disease caused by *Listeia monocytogens.*

Cinical Symptoms

Meningo-encephalitis, circling, head pressing, dummy appearance (*Nervous form*), abortion (*Visceral form*), rarely as acute septicaemia (*Trypanosomiasis and Rabies should be ruled out*).

Confirmation

Histopathological examination of brain.On necropsy microabscesses in the brain are characteristic.

Treatment

Strepto-penicillin and chllortetracycline in high doses are effective in early stage. (*For prop. preparations see under Respiratory diseases*).

Strangles (Equine Distemper)

A specified infectious, disease caused by *Strptococcus equi.*

Young equines affected. Initially high fever, nasal discharge, pharyngitis with swelling of neighbouring lymph nodes and abscess formation.

Confirmation

By examination of pus smears.

Treatment

Streptopenicillin and **Tetracycline** highly effective, if given in recommended doses.

Prophylaxis

Killed vaccine available at I.V.R.I.

Dose : 2 ml 3 ml/ 5 ml sc at weekly interval.

Imported vaccines like **"Equibac-II"** (*Fort Dodge*), **"Strepguare"** and **"Stranglevac"** (*Haver Cutter*) and **"Strepvac-II** (*Coppers/ Pitman - Moore*) are the inactivated bacterial and M-protein and extract vaccines used on stud farms. Dose is 1 ml. given at 3 months age and 2 or 3 doses repeated at 2-4 weeks interval (*detailed instructions to be followed as per product literature of each vaccine*).

Tetanus

An acute disease caused due to absorption of potent toxin produced by *Clostridiuumi. tetani.* which causes wound infection. Accident wounds and surgical wounds usually contaminated with soil is the common cause. Equines and human beings highly susceptible. Cattle, sheep, goats and dogs also suffer.

Clinical Symptoms -- Locked jaw (*trismus*), protrusion of nictitating membrane (third eyelid), hyperaesthesia, stiffness of skeletal muscles and spasms are the characteristic symptoms.

Treatment

Equines — Irrigate and cauterise the wound and dress with penicillin. Anti Tetanus Serum (ATS) in high doses (3 Lakh I.U. as an initial dose—repeated 12 hourly). **Penicillin** parenterally in high doses. Muscle relaxants (*Largactil* 5 %) 10 ml, sc. Muscle relaxants such as **tubocuraine** and **succinylcholine** as well as ataractic drugs have been employed in equines. The animal should be housed in a dark quiet room and should not be frequently disturbed so as to avoid onset of spasms.

(*see under Muscuoloskeletal system for details and doses of muscle relaxants*).

Prophylaxis

ATS 1500 - 3000 I.U. before any emergency operation or immediately after injuries in horses as a passive immunization. Tetanus toxoid 1 ml (1500 I.U.) one week before operation or along with ATS for active immunization. Annual vaccination with toxoid is also recommended. **Antitoxin** (ATS) can sometimes produce fatal serum hepatitis in equines. Hence use of *toxoid is largely preferable.*

Tuberculosis

A chronic wasting disease of animals and man. Caused by *Mycobacterium bovis.* Pulmonary involvement common.

Clinical Symptoms — Chronic cough, recurrent and slight fever, gradual loss in condition and lustre of hair coat, chronic diarrhoea (in alimentary involvement) tubercular mastitis characterised by induration developing at the base of udder.

Confirmation : Double Intradermal tuberculin test (DID) commonly performed 0.1 ml. PPD is injected intradermally (*in the thickness of skin*) on the side of neck after preparing the site by shaving on previous day. Special tuberculin syringe and needle is used. A small bead like swelling appears at the spot of intradermal Inj. if it is correctly given. Reading is taken at 48 hrs. If no clear reaction is seen 0.1 ml. injected *again at the same spot* and final reading recorded 24 hrs. after the second injection. A clear inflammatory swelling with oedema at the site of inoculation with an increase of more than 5 mm. thickness of skin is classified as a positive reaction. Retest in doubtful cases *after 6 months.*

Treatment

Streptomycin and **Para-aminosalicyclic acid (PAS).** Isoniazid,used in human medicine are effective; but prolonged and extensive course of treatment and uncertainty of complete sterility of infection are the practical limitations. Eradication of tuberculosis on the herd basis is practiced by *"Test and segregation"* method.

VIRAL DISEASES

African Horse Sickness

A highly fatal infectious disease of equines caused by a *viscerotropic virus, spread by insect vectors.*

Clinical Symptoms

Acute pulmonary from (*Dunkup*) characterized by severe paroxysmal cough, dyspnoea, nasal discharge and pulmonary oedema. Death in 4-5 days. Subacute form (*Dikkup*) is more common. Oedema of head particularly temporal fossa and eyelids. Cyanosis of oral m.m.; hydropericardium. Case lingers for 2-3 weeks.

Confirmation

Send serum for Complement fixation . test.

Treatment of no avail, isolate the animal. Control biting insects and flies.

Prophylaxis

Freeze dried polyvalent attenuated vaccine available at I.V.R.I.

Dose : 5 ml, sc. Watch for reaction till 2 weeks. Give rest for 3 weeks. *Immunity- one year.*

Blue Tongue

Principally a disease of sheep and occasionally cattle, transmitted through insect vectors. There are at least 16 antigenically different strains of the virus. Disease exists in India (6 strains identified so far) and is becoming an important problem and threat for the sheep industry.

Clinical Symptoms

Initially severe febrile reaction (5-6 days), nasal discharge, salivation and stomatitis, swelling and oedema of gums and tongue. Offensive odour from mouth, necrotic ulcers on internal surface of tongue which turns purple in colour. Swallowing difficult. Foot lesions (*laminitis and coronitis*) and lameness. Dark band above coronet is diagnostic. Mortality about 30%.

Confirmation

Send serum for C.F. test. Rule out FMD and Contagious Ecthyma.

Treatment

No specific treatment. Control secondary bacterial infections with antibiotics.

Prophylaxis

Egg- attenuated polyvalent vaccine used in South Africa. It confers immunity for 1 year. Modified liver virus vaccine used in U.S.A. Vaccination of pregnant ewes might give rise to deformity in lambs in some per cent cases. Control insect population by spraying.

Canine Distemper

This is highly contagious, air-borne disease of dogs and has worldwide distribution. Caused by a *paramyxo virus* which has also antigenic similarities with rinderpest and human measles virus. Incidence is highest in young pups ; but, adult dogs may also be affected if not exposed previously.

Clinical Symptoms

Newborn pups who have not received maternal antibodies may get a severe attack with a high percentage of morality. High fever, inappetence, respiratory distress, haemorrhagic diarrhoea and dehydration is observed.

In pups above 3 months, disease takes the typical form. Initially fever for 6-9 days; watery discharge from nose and eyes with bright red m.m. Temperature returns to normal for 2 - 3 days and then again there is secondary rise in temperature (*biphasic fever*). Secondary bacterial infection develops and dog may have bronchitis, bronchopneumonia, diarrhoea with blood, pustules on abdomen, vomiting, hyperkeratosis of footpads etc. Nervous signs appear after this stage and there may be depression, epileptiform convulsions and clonic spasms. Recovered pups may show tremors and twitching of muscles focal or diffused parts of body (*Chorea*). The animal cannot eat or drink and dies a miserable death.

Diagnosis

From clinical symptoms and history of no vaccination. In early febrile stage severe leucopenia is characteristic. In later stages it turns into leucocytosis due to bacterial inf. Cytoplasmic and intranuclear inclusion bodies are seen in epithelial cells of respiratory tract.

Treatment

Not specific. Broad spectrum antibiotics for 7 to 10 days. Vit -C (*Inj. Redoxone*) 500 mg daily for 3-4 day, given with dextrose saline iv Vitamin B-complex injections.

Intensive supportive treatment and care is necessary. Dogs rarely recover from nervous form.

Following Homeopathic remedies may be tried:
(a)   First febrile stage with thirst

Aconite - 30 X 4 hourly interval.

Distemperinum - 30 X twice daily for 7-10 days
(b)   For cough — Bryonia - 6 X 3 hourly.
(c)   For Dysentry : - Arsenic alb. 200 X one dose
(d)   For Cholera

Phosphorous *30 X* twice week is the first remedy

Right side - Arsenic, Causticum and Natr. sulph

Left Side - Cuprum or Rhododendron

In addition to this, a combination of Caleria.Phos 6, Mag.Phos. 6 and Kali Phos- 6 gives good results.

Prevention

Vaccines against distemper alone or a combined vaccine against Distemper - Hepatitis-Leptosprirosis available should be given at the age between 12 to 14 weeks. It is presumed that pup possesses maternal antibodies to protect him till 12 weeks age. This can be depended upon to a good extent if mothers are regularly vaccinated against distemper every year. This is however only an assumption and difficult to prove without serological test which is not possible easily. To avoid any risk first vaccination be done at 6 weeks age and repeated at 12 weeks of age as a booster.

It is essential to keep the pup away from contact with other dogs till it is protected against major diseases. It is also necessary to deworm the pup prior to vaccination and it should be in good health at the time of vaccination so as to develop good immune response. Annual revaccination is recommended.

Homeopathic Distemperium- 30 is claimed to be efficient as prophylactic if given twice a week till the pup reaches 6 months age.

Contagious Ecthyma (*Orf or Sour mouth*)

A highly contagious disease of sheep and goats caused by a parapoxvirus having 6 strains.

Clinical Signs

Initially pustules develop and subsequently pox like scabby lesions are produced on muzzle and lips. Animals suffer severe discomfort while suckling and grazing. Systemic reactions are rare. No specific treatment. Local application of antiseptic ointments and astringent lotions.

Cow Pox

A benign contagious disease of cattle with lesions restricted to skin of teats and udder rarely developing into mastitis. Lesions are usually observed at scab stage.

Treatment

Local application of antiseptic ointment such as **Terramycin ointment** (*Pfizer*), **SAVLON** cream (*ICI*) **BECLOSAL** (*Liva*) or **BOROLINE** oint. Turmeric (Haldi) powder in coconut oil makes a good antiseptic and emolient application. Antibiotics may be necessary if secondary bacterial infections are threatened.

Ephemeral Fever (*Three Day Fever*)

Also known as "Dengue fever" or "Tiwa". Viral fever of cattle transmitted through insect bites. Morbidity rate high. Mortality is not recorded unless complicated with bacterial infections.

Clinical Symptoms

Sudden and high rise of fever, anorexia, stiffness of muscles and lameness affecting once or more limbs, lameness sometimes shifting from one limb to another. Animal returns to normal condition on 3rd or 4th day. Secondary bacterial pneumonia is a possible complication due to exposure and infection during febrile stage.

Treatment (any of the following)

Inj. **Analgin** (*Intervet*)

Inj. **Zobid- M** (*sarabhai*)

Inj. **Paractol** (*Cadila*)

Inj. **Spasmovet** (*Wockhardt*)

Inj. **Ketop** (*Alembic*)

Rx

Sod. Salicylas	30 g
Pot. Nitras	10 g
Pot. Iod.	5 g
Spt. aether nitr.	30 ml
Aqua	Q.S.
Mft . Haust	Sig . B.D.

Homeopathic **Aconite** and **Rhus tox** of 200 potency.

Antibiotic — Streptopencillin or Long acting tetracyclines to prevent secondary bacterial infections.

Prevention and Control

The sick animal should be isolated as far as possible.

Equine Influenza (*Inf. Eq. bornchitis or cough*)

Is an infectious respiratory disease of equines with symptoms of mild fever and severe persistent cough. Although animals of all ages are affected, young animals below 2 years age are more susceptible (*adults probably develop immunity*). Secondary bacterial infections occurs very commonly. Animals become very weak (*outbreaks in equnies with close resemblance with Equine Influenza reported in Madhya Pradesh.*)

Etiology

Myxovirus – Two antigenic strains IA /E1 & IA/E2 are identified and produce slightly different clinical syndromes.

Clinical Symptoms

Initial high fever (104-106^0 F), dry cough which becomes moist later on. Animal remains ill for 2-3 weeks. Cough, dyspnoea, nasal discharge, swelling of submaxillary lymph glands, profound weakness and anorexia. Young animals may develop pneumonia due to secondary bacterial invasion.

Clinical Diagnosis

Initial leucopenia in febrile stage. Differentiate from *strangles* and *Equine viral arterities* which are much more serious diseases (*Absces formation in Strangles and severe conjunctivitis in Eq. viral arterities are the points of clinical differentiation*). Serological confirmation by laboratories where facilities exist.

(*National Research Centre for Equines - Hisar* (Haryana))

Treatment

Broad spectrum and long acting antibiotics in high doses. Intensive nursing and care. Antiseptic inhalations very beneficial.

Prophylaxis

Vaccination with imported vaccines carried out at stud farms. Inactivated vaccines like "FLUVAC" (*Fort Dodge*), "EQUI-FLU" (*Coopers Pitman Moore*) in two initial doses of 1 ml. 2 -4 weeks apart followed by annual vaccination (product literature be to followed).

Foot and Mouth Disease

Highly contaginous disease of cattle, buffaloes, sheep, goats, pigs, deers, antelopes and also communicable to man. Four major strains O, A and Asia-I and several sub-strains prevalent in India. Disease is enzootic in India. More severe in exotic and crossbred progeny and in young calves. Clinical symptoms are so characteristic that diagnosis is not difficult. For confirmation of strain send serum for C.F. test and vesicular fluid in 50% phosphate glycerine saline to I.V.R.I. or Disease Investigation Section, Pune for identification of virus type.

Treatment

Not specific. Antibiotics for control of secondary bacterial infection. Blood from recovered or vaccinated animals can be used for transfusion in severe cases particularly in young calves and save them from acute fatal attack. Levamisol.("Lemasol-75"- *Ranbaxy*) has been found to correct immune deficiency and hasten recovery.

Dose : 1 ml per 30 kg. b. wt. sc

Homeopathic drugs: Merc. sol. 200 X and **Cantheris** 200 X given alternatively for 4- 6 days @ 5 drops of tincture B.D. orally has given a favourable effect in cutting down the course of disease as well as prevention of disease at the onset of outbreak "**Khurenol**" a compound homeopathic medicine (Globulues) administered orally 6-12 globules B.D. has shown promising results. A few percentage of recovered animals suffer from "**Panting**" characterized by hyperthermia, poor heat tolerance, rough body coat etc. This is more common in crossbred cattle. Homeopathic **Natrum carb.** 1 M potency given as globules once or twice a reported to be very effective in such case.

Prophylaxis

Tissue culture inactivated vaccines incorporating all the four strains of FMD virus are now available. Vials of 30 ml. and 90 ml. available.

Intervet FMD vaccine (Intervet) vaccine	**Dose** : 2ml im for **cattle, buff.** & calves above 3 months **Sheep, goats and calves:** 1 ml im
RAKSHA-O VAC FMD (*oil adjuvant*) vaccine (*Ind. Immunological 30 ml vials*)	**Dose** : 2 ml deep 1 im for cattle, buff, calves and pigs. 1 ml im for sheep and goats.

During first year give a booster dose after 4-6 weeks. In case of Intervet FMD oil adjuvant vaccine and of primary vaccination then revaccination every 44-48 weeks after booster vaccination. However, in the event of prevalence of outbreak in the locality it is preferable to repeat vaccination. Calves as young as 4 weeks of age can be vaccinated if born from unvaccinated dams. Give booster dose at 12 weeks and again at 6 months in that case.

In case of Raksha FMD Oil Adjuvant (FMD Ovac Vaccine) first vaccination at 4 months. Booster dose 9 months after primary vaccination. Revaccination in a year.

Occasionally outbreaks the reported inspire of vaccinations (*vaccination failures*). This could be possible due to eater faulty vaccination (*improperly preserved vaccine*) or due to some new variant strain of virus not incorporated in the vaccine. In such cases strain identification is necessary.

I.V.R.I. (*Heeble-Bangalore*) also manufactures monovalent vaccine of any particular viral strain required. Substrain A-22 is found to be frequently identified by sending the material to the typing centre laboratory and get the vaccine prepared against a particular strain prevalent in the area. Second booster 24 weeks of first booster vaccination.

Haemorrhageic Gastro-Enteritis (*HGE*)

(*Canine Parvo-viral Enteritis*)

This is a viral disease affecting dogs. It is caused by *parvo virus* which is closely similar to *Feline panleukopenia virus*. A very resistant and fast spreading virus. Took a very heavy toll in big cities of India during 1978-80.

Dogs of all ages are affected but young pups and pure breeds suffer more heavily.

Characteristic clinical sign is haemorrhageic enteritis and vomiting. There is rapid loss of condition, dehydration and acidosis. In pups virus causes myocarditis and respiratory distress.

Clinical Diagnosis

Rule out Distemper, bacterial enteritis and hookworm infection. Leucopenia maybe seen in initial stage but is not diagnostic. For confirmatory diagnosis electron microscope studies and virus neutralization tests are necessary. H.A. and H.I.test on faecal matter filtrate using specific immune serum antibody ,ELISA is the highly sensitive test.

Treatment

Antibiotics like ampicillin, gentamycin, amikacin and chloramphenicol for control of bacterial invasion, correction of dehydraton and acid base balance by fluid and electroytes Dextrose potassium. Control of vomition Metoclopromide, Ranitidine

It is preferable to get estimation of *Sodium, Potassium and Chlorides* in serum as to select the most suitable electrolyte formula for administration.

High doses of ascorbic acid (Inj. **Ascorbic acid -500 mg iv** in saline), Inj. **STADREN** (*Medinex*) **BOTROPASE** haemocogulant (*Juggat Pharma*) are useful in control of intestinal haemorrahges. Inj. **BUSCOPAN** (*German Rem*) or Inj.

PERINORM are useful in controlling hyperperistalsis and vomition.

Homoeopathic remedies like **Ars, Alb** and **Ipicac** may be tried.

Prophylaxis

Vaccine against parvo virus a combined vaccine with Distemper and Hepatitis is available (**Galaxy-6 or Adenumone-7**) (*Tech-America*), **Megavac-6** (*Ind. immunol*). Principles of immunization are same as for distemper.

Disinfection - The goal of decontamination is to reduce the no. of viral particles. The best and most effective disinfectant is one part bleach mixed with 30 parts water. Apply to bowels, floors, surfaces, toys, bedding etc.

Infectious Canine Hepatitis (ICH)

Also known as Canine Adeno Virus (CAV) infection. It is specific viral disease of canines (*not transmissible to human beings*). There are 2 strains i.e., CAV-1 and CAV-2.

The CAV-1 strain causes more severe and a generalized disease, damages vascular endothelium, and liver cells. Young pups more severely affected. Recovered dogs excrete virus in faeces and urine for *several months*. CAV-2 strain produces a mild disease.

Clinical Symptoms

Fever which fluctuates without returning to normal (*saddle shape curve*), jaundice, thirst, inappetance, congestion of buccal mucosa which is very characteristic. Tenderness on abdominal palpation and tucked up appearance due to liver *enlargement and pain*. Oedema of subcutaneous tissue of head and face, corneal opacity may develop. Petechial haemorrhages and delayed dotting time.

Clinical Diagnosis

From symptoms. Rule out Canine distemper and Leptospirosis. Intranuclear inclusion bodies on H.P. examination in CD.

Treatment

Isolate the animal. Treatment not specific. Broad spectrum antibiotic coverage, treatment to support liver. *Do not treat corneal*

152

opacity with corticosteroid containing eye ointments. In uncomplicated ICH, the recovery percentage is fairly good if sustained treatment is given.

Prophylaxis A combined distemper-hepatitis vaccine *(Bivirovax, Galaxy-6Adenomune).*

Infectious Bovine Rhinotrachetis (IBR)

(Bovine Herpesvirus - 1 infection)

Is a highly infectious emerging viral disease of bovines. The virus can cause encephalitis in newborn calves, infectious pustular vulvovaginitis (IPV) in females and balanoposthitis in bulls. Transplacental transmission to foetus. Disease is also transmitted through semen.

Clinical Symptoms

Fever, congestion of nasal mucous membrane, nasal discharge, conjunctivitis and respiratory distress. Secondary bronchopneumonia may occur. The disease remains in chronic form and causes anorexia and drop in milk production. Most important effect is the abortion, followed by repeat breeding problem and infertility.

Diagnosis

Detection of virus in nasal secretions and serological diagnosis by ELISA test.

Treatment

Broad spectrum antibiotic cover for control of secondary infections only.

Prohylaxis

Vaccines are being developed. BAIF has recently developed a tissue culture, inactivated virus vaccine (IBRIVAK)

Dose : *Cattle & Buff* - (Above 300 kg) 5 ml, sc

Young animals & Calves (Less than 300 kg) 3 ml, sc

Annual revaccination is recommended.

(For details refer product literature)

Mucosal Disease

An infectious disease of cattle characterized by erosions of alimentary tract and diarrhoea.

Clinical Symptoms

In epidemic form (*virus diarrhoea*) morbidity is nearly 100% and mortality is 5-10 %. In sporadic form (*mucosal disease*) morbidity is 2 -5 % but mortality is over 90%. Clinically disease has a close resemblance with rinderpest. Young animals are more susceptible.

Confirmation

It is essential to rule out rinderpest. Send citrated blood, pieces of spleen, mesentric lymph gland on ice with special messenger for detection of virus. Serum from recovered animal for detection of specific antibody.

Treatment

Not specific. Serum from recovered animal 100- 200 ml. iv may be tried.

Bovine Malignant Catarrh (*BMC*)

It is an acute, infectious, possibly contagious disease of cattle caused by virus. Characterised by fever, catarrhal inflammation of upper respiratory tract, kerato-conjunctivitis (*corneal opacity commencing at periphery*) gastroenteritis, encephalitis, lymph node enlargement and cutaneous exantherma. Disease clinically resembles rinderpest or mucosal disease. Morbidity varies from sporadic cases to 50 per cent. Mortality 25- 30 per cent.

"*Head and eye*" form with mucopurulent nasal discharge severe dyspnoea, occular discharge oedema of eyelids has been reported in India

Confirmation — By histopathology of brain, lymph nodes, alimentary tract, liver.

Treatment-Symptomatic.

Prophylaxis— By isolation, No vaccine is available.

Rabies

A fatal disease of all warm blooded animals and man involving CNS. Transmitted by the end bite of infected animal. Most unpredictable disease with variable incubation period depending on site on bite. Dog is the chief source. *Carrier infection in apparently healthy dogs isrecently recorded although in rare cases.* The virus is maintained in wild carnivores like foxes and jackals.

Clinical Signs

Change in behaviour is the first sign . In animal becomes oversensitive, over -alert and has a tendency to attack and the even without provocations. In co-ordination of *furious form* gait and salivation. Hoarse voice which is very typical. In *paralytic form* severe depression, indifference and recumbency, profuse salivation and inability to swallow. Course varies between 1-6 days, but maximum duration being 14 days *keep the animal under observation in isolation for 14 days.*

Confirmation

Send entire head wrapped in polythene bag in ice box or Brain (*Hippocampus*) in 50% glycerine saline for biological test. Impressin smears from hippocampus for *Negri bodies* Part of brain of 10% formalin for H.P. examination.

Post Bite Measures and Immunization

Dog bite wound should be immediately washed using any ordinary soap and water and thoroughly irrigated. If this is done *immediately after bite within 10- 15 minutes almost all the virus gets flushed out of the wound and* the chances of virus getting attached to the peripheral nerve endings and the infection are minimized considerably. Cauterise the wound immediately with Silver Nitrate or Carbolic acid, so that whatever virus is left over might be killed at the spot, Late cauterization is of not of much use as far as destruction of virus from the site of wound is concerned.

Post bite vaccination (*Postbite prophylaxis*)

Antirabies Vaccine cosists of a 5% suspension of sheep brain infected with "Fixed virus "(Paris Strain)inactivated with propiolactone.

155

Manufacturers are :

I.V.B.P. Pune, I.V.R.I. Izatnagar, I.A.M.B.V. Bangalore, N.V.V.I. Hissar.

Route - Subcutaneous

Dose Schedule

Species	Dose (for animals never vaccinated)	Dose (For Previously vaccinated)
Animals weighing under 15 kg (lamb, pup, cat, dog, monkey-not below 2 months)	2 ml daily for 14 days	2ml daily for 7 days
Animals weighing 15--100 kg (dog, Calf, Sheep, Goat, Deer)	5 ml daily for 14 days	5 ml daily for 7 days
Animals weighing 100 --800 kg (Cow, Bufalo, Bullock, Horse)	15 ml daily for 14 days	15 ml daily for 7 days
Camel and Elephant	30 ml daily for 14 days	30 ml daily for 7 days

IVBP Pune supplies the BPL inactivated antirabies vaccine. The post bite schedule for:

Cattle, Baffaloes	10 ml sc for 14 days
Dogs and cats	2 ml sc for 7 days
Calves, Sheep, Goats and Pigs	4 ml for 7days
Cameland Elephant	30 ml for 14 days

Raksharab (*Indian Immunological*). An inactivated tissue culture vaccine propagated on BHK-21 cell line, manufactured by Indian Immunological at Hyderabad (A.P.).

Postbite Dose Schedule for both Above Vaccines :

(*for all types of animals*)

1 ml sc on 0 - 3- 7 - 14 - 28- 90 days as post bite course.

In addition to any of the postbite vaccination schedule, rabies specific immunoglobulin injected locally at the site of bite to neutralise the virus if the place of bite is very close to head. These immunoglobulins are costly, but not routinely available and occasionally used in human beings, pet animals and costly animals.

156

Prebite Prophylaxis (*for regular periodical vaccination*)

NOBIVAC-R (*Intervet*) Dose - 1 ml sc or im for dogs **as well as other animals.**

RAKSHARAB (*Ind. Immunol*)

RABIGEN (*Virbac-Vestas*)

ANNUMUNE (*Vestas*)

DURA-RAB (*Vestas*)

RABDOMUN (*Mallinerodit-Vet*)

Regular annual revaccination is recommended in dogs. However, immunity of 3 years is claimed in other animals (except sheep and goats).

Rinderpest

An acute, highly contagious disease of ruminants and swine. High morbidity and mortality rates. Exotic and crossbred cattle are highly susceptible and suffer a severe attack. Nationwide mass vaccination programme carried out during 1956 to 1960 has successfully eradicated this deadly disease from India. However, sporadic outbreaks are being reported during past 2-3 years and a close surveillance and vaccination has now become necessary.

Clinical Symptom

Initially high fever, lacrimation, salivation, fine necrotic ulcers on buccal m.m. resembling particles of bran, shooting diarrhoea with offensive smell, pneumonia, skin eruptions. Severe dehydration and prostration. *Atypical forms are being reported and hence classical symptoms may not always be observed.*

Confirmation

Send citrated blood, spleen and mesenteric lymph nodes on ice with messenger for virus isolation. Serum from recovering animals for C.F. test, A.G.P.T., Measles H.I. test and Immune peroxidase test etc. Counterimmunoelectrophoresis and ELISA techniques including a rapid dot-immunoassay tests are the diagnostic methods.

Treatment

Not specific. Sulpha drugs and antibiotics for control of secondary complications. Hyperimmune serum in high doses in early stage. Fluids and electrolytes.

157

Prophylaxis

Freeze dried goat tissue-vaccine (FDGTV) is very effective and a potent vaccine conferring life-long immunity (about 14 years) in indigenous cattle. For exotic and cross-breeds tissue-culture vaccine (TCRP) is used and has a 2 years immunity. TCRP vaccine is also claimed to have ability to produce satisfactory long-term immunity and as such can be employed for all types of cattle, sheep and goats.

As regards rinderpest the present state policy is not to undertake prophylactic vaccination because of total eradication of the disease.

Sheep and Goat Pox

These are the common pox diseases of sheep and goats. Typical pox lesions are produced on lips, face, udder, teats, under the tail and sometimes on the other parts also.

Pox viruses of sheep and goat are antigenically distinct although transmissible to each other.

In malignant form, mortality may reach 50%. Young lambs and kids are more severely affected. Goat pox in sheep is more severe than sheep pox.

Diagnosis

From typical lesions. Differentiate from contagious ecthyma and blue tongue.

Prophylaxis

At present only sheep pox thyroid cell culture vaccine is available. This tissue culture live vaccine available at I.V.B.P., Pune in 25/50/100 doses ampoules. This is grown on thyroid cells and is freeze dried. Can be used in clean areas as well as in outbreaks. All animals above 3 months can be vaccinated.

Dose

0.5 ml of reconstituted vaccine subcut about an inch inside the tip of ear using 21 number needle. Do not use spirit or iodine for cleaning the site. Vaccine must not enter blood vessel.

Immunity - 2 years.

Vaccine must be stored and carried on ice.

158

Vaccine also available with IAH & VB, Bangalore, as well as at Biological Products Div. IVRI-Izatnagar.

Goat pox vaccine: consists of unattenuated goat pox virus in 50% glycerine saline, and is manufactured by IAH & VB Bangalore.

The goats can be vaccinated at the face of outbreak. No clean vaccination. Observe for "TAKES" as pink raised areas and scabs at one week interval, in absence of which the vaccine may be repeated. Vials of 100/200/doses.

Peste-Des-Petits Ruminants (*PPR*) - A Goat Plague

Pest des petits ruminants (PPR) is an infectious and highly contagious viral disease of goats and sheep caused by Morbilivirus genus and is closely related to rinderpest virus, canine distemper virus and human measles virus.

Transmission occurs by primarily through direct contact with infected animals and contaminated fomites. Most infections occur by inhalation of the infectious aerosol produced by combination of sneezing and coughing. The virus spread very rapidly like RP and large amount of virus is excreted in diarrhoeic feces of sick animals.

Disease is characterized by high fever, ocuonasal discharge, ulcerative stomatitis, haemorrhagic enteritis, diarrhoea, pneumonia and death. Disease is similar to RP in many respects.

The hemogram demonstrates leukocytosis during the incubation period and leukopenia during the acute phase of clinical disease, the leukopenia is predominantly a lymphopenia.

Being viral disease there is no specific treatment of the disease. However, antibiotics are given to prevent secondary bacterial infection. Long acting OTC, astringents and expectorants can reduce mortality rates. Supportive therapy (B-complex and dextrose saline) for 5-7 days in recommended.

Prevention - Live attenuated PPR vaccine 1 ml sc

Swine Fever (*Hog Cholera*)

An acute septicaemic disease affecting only pigs. Spread rapidly and rate of mortality is very high. It is a big threat to pig industry. Pigs of all ages are affected. Virus is very resistant and spreads through food and water. *Salmonella cholerae suis* is commonly associated with the disease.

Clinical Symptoms

In peracute cases young pigs die without any premonitory symptoms. In acute cases, which are common, the temperature is very high (105–107°F) and the animal becomes dull. Severe conjunctivitis with purulent discharge. Nervous signs like convulsion, tremor etc. are seen followed by terminal coma.

Clinical Diagnosis

Morbidity - mortality pattern is very typical. Symptoms are very diagnostic. Severe leucopenia in early stage is characteristic. Post mortem examination shows petechial haemorrhages in submucosa, serosal surface, under the capsule of kidney and on ileocaecal valve. In chronic cases necrotic ulcers, non-suppurative encephalitis. For confirmation send blood, serum and tissues for transmission test and C.F. test.

Treatment: Hyperimmune serum in early stage.

Dose: 50-150 ml

Prophylaxis

Crystal violet vaccine (*Killed virus*) safe and efficient. (*Immunity: One year*)

Dose: 5 ml for young and 10 ml for adult (above 30 kg). It takes about 12 days for **production of immunity**.

Live tissue culture or attenuated vaccine are not free from risk and in the event of outbreak have to be used in combination with serum. ***Pregnant sows in first third of gestation should not be vaccinated*** because of possibility of product in congenital abnormalities.

Freeze dried Swine Fever vaccine now available with I.V.B.P., Pune in 5 dose packing. Vaccine must be transported and stored on ice.

Dose: 1 ml of reconstituted vaccine a subcut inside thigh.

Immunity: One year

Live attenuated virus (*freeze dried*) from BAIF available in 5/10/25 doses along with dilution.

Dose : 1 ml im for all age groups once in a year. Vaccine to be stored at -20°C or in freeze chamber.

General Precautions for Carrying out Vaccinations

1) A veterinarian first, must decide as a matter of policy whether to carry out vaccinations or not. There are two types of situations A) area is endemic but presently there is no disease prevailing. and B) at the face of an outbreak.

   All types of vaccines cannot be used at the face of outbreak. The choice of vaccine is important on such occasion. Therefore, study of literature is advocated at such a time.

2) While carrying out vaccination (either at a village level or at an organized farm), cent percent animals in the viciity are to be covered to avoid the animals left at risk.

3) Conduct preliminary enquiries from the farmers regarding the type of animals, their age groups and if any recent vaccinations are carried out. If any other recent vaccination are done, it is advised to give a gap of 15-21 days for FMD vaccination.

4) Transportation and storage of vaccine must be made between 4 to 10 degree centigrade. Vaccine must never be exposed to direct sunlight in any case and multidose vials must be utilized within the stipulated period.

5) Instructions on the label must be rigidly followed and the vaccine containing aluminium hydroxide gel must be frequently shaken before filling the syringe.

6) The leftover vaccine and the containers must be destroyed after the use.

PROTOZOAN DISEASES

Anaplasmosis

A haemoprotozoan disease of cattle, sheep and goat caused by *A. marginale* an intra-erythrocytic protozoan transmitted principally through tick bites. Indian breeds of cattle are carriers. Disease is severe in exotic and crossbreeds.

Clinical Symptoms

Continuous high fever, rapid and progressive anaemia, icterus (not a constant symptom) with presence of Anaplasma bodies within the RBC.

Confirmation

Send blood smears, blood for animal inoculation. Serum for C.F. test and capillary agglutination test.

Treatment

TERRAMYCIN (*Pfizer*) or
@ 10 mg./kg b.wt for 5-7 days

OXYSTECLIN (*Sarabhai*) or

INTAMYCIN (*Intas*)

WOLICYCLINE (*Wockhardt*)

EMBACYCLINE (*Rhone P*) or

ALCYCLINE (*Alembic*)

All tetracyclines are equally effective. That Oxytetracycline hydrochloride, (*Terramycin*) given @ 22 mg/kg dose rate for 5 days is found to be highly effective and elminates carriers.

Other drugs recommended after are :

GLOXAZONE - Single dose therapy @ 5 mg/kg iv or IMIZOL - 5 mg/kg. im 2 doses at 7 days interval.

Supportive Therapy

Nutritious feedings Inj. BELAMYL or LIVADEX @ 5-10 im twice in week for 3 weeks. Inj. IMFERON FERITAS 10 ml im twice a week.

(*Virback*) 10 ml daily for 10 days in feed or water.

VITAFERRON (*Univ. Ayur*) 20 g B.D. for 10 days.

Prophylaxis

Control of ticks. A killed vaccine is insured in African countries. Vaccine productions under trial stage in India.

Babesiosis (*Tropical red-water of cattle*)

A tick transmitted disease of bovines, horses and dogs. Recovered animals remain carriers.

Clinical Symptoms—: High fever, haemolytic anaemia, haemoglobinuria (coffee coloured urine) and some times jaundice.

Confirmation : By exam. of blood, smear collected at the height of fever.

Treatment : For Bovines and Horses: (Adult doses)

TRYPAN BLUE 1 % sol 80 - 100 ml slow iv

ACAPRIN (*Bayers*) - 6 ml im single dose.

BERENIL (*Intervet*) - 1.6 gm for 100 kg b.wt. by deep im Average dose 4-5 gm. for adult cattle.

BERENIL (*Intervet*) - 6 mg/kg b.wt. im

For Dogs : 3-4 mg/kg b. wt. im

Babesan (*ICI*)

Cattle - 1 ml of 5% soln. / 50 kg sc

Horses - 0.6 ml of 5 % soln. / 50 kg sc

Dogs-0 .25 ml of 0.5% soln. / 4.5 kg sc

Supportive therapy : As under Anaplamosis

Coccidiosis

Caused by Eimeria Species. Principally a contangious enteritis of young calves below 6 months age.

Clinical Symptoms

Sudden onset of severe diarrhoea faeces containing mucus and blood. Anaemia, dehydration and weakness. Rule out concurrent parasitic infection and bacterial scours.

Confirmation

By faecel examination.

Treatment

Sulphamezathine (*ICI*)   Orally
Diadin (*Pfizer*) or other   sulpha @ 5 gm. tablet for 40 kg. b.wt.
drugs (see under resp. dis.)   for 3 days.

Amprolsol-20 % (MSD) 4 @ 50 to 100 mg kg bwt daily for 4 -5 daily for 4 - 5 days in water.

163

NEFTIN (*SKF*) 100 mg tablets 1- 2 tablets daily for 3 - 5 days.

Supportive : Inj. **Prepalin** (*Virback*) 2 ml im or **VITABLEND-WM** forte (*Virback*) **ROVISOL-100** (*Roche*) or **VIMERAL** (*Virbac*) 2 ml daily in milk or water.

Theileriasis

An important disease of exotic and cross bred cattle. Caused by intraerythrocytic pleomporphic bodies. *Th. annulata and parva* transmitted by ticks indigenous cattle remain as carriers and source of infection.

Clinical Sympoms

Persistant high fever, capricious appetite, enlargement of superficial lymph nodes, progressive anaemia, secondary bacterial infections common.

Confirmation

Exam. of B.S. during febrile stage *Koch's blue bodies* in lymph gland smears, severe drop in haemoglobin conc. and anaemic anoxia. Serodiagnosis using Capillary-Agglutination (CA) test and C.F. test possible.

Treatment

Inj. **TERRAMYCIN** (*Pfizer*)	@ 5 -10 mg/kg
or Inj. **STECLIN** 1/m. (*Sarabhai*)	b.wt daily for 6
or Inj. **ALCYCLINE**(*Alembic*)	days.
or Inj. **INTAMYCIN**.(*Intas*)	

combined with **BERENIL** (*Hoechst*) 4- 5 gm im and **NIVAQUIN** (*Rhone P.*) 20 - 30 ml im daily for 3 days. **TERRAMYCIN** in high dose @ 15 - 20 mg/kg b. wt. given daily for 4 - 5 days has been reported to be very effective. **Chloroquin phosphate** (*Resochin or Avlochor*) 2400 mg im along with quinine dihydrochloride 3 g in (30 ml iv) once daily for 4 days.

Other drugs used for Theileeriasis are as under :

(1) **MENOCTONE** (*Welcome Foundation : London*) (*2-8 Cyclohexyloctyl -3 - hydroxy -1 4, napthoquinine*) @ 12.5 mg/ kg bwt in 4 divided doses im has an antimetabolite activity which blocks enzyme 'Q'.

(2) **CLEXON-4** An antimalarial drug. Given as a single dose @ 20 mg /kg im or double injection @ 10 mg/kg im repeated after 48 hrs.

(3) **BUPARVAQUONE**

(*Butalex- Cadila*) (20 ml vial 50 mg/ml conc) Zubin (*Intas*), Butawock (*Vetoquind*).

Given @ 2.5 mg/ kg body wt (1 ml/ for 20 kg bwt) as a single injection im. Milk be withheld for 2 days in lactating animals.

(*Effective against all stage of various strains*)

(4) **HALOFUGINON LACTATAE**

(5) **PROTOCIDINE** are under trial

Success in the treatment of theileriasis depends on effective supportive therapy. For supportive treatment see under *Anaplasmosis*. Blood transfusions may be given and have been found very useful in extremely anaemic patients.

Prophyaxis

Control of ticks.

A cell culture vaccine is developed by National Dairy Dev. Board and successfully tried in the field. The vaccine is manufactured and marketed by *Indian Immunolgical Hyderabad* (*unit of N.D.D.B.*) as **"RAKSHAVAC-T"** for prophylactic vaccination against tropical theileriosis (*T. annulata infection*) in cattle. The vaccine is stored in *liquid nitrogen* and after thawing is to diluted with the diluent provided along with vaccine.2 and 5 doses vials available 5 ml diluent available is added to a 2 dose vial. This makes total volume of 6 ml. Dose is 3 ml subcutaneously, on neck region (5 dose vial is mixed with 12.5 ml. diluent to makes total volume of 15 ml. Reconstituted vaccine is used immediately and not frozen again. *Animals in advance pregnancy are not vaccinated.*

Immunity- one year.

Trypanosomiasis (Surra)

A disease caused by *T. evansi* - a flagellate extracellula protozoan. Disease more widely prevalent in forest areas du to heavy population of bitting flies. Disease is endemic in certain areas of high rainfall and forests. A high proportion of buffaloes transported from North India are detected as carriers.

Clinical Symptoms

Disease is very chronic in camels (*Tibersa*) and also in equines and elephants. Cattle and buffaloes relatively resistant and remains carriers. Occasionally acute disease occurs in cattle and buffaloes, with high rate of mortality. Acute and chronic atypical form of the disease is common in buffaloes.

Horses: Intermittent fever, progressive weakness, anaemia, patechial haemorrhages on conjunctiva, swelling on scrotum.

Cattle : High fever, nervous symptoms, inco-ordination, circling head pressing etc. The disease may coexist with *Babesiasis* and parasitic infections and present an atypical clinical picture of chronic recurrent indigestion, drop in production and general loss of health.

The disease also occurs quite commonly in dogs and cats. Fever, nervous sign, head pressing, blindness with corneal opacity, petechial haemorrhages on sclera, oedema of face and limbs, splenomegaly are the clinical signs which should arouse suspicion.

Confirmation

By blood smear exam. at the height of temperature. The disease occasionally occurs in a typical form. Response to treatment gives confirmation in such cases. When it is not possible to demonstrate trypanosomes, in blood smear in all cases. In endemic areas the disease is usually diagnosed by symptoms without much difficulty. Inoculation of blood from suspected animal into mice is a very useful biological test for confirmation. Inoculated mice die within 72 hrs. and trypanosomes demonstrated in its blood in positive cases.

Treatment

Horse & Cattle: ANTRYPOL (*ICI*) : 3 g in 30 ml iv repeated on 8th and 15 th day at half the above dose in equines and on 14 th day in cattle.

Camels : 6 g on Ist day and 2 g on 8th and 15 th day.

A combination of *Quinapyramine sulphate* and *chloride* is found very useful as curative as well as prophylactic against trypanosomiasis. *Q. sulphate* is quickly absorbed and has a curative effect whereas Q. Chloride is less soluble, slowly absorbed and has prophylactic value. The above combination are commercially available as **ANTRYCINDE** Prosalt (*ICI*), **TRIBEXIN** (*IDPL*), **TEVANSI** (*Ranbaxy*), **TRYPNIL** (*Merind*), **TRIQUIN** (*Wockhardt*) and **CORRIDAN** (*Hind. Antibiotics*). The above drugs are in powder form and are to be suspended in sterile distt. water and injected subcutaneously. The average dose for adult bovines is 2 to 2.5 g suspended in 15 ml. dist. water. This is a single dose treatment and in endemic areas should be repeated after 3 to 4 months. A small swelling way be produced at the site of injection which subsides after a few days.

SURAL (Alembic) contain Isometamidium chloride HCl is a effective trypanocidial at low dose. No resistance yet reported. No milk withdrawl prediod. 250 mg of the drug has to be dissolved in 25 ml of FFSWFI Dose - 0.5 mg/ kg b.wt. by deep im prophylaxis 1 mg/kg bwt by deep im.

BERENIL (*Intervet*) or **PRONIL-H** (*Merind*) and **BATRYZINE** (*Torrent*) Bilbery (Intas), Dimaze RTU (Vetoquinol) another chemotherapeutic agents effective against Trypansomiasis as well as babesiosis. They contain Diminazene aceturate. Average dose is 3.5 mg/kg for all species and given deep im.

Dose for Berenil: 0.8 to 1.6 g/ 100 kg given by im route as a single dose. These are in the powder form and to be dissolved in sterile dist. water.

For treatment of dogs.

"Berenil" is found to be quite effective and usually well tolerated. A very small dose of 0.1 to 0.2 g dissolved in 2 ml. dist. water is given by intramuscular route. Sometimes a transient reaction is produced after injection but can be controlled by prompt administration of antihistaminic

TARTAR EMETIC (*Sodium antimony tartrate*) is the old and effective treatment but less preferred by clinicians now a days as better drugs are now available.

Dose : 1.1.5 g in 100 ml dextrose saline by slow iv route given carefully ensuring that drug is not injected subcutaneously. The injection may produce reaction in some animals. **TARTAMETIC** 2% and 4% (*Ethicare*) ready to inject solution is also available.

SAMORIN (*Rhone P*) 0.25 mg. per kg. wt. as 1% solution in sterile dist. water given as a single dose intramuscular injection has been found highly effective against *T. evansi.*

GILPOL (*G. Loucatos & Co.*) This is 'suramin' 1 g vial given intravenously after dissolving in 20 ml distt. water. Average. single dose for adult cattle is 2 g.

In all cases, administration of 25% dextrose soln. is recommended as supportive therapy because the trypanosomes produce hypoglycaemia.

If any animal in a dairy herd is confirmed as case of trypanosomiasis it is necessary that blood smears of all other animals in contact be examined for carrier infection. Control of biting flies by regular periodical spraying of cattle shed.

Bovine Ehrlichiosis

Is a tick-borne rickettsial disease of cattle caused by *E. bovis* characterized by irregular fever, lymphadenosis, depression and loss of condition. Recovered animals if stressed develop severe illness that may end fatally.

Diagnosis

The history, clinical signs, examination of blood smear.

Treatment

Tetracycline formulations are effective.

Canine Ehrlichiosis

An acute syndrome occurs in dogs caused by *E. canis.* The onset of illness is sudden and is manifested by depression, anorexia, fluctuating fever and vomiting. Splenomegally and lymphadenitis, mucous membranes may be pale or congested. Some dogs develop uremia manifested by poly urea, polydipsia.

Diagnosis

Depends on the detection of *E. canis* in blood film.

Treatment

Tetracycline is the drug of choice. Uraemic cases may not tolerate oral tetracyclines and they should be switched to doxycycline. Imidocarb dipropionate is also advocated.

PARASITIC DISEASES

Endoparasitic infections are of great economic importance. Chronic debility, diarrhoea,stunted growth, anaemia, uneconomical milk production, rough coat as well as poor working capacity of bullocks should arouse suspicion of parasitic infection. *Confirm by faecal examination.*

The parasitic infection, could be due to any of the several species of worms. Some of them are sucking worms. (*Hemonchus, Bunostomum, Ancylostomes etc.*) Animal may appear healthy in spite of harbouring worms, if level of nutrition is good. In any case, worms do utilise nutrients from the host animal and cause economic loss by way of low growth rate in young animals and efficiencies leading to low production of milk, mat wool etc.

Fascioliasis & Distomiasis (*Cattle, Sheep, Goat*)

More common in certain areas where there are more tanks and ponds. Intermediate host is snail (*Indoplanorbis*). Infections occurs after growing on pasture contaminated by infective metacercariea present on grass blades.

Clinical Signs: Chronic diarrhoea, debility, faeces black, anaemia, submandibular oedema (*bottle jaw*), razor back and pot belly (*asictes*). These are the signs of hypoproteinaemia. **Confirmation :** By faecel examination.

Treatment:

DISTODIN (*Pfizer*) 1g tab.

Cattle : 1 g tablet for 100 kg body wt.

Average dose 2 tablets *Only once.*

Sheep and Goats 100 mg tablets (1 - 2 tab. only once)

FASINEX (*Ciba-Geigy*) *Triclabendazole* : A new generation flukicide safe and effective against all stages of flukes, 5% suspension and 250 mg /900 mg bolus.

Cattle : 900 mg bolus per 75 kg body wt.

Sheep/Goat : 250 m, bolus per 25 kg body wt.

ZANIL (*ICI*) good for distormiasis.

Dose : 30 ml per 100 kg (*max. dose of 100 ml. for cattle*)

RANIDE (*Refoxanide M.S.D.*) 20 % water dispersible powder. A highly effective flukicide (including immature flukes) 10 g powder is suspended in 80 ml water.

Dose: Young animals : 20 to 50 ml   given

Adult : 75 - 80 ml   only once.

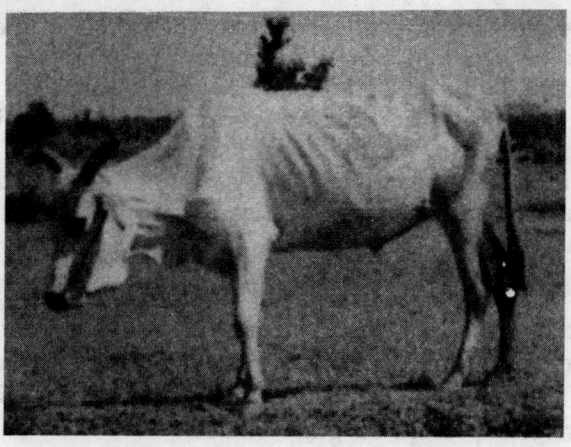

Fig. 13. Razor back, Bottle jaw & Pot belly are the typical signs of worm infection and anaemia.

TOLZAN-F (*Intervet*) (*Oxyclozonide 3.4% suspension is a new flukicide*).

TRODAX (*Rhone P.*) **Single injection.**

Cattle & Sheep : 1 ml/20 kg *subcutaneously.*

Milk from treated animals not to be used for human consumption for 3 days after injection.

ALBENDAZOLE (*Analgon, Albomar, Labenzole* etc.) @ 10 - 15 mg is also claimed to be effective against flukes.

EXINOT (*Cadila*) Closantel 15% oral solution. New single dose treatent eradicates liver flukes, nematodes, cestodes as well as ectoparasites. Effectively prevents reinfection for 7 weeks. Available in 30 ml and 500 ml bottle.

Supportive Therapy

Inj.**Levadex,**(*Virback*) **Beekom-L** (*Wockhardt*) **Leviplex** (*KTS*) or other similar products 5 - 10 ml twice a week.

Liv- 52 or **Tefroli** powder for 10 days.

Prophylaxis

Control of snails by duck rearing, giving stored water for drinking and by regular periodical deworming. Hand picking of snails in and around small ponds which get partially dried up in summer helps in reducing incidence.

Nasal Schistosomiasis (*Nasal granuloma*)

A disease of cattle transmitted by the intermediate host snail.

Clinical Symptoms

Granulomatous growth in nasal chambers, stenotic (Snoring) sounds, respiratory distress and poor production.

Confirmation

By faecal examination as well as examination of nasal discharge for typical spindle shaped ova.

Treatment

ANTHIOMALINE (*Rhone P.*) or **Lithium antimony thiomalate** 6% soln. (*Ind. Immunol*) 15 ml deep im repeated 3 - 4 times, alternate day.

Sodium Antimony tartarte (*Tartar Emetic*) - 0.5 to 1 g in 100 ml dextrose saline by slow iv route.

Although the treatment with tartar emetic is highly effective, it is likely to produce undesirable shock-like reaction which may be sometimes fatal. Drug entering outside the vein may cause sloughing of tissue.

Tape Worms

Common in calves and dogs. Difficult to eradicate as compared to worms. Cucumber seed-like segments seen in faeces. *Rubbing of anus on ground is the typical symptom in dogs.* Some tapeworms of dogs (*Taenia and Echinococcus Spp.*) can be potentially harmful for other animals as well as human because the intermediate stage of cysts develop in any organ of animals and who get infected by ingestion of infective ova from close contact of dogs.

Treatment

(i) **NILTAPE** (*Ethicare*) 20% Powder of lead arsentate

Dose : Calves, sheep, goats : 2.5 g to 5 g

(ii) **NICLOSAN** (*Niclosamide*) or **NICLEX** (*Alved*)

Dose : @500 mg/ 3 kg bwt for dogs.

(iii) **DRONCIT** (*Bayer*) or praziquintel 50 mg tabs.

Dose 1 tab. per 10 kg body wt

(iv) **PRAZI - Plus** (*Vetcare*) used in dogs, cats, sheep and goats, Repeated at 6 weeks interval. Dose -as above.

Ayurvedic and Herbal preparations

ARECANUT (*Supari*) : 2- 3 g in powder form given to dogs and other small ruminants from 10 -15 days is reported to be effective.

Round Worms *(in young calves and dogs)*

Round worms of Ascaris, Neo-ascaris and Toxocara spp. are very common in young animals. Faecal exam.should be done periodically. Verminous bronchitis and pneumonia may occur.

Clinical Symptoms

General unthriftiness, diarrhoea, stunted growth, pot belly, stairing coat, grinding of teeth, Sometimes convulsions and fits in severe infections. Vitamin A deficiency and hyppoproteinemia are also associated with worm infection.

Treatment

(*Any of the following*) :

(i) **PIPARIZINE** (Adipate or Citrate powder)

Calf : 8 - 10 g mixed in feed.

Repeat at 15 days interval till 3 months age.

Dogs : 0.1 g/kg in food or milk.

(ii) **PIPARAZINE** Liquid (*Virback*) vety. 45% sol.

172

Dose : @ 4 ml/10 kg bwt for calves 1 ml/5 kg bwt for dogs.

(iii) **VERMEX** (*Pfizer*) @ 5 ml per 100 kg b. wt. to calves.

(iv) **PIPEREX** (*Sarabhai*) 1 - 2 g in food or milk.

(v) **BANMITH forte** (*Pfizer*) A broad spectrum anthelminitic. 200 mg. tablets for calves @ one tablet for 40 kg body wt. Liquid also available.

(vi) **ALBOMAR** (*Virback*), **ANALGON** (*Wockhardt*), **PANAUR** (*Hoechst*) etc. are the broad spectrum anthelmintics and are given @ 5 - 10 mg kg b.wt.

(vii) **HELATAC** (*SKF*) @ 15 - 30 g for calf once in 3 months.

Worm Infection in Adult Cattle & Sheep

(viii)**NILVERM** (*ICI*) powder. (*Tetramisole*) single dose pack.

(ix) **CURAMINTH** (*Sarabhai*) bolus contains Fenbendazole 1.5 g effective as broad spectrum anthelminic.

Dose: for cattle : 1 - 2 boluses. Sheep : 1 - 2 g

(x) **THIOPHANATE** (*Rhone. P.*) A broad spectrum anthelmintic cattle & Buff : Av. single Dose 10 - 20 g powder.

Sheep Goat : Av. single dose 3 - 5 g powder.

(xi) **ROBENDOLE** (*TTK*) 2 g bolus and powder

Dose : 2 boluses for adult.

(xii) **LABENZOL** (Albendozole - Torrent)

12 %powder and 2.5 % suspension.

Dose : @ 5 mg/kg b.wt. for roundworms.

10 - 15 mg/kg for liver flukes.

(xiii)**VALBAZEN** (*SKF*) 600 mg bolus and tablets.

(xiv)**FENCUR** (*Fenbendozole-Torrent*) 25% granules @ 5 mg/kg body weight. Effective against gastrointestinal round worms and lung worms.

(xv) Inj. **IVERMECTIN** (*Ivomec-MSD*) @ 1 ml/50 kg sc single injection.

(xvi)**XYCLOZ** Closantel (*Cadila*)- A new generation Ectoendoparasiticidal effective against trematodes,

173

nematodes, cestodes & ectoparasties is recently introduced for all species as a broad spectrum anthelminitc.

(xviii) **ENDOBAN** (*TTK*) for control of all endoparasties (available in the form of suspension @ 125 mg/5 ml. and bolus with 750 mg/per bolus).

(xix) **ALZOEX** (*Neospark*)-Albendazole suspension and tablets (150 mg & 600 mg)

Herbal Products

(i) **CRUMINIL SYRUP** (*Charak*) 100 ml in 2 divided doses. Repeat after 1 week.

Hookworm Infection in Dogs (*Ancylostoma spp.*)

Very common in dogs, cats and carnivores of zoo.

Clinical Symptoms

General condition emaciated, body coat rough, anaemia, itching of skin with heavy loss of hair, indigestion, diarrhoea with black faeces, dysentery (haemorrhageic enteritis)

Confirm

By faecal examination.

Treatment

ANCYLOL (*Cynamid*) Disophenol Injectable.

Very effective drug for hookworms.

Dose : 0.22 ml. per kg body wt. *subcutaneously*. Repeat after 21 days for the drug doesn't act against larvae. Work out doses correctly and dilute with distilled water while using in very young pups as the injection is very painful.

Mebendazole and allied compounds which are broad spectrum anthelmintics used in human medicine, are commonly used in canine practice and are found to be reasonably effective in most types of round worms and hookworms also. The common proprietory preparations are :

ALBRODO (*Shalax*) 25 —50 mg/ Kg, P.O, b.i.d.

MEBEX (*Cipla*)	Av. dose for adult dog over
IDIBEND (*IDPL*)	20 kg body wt. is 2 tablets
ELZOL (*Camlin*) 100 mg.	B.D. for 3 days.
WORMIN (*Cadila*)	For young animals and
PANTELMIN (*Ethnor*)	smaller breeds half the
MINTEZOLE (*MSD*)	above dose

Pyrantel pamoate (*Combatin Pfizer*) 200 mg tablets or **Thalmax** (*BPL*) suspension and tablets.

Dose @ 5 - 10 mg / kg b.wt. P.O. Single Dose.

Drontal Plus (*Bayer A.G.*) @ 1 tab. per 10 kg body wt. is the new anthelmintic effective against both, roundworm as well as tapeworm .

Inj. **Ivermectin (IVOMAC**-*MSD*) @ 200 microgram/kg single dose as subcut injection. Repeat after a week if necessary.

Supportive : Inj. of Liver ext. with B-complex 1 - 2 ml and iron preps. like **IMFERON** with B_{12} injections alternate daily for 1 - 2 weeks to cure anaemia.

Fesovit or **Rarical** (*Ethnor*)1 tab. B.D. x 6 days. Liv-52 or Valiliv tablets or drops from 15 days. **Sharkoferrol** (*Alembic*) is very good oral tonic for dog.

Filariasis (*Heart Worm*) in Dog

Dirrofileria immitis is transmitted in larval form by mosquitoes. Larvae develop and migrate to right side of heart and lungs.

Diagnosis & Treatment

By blood smear exam. for microflariae. **Caricide** (*Cynamid*) 400 mg tablet. one tab per 7 kg bwt. Repeat after 20 days.

Control of Ectoparasites (*Ticks, Lice and Fleas*)

A very important and a common problem and may become a nuisance if not controlled in time. Apart from constant irritation, itching, loss of hair, ticks transmit protozoan infections and cause anaemia. Fleas also produce allergic dermatitis.

Dust the animal body with **Gammexine** 5% powder. D.D.T. soln. 5% or spray **BUTOX** (*Intervet*) @ 2 ml per litre water in the animal houses and cattle sheds.

Malathion 50% w/v. 0.1% soln. for spraying over animal body. 2.0% soln. for spraying cattle-sheds.

Do not spray over grass, hay and in mengers.

Sumithion (Tata - Fision) 50% w/v for spraying.

50 ml in 20 litres of water for lice, fleas and mites.

100 ml in 10 litres for ticks. (useful for poultry).

"Butox" (*Hoechst*) Deltamethrine

For spraying : on animal body   @ 1 ml/litre water

For spraying : in cattle shed   @ 2 ml/litre water

"Notix" shampoo, Powder (*Vetcare*) is useful for small animals.

"Cyprol" (*Intax*) ecotoparasitic spray

@ 1 ml/litre water reportedto be effective.

Follow the instructions for its use. Caution the owner about handling and storage of drug and keep the antidote ready at hand. (See product literature).

Antidote : (*For organophosphorus compounds*)

Atropine sulph. 50 - 100 mg for adult cattle and 0.6 mg for dogs. Always keep at hand.

Pestoban (*Indian Herbs*) An Ayurvedic herbal compound effective and safe for external application after dilution 30 - 40 times with water.

Chapter 13

Dairy Farming

Dairy farming is the basic production industry with which a veterinarian is directly connected and concerned regarding it's welfare, scientific management and development. It is by virtue of this industry that the national development, food crisis, the rural economic stability and the general health of growing children is augmented. It is the veterinarian working in rural and the urban areas of India whose efforts and the contribution that are responsible to take the nation to the top position in the total milk production. This achievement is due to the large number of average milk producing cows and buffaloes producing under most average conditions of feeding and management. One can imagine the picture, if these animals are judiciously selected, managed and fed in ideal conditions !

Government of India has several schemes for promoting Dairy industry through the agencies of State Animal Husbandry Department, Zilla Parishads and also through agencies like NABARD which offers affordable loan at very low rate of interest as well as subsidies. Some schemes of NABARD offer 50 % of the project as interest free loan. Dairy farming is a *safe business* because of the following:

- It is eco-friendly and does not cause environmental pollution as compared to other industries.
- Dairy product market is active throughout the year.
- There is minimum requirement of the highly skilled labour.
- The entire establishment can be shifted to a new location if need arises due to fire, floods etc.
- Energy requirements are less as compared to other industries. Biogas plant and compost manure are useful.

- Disease control is easier by prophylactic vaccinations and proper management practices and the insurance of animals can also minimize the risk.

Limitations and Constraints

Regular breeding of animals and getting expected quantity of milk yield is a biological phenomenon, which depends on various factors which need a meticulous management.

Inadequate management of feeding, herd health cover and lack of quality control in handling and distribution of milk can cause major loss affecting profitability of the entire project.

Besides good planning, the dairy business needs a hard working resourceful reiliable and alert manager. In India the household family members can participate in the industry to safeguard these aspects which are very important.

Proximity of market , reliable and hard working servants, prompt and efficient record keeper are the important assets.

Important Considerations for Starting the Dairy Farm

- One must first decide the aims and objectives of the farm. Every year there must be progressive aim of breeding and the number of animals to be maintained and production of milk that is to be handled.In other words the size and the capacity of the farm must be decided in the mind.
- It is better to visit some established commercial farms and discuss with farm owners. You need not rely on the experiences of others but should analyze the situation and if needed the veterinarian be consulted for more information.
- If you are going to manage the farm yourself, then it is better to look for getting the work experience fo at least 6 months at the existing farm.
- Develop interest and study the feed and fodder situation and market, in relation to various seasons.
- Manage a good team of labourers . You need to have a good team of reliable and hard working labourers, preferably with some previous experience. You can also train them for specific jobs .

- You must visit the cattle markets occasionally, observe animals on sale and talk with animal traders.
- You must read the magazines on Dairy Industry and keep yourself informed. If possible get some professional training available at Veterinary Universities, Krishi Vigyan Kendras, State Animal Husbandry Department or Non Governmental Organizations. It is better to have such training in management and rearing of dairy animals and also on manufacture of milk products.

Selecting Animals for your Dairy. (COW V/S BUFFALO)

COWS

- Good quality cows are available in the market at the cost around Rs. 1200 to 1500/ per litre milk per day. Average cost of a cow with 10 lit. capacity would cost approx. 12000 to 15000/
- In ideal management and care a cow regularly gives a calf every 13-14 month interval, and feed requirements are economical.
- Cows are more docile and easy to handle. Good yielding crosses of Jersey or Holstein have well adapted to Indian conditions. However, good Indian breeds like Sahiwal, Gir, Red Sindhi or even selected Gaolao breeds are also worth consideration.
- Cow milk has a fat percent ranging from 3.5 to 5 % and is preferred for children and elderly persons in a family who are health conscience and prefer low fat diet.

BUFFALOES

- In India, Murrha and Mehsana are the two breeds that are preferred for the Dairy industry and are suitable.
- Average cost is around Rs. 18000 to 22000 per animal giving approximately 12 to 15 litres of milk initially.
- Buffaloes usually mature late and give a calf at the interval of 16 to 18 months. Female calves if reared carefully for first 3 months, can be available as a breedable animal at her age of about 3 years.

- Buffaloes can be maintained on more crop residues so as to reduce feed cost, but the feed requirement is more than a cow.

- Buffalo milk with 6 to 8 percent fat is preferred for tea , butter and ghee making and for bye products like sweets and has a better market in most parts.

Buffaloes need more water for wallowing tank and for showering as basically it is a semi aquatic animal.

Some Suggestions for Deciding Selection of Animals

Most of the middle class, health conscious Indian families prefer low fat milk for consumption and buffalo milk has a good market. Hence, it is better to have a commercial farm of a mixed type. High yielding cross bred cows and buffaloes be kept in separate rows in one shed. Conduct a thorough study of the market where you are planning to market your milk. You may mix both types of milk as per the need. Hotels and some customers prefer pure buffalo milk,whereas hospitals and sanitoria prefer pure cow milk. It is better to earn confidence of the customers for supply of unadulterated milk.

Popular buffalo milch breeds are Murrah, Surti, Mehsana, and selected Nagpuri/ Padharpuri.

Indigenous Cow breeds are Gir, Sahiwal, Red Sindhi, Gaolao and Tharparkar. The Exotic breeds are Jersey, Brown Swiss and Holstein Friesian.

Economic life of a buffalo is 5 to 6 lactation and that of a cow is 6 to 7 lactation.

The minimum economic size of a commercial dairy farm should be 20 animals (10 cows and 10 buffaloes) and this strength can be increased to 100 animals in the proportion of 50:50 or 40:60. After this you need to survey the market situation before going for expansion.

Infrastructure and Manpower Requirements

The space requirements per animal is 40 sq. ft. in the shed and 80 sq.ft. open space. In addition you need :
- One room 10' x 10' for keeping implements.

- One room 10' x 12' for milk storage.
- Office cum living room of suitable size.
- Water tank with a capacity to store 2000 litres.
- A good borewell or any other good watersupply.

The total land require for 20 animals to start with is about 3000 sq,ft. with enough scope for expansion up to 100 animals which will need total space of 15000 sq.ft.

You must also make a contractual arrangement for regular supply of about 400kg of Lucern/Barseem and 300 kg of maize fodder per day, and for meeting the requirements of 100 animals. In due course, you need to have land of 15 -20 acres with irrigation facility for fodder cultivation. (One acre land needed for 5 animals as a thumb rule). The economics of the dairy industry depends on the economy of home grown fodder so that cost of concentrate feed can be reduced substancially.

Labour strength on the farm depends on the number of animals. The common thumb rule is one labour for every 10 animals in milk, or 20 dry animals or 20.young stock.

All said and done, you need to calculate the requirements of the cost of agricultural land utilized for fodder cultivation, investment for infrastructural facilities, market price of feeds and fodder, labour charges, processing, transport of milk, veterinary aid and medicines and the depreciation of value of animals as well as buildings etc. for working out the cost of milk production so as to decide the sale price of milk. The assets of organic manure, cost of biogas produced and cost of animals born and reared for replacement, cost of animals sold etc. also will have to be taken into account for preparing the balance · sheet of profit and loss account of the industry.

The small dairy farmers must form a strong union and decide some common operational plans and approach the concerned Government authorities to grant subsidies and give proper purchase rates for milk, based on the actual cost of milk production so that the dairy units will come up rapidly and the dairy industry will get boosted up and new entrepreneurs will be attracted to this very useful and prestigious industry which is presently grossly ignored.

Chapter 14

Poultry Medicine

Poultry has developed fast as a big industry in the recent past.

Breeding, housing, rearing, feeding, management and marketing of Poultry is now collectively recognized as an independent science.

Scientifically managed poultry farms lead by qualified veterinarians specially trained in nutrition and business management are coming up with big investments around cities which provide regular market round the year. Average size of such farms provides housing capacity of 10 to 50 thousand birds. Ancillary industries such as feed manufacturing factories, transport agencies have simultaneously found new avenues and also biological competition to produce new and effective vaccines, antibiotics, vitamin and mineral supplements which have actually flooded the market.

Apart from these big poultry farms, small units of 50 to 500 birds are also coming up in rural areas is a boon for a landless labour and unemployed youth who can earn their livelihood in a better way. They need to be supported by some training and financial assistance from government and banking sector. Average veterinary graduate is usually consulted by these small and medium size poultry units.

Poultry farming needs comparatively lesser investment and space and can be a good source of regular earning. It is a good source of high quality manure for agricultural land. Poultry industry gives quick returns and helps solving problem of quality protein food for young and growing individuals.

Poultry farmers' success depends on the following five important factors and deficiency of any one factor can offset the anticipated progress,

(1) Strain (2) Feed (3) Management (4) Health control and (5) Marketing

Feeding and management including housing are the important factors governing the health aspects of the poultry.

Before starting a Poultry business one has to decide whether to go for :

(1) Establishment of a 'layer' *farm*.

(2) Establishment of a *'broiler' farm*.

A *layer* farm needs a long term flock management and care to keep production at the optimum level of average 70% and above, for getting good profits. The birds must be properly selected and must be in best health and productivity. Small efforts in feed quality and management can cause enormous losses.

Broiler farming is comparatively a short term business and one gets full returns within only about 6 weeks from the beginning. Birds are to be looked after for a brief period and this reduces concentration over management and care.

Important Rules for Keeping Diseases Away

Whether you plan for a 'layer farm' *or a* 'broiler farm'

(1) It is always preferable to start by rearing from day-old chicks obtained from a hatchery known and certified free from Salmonellosis, ALC and Marek's disease instead of getting grown up pullets.

(2) Ensure that day-old chicks that you are purchasing, are protected with either LaSota or F_1 strain against Ranikhet and vaccinated against Marek's disease. Brooder life is important for broilers.

(3) Do not forget or postpone vaccination with *Mukteswar* or R_2B strain or Ranikhet disease vaccine and fowl pox vaccine at 6 weeks age.

(4) Keep a close watch on quality of feed and ensure that it provides at least 21 - 20% proteins and adequate vitamins and minerals and added to it. This will ensure proper growth, economical laying and prevent deficiency diseases. Good quality cf feed is very essential for broliers.

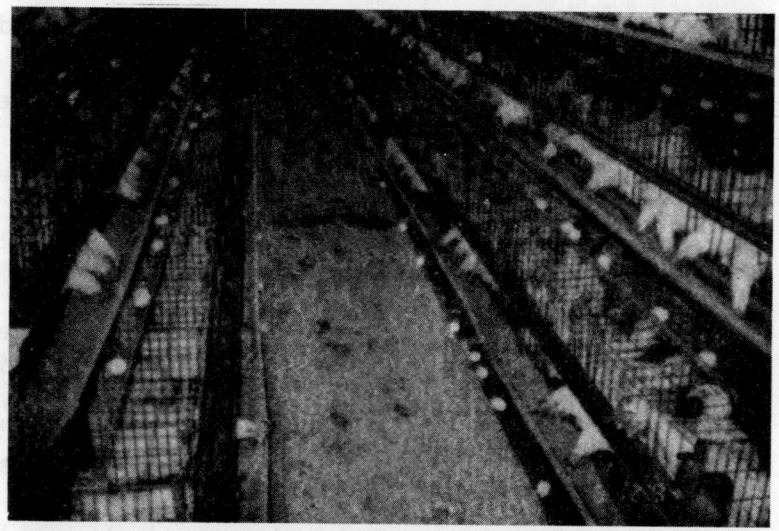

Fig. 14. Commercial Poultry Farm.

(5) Ensure incorporation of coccidiostat in the feed particularly for starters and growers.

(6) Provide disinfectant foot-bath at the entry of the flock house and make its use a practice. Do not allow entry to visitors near to or inside a flock house. This will prevent mechanical transmission of disease.

(7) Keep the deep litre dry by regular raking and periodical change. Avoid spilling of water.

(8) Ensure free ventilation. Stuffy feeling with amoniacal smell on the entry into flock house indicates bad ventilation.

(9) Follow a regular deworming schedule.

(10) Get your layer birds tested for Salmonellosis and CRD at 16 weeks age and maintain the flock *certified free* based on two consecutive negative testing reports.

(11) Be watchful and control tick infestation. Carry out periodical spraying of houses. Undertake vaccination against spirochetosis, if there is a history of outbreaks.

(12) Dispose off the carcasses of birds suspected to have died due to any disease, either by *burning or burial*.

(13) Get prompt disease investigation service as soon as any health problem crops up. Send a *freshly dead* bird on ice or few ailing birds to the nearest Disease Investigation Laboratory for timely diagnosis.

(14) Never exchange or mix birds from outside with your flock even your own *birds if* they had been taken out for a show or exhibition until they are observed in isolation for a week.

(15) Fumigate incubators before setting up a new hatch. (75 ml formalin + 50 g Pot. permagnate for 100 cubic ft. space).

Chick Mortality

(1) Check brooder temperature and possible overcrowding.

(2) Arrange to send a few chicks in extreme condition to the nearest disease investigation laboratory with a messenger. Request cultural exam. for Pullorum disease and to rule out Marek's disease by careful p.m. studies.

(3) Isolate the sick chicks.

(4) Rule out Ranikhet, Fowl pox. Check up vaccination dates. Critically examine for IBD (*enlarged and haemorrhagic bursa is an important observation*).

(5) Test the adult flock for carriers of salmonellosis to rule out egg borne infection.

(6) Clean and disinfect the feed and water utensils by using boiling water. Check up feed also.

(7) Critically examine for coccidosis by faecal examination for oocysts as well as exam. of intestinal scraping for merozoites in peracute cases.

Till the time you get a laboratory report and confirmed diagnosis, give **any of the following** for 3 -4 days , to all the birds as a water medication.

(i) **HOSTACYCLIN** water soluble powder (*Intervet*) @ 2 teaspoonful in 4 -5 litres water.

(ii) **AUREOMYCIN** (*Cyanamid*) soluble powder @ 4 teaspoonful in 5 litre water.

185

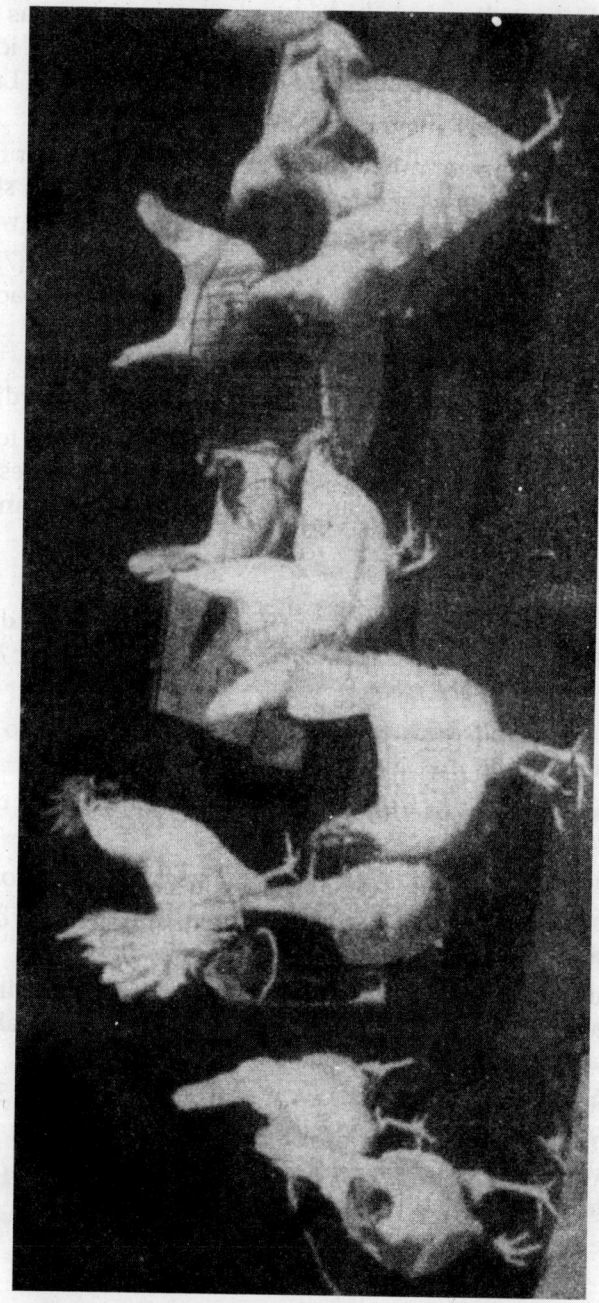

Fig. 15. A flock of white leghorn in a house.

Supportive : VITAMBLEND *wm−forte* or VIMERAL (*Virback*) or VITADEC (*BAIF*) or WINSTRESS (*Cadila*)

@ 2 ml per litre drinking water for 15 days.

Colisepticaemia

Colisepticaemia is a disease of chicken generally 4 to 10 weeks of age but can be seen in adult flucks too. Broiler and growers show depression loss of appetite and dyspnoea. Post mortem often reveals pericarditis, perihepatitis with thick and cloudy air sac membrane.

Omphalitis

This is again a very important disease causing heavy losses in newly hatched chicks. Main gross lesions are unabsorbed, congested and foul smelling yolk.

A key to get rid of E. *coli* infection at the farm is to avoid stress of any kind and provision of clean water and quality feed. But, its better to go for culture and drug sensitivity test as in case of E. *coli* infection drug resistance is fairly common.

Pullorum Disease (*Bacillary White Diarrhoea*)

A highly infectious disease principally of young chicks of brooder age. High rate of mortality.

Clinical Symptoms

Sudden deatlh due to septicaemia, white diarrhoea. viscera congested. Infection also- egg borne. Recovered birds remain as adult carriers and uneconomic layers. Ovaries cheesy, misshapen and pedunculated.

Confirmation

By cultural exam, in chicks, By serological test in adults. (Rapid whole blood plate test with coloured antigen is the field test).

Treatment

NEFTIN (*SKF*) powder in feed at curative level (one tin of 454 gm in 50 kg mash) or **Nefrazone-200** (Wcohardt) curative level @ 200 g/100 kg feed for 10 days. Water medication with any of the drugs prescribed under *"Chick-mortality"*.

Dose : 1 g in 2 litre water for 3 to 5 days.

Prevention

NEFTIN (*SFK*) **NEFRAZONE** (*Wockhardt*) in feed at *preventive* level for 10-20 days to newly hatched chicks. **Furex-20** (*BAIF*) for mixing in feed @ 25 g per 100 kg. feed to be gien regularly. Periodical testing of layer flock, fumigation of incubators and other hygienic measures.

Fowl Typhoid

Usually a disease of young adults (pullets) caused by *Salmonellall gallinaru:n.* Can also cause septicaemia and heavy chick mortality as in pullorum disease.

A greenish-yellow diarrhea appears early. Birds are intensely thirsty. Affected birds breath faster. In acute fowl typhoid, the comb and wattles may become dark.

Confirmation

Treatment & Prophylaxis: As in pullorum disease.

Fowl Cholera

A fatal speticaemic disease caused by *Passteurella multocida* (*avain strain*) affecting birds of all age groups.

Clinical Symptoms

In per acute type -sudden deaths without apparent illness.

In the acute form, many birds in the fluck become sick at the same time. The comb face, and wattles may be a purplish colour.

In the chronic form diseas will localize, causing a swelling of the face and wattles- the wattles may be fiery red and hot to the touch.

Confirmation

By bacteriological and cultural exam.

Treatment

Sulphamezathine (*ICI*) 16% or **Diadin** (*Pfizer*) 16%	30 ml in 4 litres water for 2 - 3days followed by half the dose for 4 days

Prevention

A matter of sanitation and building resistance. Clean feeding and watering equipment. Dispose of carcasses of birds promptly.

Treatment

DIMDIM (*Ar-Ex*) 16% powder is also recommended.

In addition, any of the drugs prescribed under "Chick Mortality".

Prophylaxis

Fowl Cholera vaccine availeble at I.V.R.I. or. I.V.B.P. Pune, **Dose : 1 ml Immunity : 6 months.**

Infectious Coryza

A respiratory disease caused by *Haemophillus gallinarum* with high morbidity, but low mortality.

Clinical Symptoms

Nasal discharge, sneezing, soft swelling and odema of face which contain fluid. Occasionally become similarly swollen wattles. Sharp drop in egg production. Recovered birds remain carriers. Infectious coryza, spreads rapidly within a flock.

Confirmation - By cultural examination.

Treatment

Sulphamezathine (*ICI*) 16% 30 ml in 4 litres water
Diadin (*Pfizer*) 16% for 3-6 days (*Give*
Sulmet (*Cynamid*) 16% **Vetydine** *medicated water only*)
(*TCF*) 16%

AVISOL (*Rhone P.*) 40 ml in 4 litres for 4 - 6 days.

DIMDIM (*Ar-Ex*) 16% powder is also recommended.

(*Response to sulpha drugs indirectly confirms diagnosis*)

Supportive: Vitablend-Wm forte. **Vimeral** (*Virbac*) in water.

Prophylaxis

A killed vaccine manufactured by Ventri Biologicals available (200 and 500 dose vials)

Dose : 0.5 ml sc. Vaccinate birds above 8 weeks age. Repeat vaccination after 3 - 4 weeks as booster for better protection.

Immunity - About one year.

Chronic Respiratory Disease (CRD)

A chronic disease caused by *Mycoplasma gallisepticum* (Pathogenic strain). Usually a concurrent infection with *E. Coli* or infectious coryza.

Clinical Symptoms

Drop in egg production, chronic coryza and rattling sounds (tracheal rales) and cough. Mortality upto 20% in young lot. Disease transmitted through eggs.

Confirmation

By histopathological exam. of respiratory passage and air sac membranes, Serological test. (*Plate or tube agglutination test*) using S-6 strain antigen is possible. Cloudy air sacs with cheesy material on post-mortem should arouse suspicion.

Treatment

TYLOSIN or ERYTHROMYCIN	3-5mg/kg subcutaneously is *highly effective.*

Dynamutillin (*Ciba-Geigy*) a highly effective antibiotic active against **CRD** (*Tiamulin hydrogen fumarate*)

As curative : 100 mg in 180 litre water for 3 - 5 days

As routine : 100 g in 360 litre water for 3 - 5 days

Water medication as prescribed under "Chick-Mortality" along with supportive treament.

Prevention- Strict isolation and hygienic measures. Test the layer flock. Dipping the eggs in solution of Tylosin or Erythromycin (400 - 1000 ppm) before hatching reduces the chances of egg tranmission.

Spirochetosis

A febrile, septicaemic disease of poultry caused by various strains of *Borellia anserina*, transmited by tick bites. (*Argus persicus*) . High rate of mortality.

Clinical Symptoms

High fever, greenish diarrhoea, drowsiness and death in 2 - 4 days. Mottled and enlarged spleen on p.m.

Confirmation

Examination of blood smears, impression smears of spleen and bone marrow, histopathological examination of spleen.

Treatment

Penicillin 200 i.u. per bird as Inj. **(Pronapen or Crys-4)** or **Tetracyclines** Injectable **(Terramycin, Oxysteclin)** 1 ml per bird for 3 days, is effective.

Proplylaxis

Formalin- killed vaccine preferably prepared from the same prevalent strain is highly effective. Vaccine available from I.V.R.I. or I.V.B.P. Pune. **Dose:** 1 ml sc.

Immunity

One year. Control of ticks is the imporant prophylactic measure.

Necrotic Enteritis

An acute enterotoxaemia characterized by sudden onset of mortality is caused by *Clostridium perfringes* type or c. It primarily affects chicks between 2 to 13 weeks of age and seem most frequently in broiler houses with old built up litter.

Enterotoxemia is likely to occur when gut micro ecology is altered drastically by variation in feed, aggressive pathogen and by toxins. These changes may promote clostridial colonization and toxin production.

Depression along with diarrhoea and dehydrated breast are common features. Lesions include yellowish brown and dry intestinal mucosa with necrotic spots and foul smelling brownish fluid.

Strict sanitation and efforts to prevent coccidiosis, salmonella and other intestinal infection minimize the risk of necrotic enteritis. Use of good quality feed and supplementation of bacitracin methylene disalicylate and lincomycin is reported to be effective against the disease.

191

Infectious Bronchitis (IB)

Highy contagious the most widespread virus respiratory disease

Clinical Symptoms

A very short incubation period (18- 36 hrs). is very characteristic, high morbdity but low mortality (25% in chicks), nasal discharge, gasping, rales and coughing. Layers produce misshapen, soft and deformed eggs. The birds are tending to huddle near the brooder.

Confirmation

Send serum for S.N. test, trachea and oviduct in 10% formalin for histopathological examination.

Treatment

Not specific. Give water medication as prescribed under "Chick Mortality" along with supportive treatment.

Prophylaxis

Modified virus vaccines are used along with Newcastle Disease vaccine. Live attenuated freeze dried vaccine (*mass strain*) available with *Ventri Biologicals* and Glaxo-SKF. Use intranasaly in chicks at 3 - 4 weeks age and again at 16 - 18 weeks age. Similar vaccine developed by Ventri Biological lab. Pune is available and used by intraocular or drinking water method (*see chart VII for details*).

Infectious laryngo tracheitis (ILT)

Acute contagious respiratory disease usually of grown up birds, caused by a virus.

Clinical Symptoms

Gasping, rales and coughing, and difficult breathing, especially at night. Stretching the neck when inhaling is a characteristic symptoms. Birds frequently emit a cawling sound and expell bloody mucus in the act of coughing. Drop in egg production. Mortality about 20 - 30 %.

Haemorrhaegic tracheitis seen on p.m. *is diagnostic.*

Confirmation

Histopathological examination of trachea. Send material containing virus (*respiratory organs*) in glycerine-saline for biological test and egg inoculation.

Tratment

Not specific. Water medication and supportive therapy as prescribed "Chick Mortality".

Prophylaxis

Egg propagated live virus vaccine administered on cloaca with a brush. Not routinely prescribed in india.

Ranikhet Disease (RD) Newcastle Disease

A highly infectious and contagious, fatal disease of poultry with a high morbidity and mortality. Spreads very fast.

Clinical Symptoms

Acute respiratory distress, gasping and tremors. Diarrhoea, nervous signs (*torticollis*) and paralysis. Mortality 90 to 100%. Pin-point haemorrhages on the tips of proventricular glands and ulcers on ileocecal valve are characteristic lesions observed on autopsy.

Confirmation

Send citrated blood on ice for H.A. and H.I. test, brain, liver, spleen, lung in 50% glycerine and 10% formaline *separately*. Serum from recovering birds.

Prophylaxis

Lasopta or F_1 strain intranasal vaccination of day- old chicks. Revaccination at 6 week age with Mukteswar strain or R_2B strain (*Ventri*) by sc inoculation. Give a second booster with R2B strain at 16 weeks age. A new CDF stran developed at Mhow is a live, attenuated vaccine. This can be used in day old chicks (*orally*) as well as adults (sc).

Immunity- One year. VENTRI Biological Lab has developed an inactivated (*Killed*) vaccine (R_2B strain) which is safe and convenient for use in adult layers on the face of outbreks without affecting production. Give **Vimeral** (*Virbac*), **Rovisol** (*Roche*), **Aureomycin Nutritional formula** (*Cyanamid*) or

Winstress (*Cadila*) as antistress factor after vaccination and during outbreak.

In the face of outbreak extra efforts to be taken as:

1. Strict sanitory measures should be implemented.
2. Spray antiviral disinfectants (Aldepol/Disfect) in affected areas.
3. Placement of new lot is advisable after a month.
4. R2B is not safe in birds below 6 weeks of age.

Fowl Pox

A contangious viral disease. Mild in adults but severe in young chicks. Typical pox lesions seen on featherless parts (comb, wattles) but also may appear on the legs and feet of adult. Diptheretic depostis on throat in young chicks. Lesions in eyes may cause blindness. Breathing may become difficult.

Confirmation

By Chorio -Allantoic membrane inoculation and exam. for inclusion bodies under microscope.

Treatment

Not specific. Water medication and supportive therapy as prescribed under "Chick Mortality".

Prophylaxis

Fowl Pox vaccine (*live*) to chicks at 6 weeks age by cutaneous scarification. (*Reconstitute the vaccine away from brooder house*). Pigeon pox virus vaccine by feather-follicle method be to used in chicks below 6 weeks age when outbreak is threatened. 'SRINI' vaccine containing live virus strain is also available and is used by wing web puncture using the lancet.

Avian Leucosis Complex (ALC)

A neoplastic disease of poultry. A problem in exotic breeds of poultry bred for high production. Some types (Visceral form) have a viral etiology and endemic.

Drop in production and deaths due to functional disturbances of vital organs due to metastasis. Diagnosis during life is difficult.

Liver and kidney mainly are involved. Liver may fill the entire fron of the body cavity, dots on its surface, giving it a marbalized appearance. The spleen may be enlarged.

Confirmation

At P.M. By histopathological examination. Send the affected tissues in 10% formalin. Liver and kidneys mainly are involved. Liver may fill the entire front of the body cavity, dots on its surface, givng it amarbalized appearance. The spleen may be enlarged.

Prophylaxis

Breeding for resistance and hygiene. Vaccine not available

Young chicks should be isolated from adult birds. An insect control program is necessary. Disinfectant foot baths should be placed in the door of each building.

Marek's Disease

Is one of the most ubiquitous avian infections. A viral disease very closely resembling neurolympho-matosis — a type of ALC.

Clinical Symptoms

Lameness, limping and ultimate paralysis of legs. More severe in young lot (3-6 months of age).

Confirmation

Rule out Vit. B. group deficiency which produces identical signs. Response to the treatment is the simple way to know this. Nodular lesions in sciatic nerves of leg, brachial nerve of wing or vagus nerve along neck. The nerves are thickened (3-4 times) similar to those seen in Neurolymphomatosis. Send affected pieces of nerves in 10% formalin for histopathological examination and confirmatory diagnosis.

Prophylaxis

An imported vaccine is presently used for day-old chick by commercial poultry breeders. Observe hygienic meausres and isolation etc. A "HVT" strain live attenuated free dried vaccine is now available. Vaccination of day old chicks @ 0.2 ml. by sc route under skilled supervision. *"Ventri Biolgicali"* and

BAIF also now have the vaccine containing FC-126 strain of turkey herpesvirus propogated on chick embryo cellculture.

Dose : 0.2 ml sc to one-day old chicks.

Avian Encephalomyelitis (*Epidemic tremors*)

Is a viral disease of young chicks between 1 - 4 weeks age. There is leg weakness and fine tremors of head, neck and legs. Causes 10 -15% mortality in young chicks. Adults do not show clinical symptoms but remain carriers and transmit infection through egg. Hence a problem for a hatchery.

Confirmation

Rule out Vit. E. deficiency by treatment. Send brain for histopathological examination, and serum from adult laying flock.

Prophylaxis

A live freeze dried vaccine is recently introduced. All the birds between 13 - 14 weeks age in the hatchery should be vaccinated. Vaccine given in cold drinking water orally (Refer Literature).

Avian Influenza (Bird Flu)

Is a contagious disease caused by virus that normally infect only birds and less commonly pigs.

Influenza virus is a single standard RNA virus. In domestic poultry infection is caused by Avian influenza viruses.

Faeceal to oral transmission is the most common mode of spread.

Clinical Symptoms

The signs of disease are extremel variable. High temperature, marked depression, loss of appetite, mild to severe respiratory signs, coughing, sneezing, rales and excessive lacrimation. The conjuctivae are congested and swollen and occasionally haemorrhegic. Swollen combs with cyanotic tips and haemorrhogeic surface. Oedematous wattles and oedema around the eyes and neck. Torticolis and ataxia may be seen.

Confirmation

HA will be positive for Avian influenza. H.I., AGPT, FAT, ELISA.

Treatment - Not specific

Porphylaxis - Immediate depopulation with burial of the infected or exposed birds. Restrictions on the movement of live poultry both with in and between countries. Rigorous disinfection of farms. Common disinfectants such as formalin and iodine compounds. Keep all-in-all out philosophy of flock management.

Infectious Bursal Disease (IBD)

(*Gumboro Disease*)

A disease first recognized in poultry in 1957 in Gumboro island in USA. Caused by RNA virus belonging to Avian reovirus group. Probably two antigenic strains reported varying in pathogenicity and virulence. The virus selectively destroys the Bursa of Fabricius which is an important lymphoid organ associated with production of immunity.

This viral disease identified in India in 1971 onwards usually affects chicks between 4 - 8 weeks age. The chicks become very weak with ruffled feathers. The resistance is reduced and immunological mechanism is shattered due to destruction of bursa and they become susceptible to other diseases. There is breakdown of immunity and vaccinated birds suffer and die due to Ranikhet disease. The bursa is usually enlarged, has haemorrhageic striations and filled with caseous mateial. Kidneys are pale and tubules filled with urates. Mortality about 80%. Confirmation by serologial test, chick embryo inoculation and histopathology.

Treatment

No specific treatment. Give vitamins in feed/water, improve hygienic conditions.

Homeopathic Remedies— Lachesis- 200 followed by **Gelsemium**-30 and **China**-30 used as tinctures in drinking water @ 10 ml/100 birds is reported effective (*Sahnbi & Grewa-Jalanadhar*). These drugs may be given a trial.

Prophylaxis

A live mild strain (Lukert type) vaccine is produced by Ventri Biolgicals and used as primary vaccination in young chicks (*14 -16 days*). A killed vaccine is also available for use as a booster at 16-18 weeks age, **Dose -0.5 ml subcut on the neck.** (*See chart no. VII for other vaccines*).

The key to success of IBD control is strict parent breeder vaccination schedule followed by regular monitoring of day old chick for maternal IBD antibody titre by ELISA.

Hydropericardium Syndrome (Leechi Disease)

A comparatively new disease of poultry it was first recorded from Angara Goth in 1987 and was hence named as "Angara Disease". It knocked Indian doors in Jammu area in 1993-94 and the poultry farmers in the area called it "Leechi Disease" due to its resemblance to the leechi fruit.

It is basically a broiler problem but has also been seen in layers where broilers and layers are reared together or where layers are surrounded by broiler population.

The disease usually affects well nourished healthy birds. The birds die sudden death in a typical "leg facing up" posture with impacted crop full of feed. Initially huge losses upto 90% were noticed but following introduction of auto vaccination, the mortality rate has dropped considerably. Gross lessions include a straw yellow coloured fluid around the heart giving it an appearnace of "Leechi" with enlarged liver.

Chicken Infectious Anaemia

Also called Blue Wing Disease, is snailing its way to poultry industry. It is caused by adeno associated DNA virus.

Mostly broiler chicks between 2 to 4 weeks of age are affected and the disease is transmitted vertically. This is immunosuppressive disease and is characterized by anorexia, lethargy, depression, anaemia and haemorrhages (cutaneous, subcutaneous and intramuscular). Watery blood and reduced hematoerit values. Mortality upto 50% has been noticed.

Breeder Flock vaccination around 13 to 15 weeks age is recommended but a fixed and effective vaccination schedule has to be worked out.

Coccidiosis

A most important disease of the poultry primarily of young birds causing considerable economic losses mortality. Caused by protozoa, *Eimeria necatrix* (intestinal and doudenal) and *E. tenella* (caecal) are the common species. Basically a self limiting disease due to developmenet of resistance in grown up birds. Poor hygiene, dampness of litter, overcrowding and deficiency of Vit.-A are the predisposing causes for a severe outbreak of coccidiosis.

Clinical Symptoms

Haemorrhageic enteritis and bloody droppings and considerable mortality.

Confirmation

By faecal examiation for oocysts. Examination of intestinal scrapings necessary to demonstrate merozoites when deaths in acute stage without bloody droppings as a clinical sign. Coccidoisis is the disease which should be first ruled out in the event of chick mortality.

Treatment

SULPHAMEZATHIN (*ICI*) 16% soln.   @ 30 ml in 4 l
DIADIN (*Pfizer*) 16% soln.   drinking   water
SULMET (*Cynamid*) 16% soln.   for 4 days
VETYDINE (*ICI*) 16% soln. **DIMDIM**
(Ar-Ex) 16% powder is also recommended

AMPROSOL 20% (*MSD*) 30 gm. in 25 litre water 5 to7 days *Give only mediacated water duing period of treatment.*

Embazin (*Rhone P.*) soln. for water medication

Caecal coccidiosis: 50 ml in 10 litres water
3 - 2 -3 schedule

Intestinal coccidiosis   50 ml in 15 litre water 3-2-3-2-3
i.e., (3 days medication 2 days
gap and 3 days treatment.)

BIFURAN (*SKF*) tablets (1 tab in 1 litre for 7days).

CODRINOL (*Hoechst*) A very effective remedy @ 4 g in 1 litre for 4 -5 days

Supportive- High dose of Vit. A presribed under "Chick Mortality".

Prophylaxis (*Coccidostats*)

(i) **EMBAZIN** Premix (*Rhone-P.*) @ 50 g per 100 kg feed to be given during first 8 weeks of life.

(ii) **BIFURAN** (*SKF*) @ 1 tablet in 4-5 litres drinking water.

(iii) **CODRINOL** (*Hoechst*) @1 g in 1 litre water for 10 days.

(iv) **AMPROSOL** 20% (*MSD*) @ 30 g in 100 litres water till outbreat exists.

(v) **COCCILUM-Premix** 25%(*Wockhardt*)@ 500g in a ton feed.

(vi) **COYDEN** (*M.J. Pharma*) Feed mix also found effective.

(vii) **COCCIWIN** (*Sarabhai*) or **COCCINIL** (*Vetcare*) @ 1 kg per 2 to 3 tonnes feed till about 12 - 14 weeks, age.

(viii) **COBAN-100** (*Ventri chemicals*) contains **"Monesin sodium"** and to be used very cautiously as feed mix strictly as per directions of manufacturer.

(xi) **VELODIT** (*Ventri Chemicals*) containing *"Dintolmide"* as a coccidiostat. To be used as per directions.

(x) **COXIDOL** (*Ventri Chemials*) contains *"Clopidol"* Mixed @ 500 g per tonne of feed.

(xi) **CMP-1** (*Diclazwil*) is a new product which interrupts the life cycle easily. Introduced by **Venkys** (*Ind.*) Given by mixing in feed @ 1 kg in per ton of feed.

Worm Infestation in Poultry

Round worm infestation with *Ascaridia galli* is a common problem of poultry. In heavy infection, live worms are passed in faeces and worms sometimes obstruct the lumen of intestines as revealed at p.m. examination. Produce severe anaemia and drop in egg production.

Worm infection causes retardation of growth and economic losses. Deficiency of Vit.-A in the diet is usually associated with heavy worm infection as well as coccidiosis. Periodical faecal examination of few random samples from flock should be conducted regularly so that intensity of infection could be known.

Treament

Piparazine compounds are highly effective. Repeat once a month (*any of the following*) regularly.

1. **WORMEX** (*Pfizer*) liquid- 4 - 6 weeks age 30 ml per 100 birds in 3- 4 litres water. Above 6 weeks - 60 ml per 100 birds in 4 - 5 litres water.

2. **PIPARAZINE ADIPATE** (*ICI*) @ 100 g in 35 kg feed.

3. **PIPARAZINE** (*Virbac*) 45% soln. @. 5 ml for 10 birds.

4. **Piparazine** (*Sarabhai*) 34 g (one bottle) for 300 chicks below 12 weeks or 150 aduls in drinking water.

5. **VERBAN** (*Cyanamid*) soluble powder. 60 g in either 13 litre water or 7 kg feed. (This is sufficient for 300 chicks below 12 weeks, or 150 adult birds).

6. **ARPEZINE** (*MSD*) 40 % sol. of piparazine hydrate. 30 ml per 100 chicks and 60 ml per 100 adults.

7. **L-MEZOLE** (*Vetcare*) is a broad spectrum dewormer 5-10 g for 300 chicks for 100 adult birds in drinking water once in 12 months.

8. **TINEACARE** (*Vetcare*) for poultry tapeworms, single dose treatment 1.5 g /kg body wt. in feed.

For Faster rate of growth, Prevention of diseases and Optimum Egg Production.

Optimum growth, freedom from disease and high level of egg production are the outcome of cumulative factors like ideal mangament, housing, feeding, and high standards of hygiene provided to the best lot of chicks having high genetic potentiality for the particular trait (*i.e.*, *meat or eggs*).

With increase in cost of good quality feed and overheads a high quality of vigilance and technical supervision is essential to maintain the affordable profit-margin in poultry industry. There cannot be one simple solution to achieve this perfection. Having taken for granted ideal breed, feed, management, regular prophylactic vaccination and parasitic control, here are some of the supplements which could correct the deficiencies of essential factors whose estimation may not be always possible at every place.

(*Any of the following may be tried*)

(1) **TERRAMYCIN** (*Pfizer*) Egg formuala- 1 teaspoonful in 4-5 liters water during stress period, outbreaks, vaccinations,

etc. and 1teaspoonsful in 45 litres water for maintenance of full production.

(2) **POULTRYMIN** (*Aries*) An ISI approved quality balanced mineral mixture 2% level in feed.

(3) **STECLIN** Egg formula (*Sarabhai*) Dose rate same as Terramycin Egg formula.

(4) **Aureomycin** *(Cyanamid)* Nutritional formula.

1 teaspoonful in 5 litres drinking water during stress and 1 teaspoonful in 10 litres drinking water during laying period.

(5) **VITABLEND WM** forte (*Virbac*) or **Vimeral** Liquid (*Virbac)* 2m. in 1 litre drinking water.

(6) **VITABLEND AD₃** *(Virbac)* 100 g in 100 kg feed.

(7) **AVLOMIN** (*ICI*) Mineral supplement for poultry to be mixed in feed @ 2% for layers and @ 2 % for chicks.

(8) **FLEXAID** (*MSD*) an antibiotic vitamin combination.@ 60 - 80 gm. in 100 litres drinking water for 1- 2 weeks.

(9) **YOLK -O- GOLD** (*Aries*) A poultry feed supplement containing essential amino acids (Lysin, Methionine and Vitamins) @ 1-2 % in the feed.

(10) **ARIES** *"formula-100"* @ 1 kg in a ton of feed for layers.

(11) **PLYYMIX-L** (*Ar-Ex*) @ 2 g mixed with 10 kg poultry mash for 2 weeks.

(12) **CHQ-60** (*Sarabhai*) a non-antibiotic feed additive growth promoter @ 1 kg per tonne feed.

(13) **ZB- 80** (*Sarabhai*) Zinc, Bacitracin @ 250 g per 1000 kg feed.

(14) **AKTIVIT** Forte (*Vetcare*) Mineral vitamin premix @ 100 mg per tonne feed.

(15) **G-PRO** (*Vetcare*) a non-antibiotic water soluble growth promoter contains essential amino acids @ 250 g for 1250 birds daily in water twice a week.

(16) **ALBAC** (*VentriChemicals*) Zinc. Bacitracin. A poweful antibacterial and egg and growth promoter @ 100 to 300 g per tonne feed.

(17) **ALVITE -M** (*Alembic*) Layers: @ 2.5 kg per tonne fed. Starters/Broilers @ 5 kg/tonnes feed.

(18) **VITADEC** (*BAIF*) Water soluble - @ 2.5 ml per 100 birds.

(19) **VIMICON** (*BAIF*) feed concentrate-@ 250 -300 g per 100 kg feed.

(20) **AMNOVIT** (*BAIF*) Vitamins & amino acids- @ 10 g per 10 kg feed.

(21) **ROXOLIN**-300 plus (*Ciba-Geigy*)-@ 1 – 2 kg per tonne of feed.

Chapter 15

Emu Farming

Emu farming is emerging as a nonconventional industry to which the Indian farmers are getting attracted. Ostrich is a very big non flying bird mainly from Africa. Emu is slightly smaller in size and has origin in Australia and New Zealand. The first ostrich farm was started in South Africa in the year 1860 and after observing it's success, this farming was started in several other countries like Egypt, Australia, America,and recently in India also as a profiteering business. Commercial Emu farming was first started in Texas in 1989 and since then pursuing the trend are the countries like Canada, China, Southern Russia, Belgium, France and many more European coutries and middle east.

This bird is known as "Emu" in Australia , " Casovery" or " Kiwi " in New Zealand, and "Reha" in U.S.A. and "Shahamrug" in India. It belongs to the "Retit" family of Australian desert. Due to low fat content, the Emu meat is recommended by the American Cardiac Association. Emu meat has a tremendous world market and due to it's taste it is considered as a delicacy in multi star hotels in India and abroad. Emu meat. which was being exported till recently, has good demand in local market too. There are nearly 100 Emu farms in India at present, and Andhra Pradesh is leading. There are over 50 Emu farms in Maharashtra in Beed, Phaltan, Ahmadnagar, Potada and Satara.These farms are also established in and around Baramati,in Pune district, and also in Wardha, Chandrapur , Akola, Buldhana and Bhandara districts of Vidarbha. The Association of Emu breeders has also been established with it's headquarter at Malegaon in Baramati taluka of Pune district. This association guides the member farmers in respect of sale-purchase of birds, it's meat, eggs, feathers and other bye products

Classification of Emu

In the animal kingdom Emu classified as below:

Kingdom	-	Animalia
Phylum	-	Chordata
Subphylum	-	Vertebrate
Class	-	Aves
Subclass	-	Neomithes
Super order	-	Ratitae
Order	-	Casuariformes
Family	-	Dormaidae
Genus	-	Dormaeus
Species	-	Dormaius novaehollandiae

Features of Emu

The emus are second largest bird of the world belong to an order ratite i.e. flightless birds with flat breast bone. Though these birds can't fly but can run upto 30 mph. Emus also swim very well.

These huge brids are native of deserts and wood lands of Australia live in flocks 25-40 birds.

Emu has long neck, relatively small naked head, long legs with three toes and body covered with feathers. Birds initially have longitudinal strips on body (0-3 months age) then gradually turn to brown by 4-12 months age. Mature birds have bare blue neck and mottled body feathers. Adult bird height is about 5.5 to 6 feet with a weight of 45 to 60 kg. Legs are long covered with scaly skin adaptable to hardy and dry soil. Birds sit on their haunch and also walk frequently along the fence.

Natural food of emu is insects, tender leaves of plant and forages on different grasses, Cats different kinds of vegetables and fruits like carrot, cucumber, papaya etc.

Air sac hangs down loosely in females and is prominent during breeding season, gives booming sound where as males do grunting sound. Female is the larger of the two especially during breeding season when the male may fast. The male emu sits on nest. Emus live for about 30 years and may produce eggs for more than 16 years.

Important Characteristics of Emu bird

Due to peculiarities of vertebral column, flat sternum, heavy body with 2.5 meters height ,wings are not developed with strength for flight, but has immense capacity and strength to run at a speed of 60 to 70 kilometers per hour. Average body weight of 2 year old Emu bird is around 60 to 70 kilograms. The breedable age is about 18 to 20 months when the female starts laying eggs. The total length of oviduct is about 118 centimeters and and the last segment has calciferous secretary glands where the egg shell is formed the average weight of egg is about 600 to 700 grams and is greenish in colour. The female lays about 6 to 8 eggs per season in the beginning and egg laying increases to 20 to 28 eggs per season(November to March) after 1 to 2 years of laying.Emus usually remain in pairs.(1 : 1) Female is rather bulky as compared to male. The male has a phylus (penis) which is about 10 cm.long and is folded when not erect.It projects at the time to allow defecation and urination. Female has a demunitive phyllus.

The incubation period of eggs is 50 to 52 days and it is the male Emu which hatches eggs by covering around them. The chicks after hatching are kept in a brooder and temperature of about 30 degree gradually reducing to 28 to 24 degree,@ 2 degree everyweek.

Emusing Secrets

1. Eggs used as table delicacy having a pleasant taste. Storage life is longer due to it's chemical composition.

2. Infertile as well as broken eggs are used to make attractive painted and carved ornaments sold as special gifts, as works of jewellary arts and crafts.

3. Emu meat (Gourmet) is dark red in colour, lean and tender in texture with a delicious taste, and the thigh muscle is an excellent alternative to beef as per taste and texture due to high protein and less calories and sodium. Fat is 10 times less in fattyacid than beef. The Cholesterol is also less than 0.5 %(45% mono-unsaturated LDL cholesterol). Calories are also 4 times lower than beef. Low fat meat

loses quickly moisture,so it is advisible to moist heat cook. Vitamin C is also more than any other meat. Gourmet is sold approximately at the rate of Rs. 250/- to 300/- per, Kilogram.

Emu Oil

About 4 litres of oil can be derived from 14 to 18 month old Emu bird from the fat only once. There is a thick pad of fat on the back initially provided by Nature to protect the bird from extreme temperature. The crude oil when processed is stabilized. The animal trials have indicated that Emu oil has properties of lowering cholesterol, reducing inflammation (anti inflammatory) and non pore clogging properties. The oil is absorbed by the skin easily without greasy feeling which makes it's use very beneficial in moisturing and emollient applications making the skin soft and supple. Emu oil also reduces inflammation and pain from joints and muscles and helps in healing the scars. Oil is also used as a base for hair conditioners and shampoos. Emu oil is sold at approximately the rate of Rs. 2500/ to 3500/ per litre.

Emu Feathers

Feathers are very attractive and are used in craft industry and are in great demand.

Emu Leather

Is used for leather belts, purses, jackets, valets and other gift articles. So also Emu bones are also used for various artistic purposes.

Digestive System

The gizzard contains stones and pebbles for grinding food as in chicken. The average productive age of the Emu bird is over 30 years.The average price of Emu egg is about Rs. 600 to 700 and the meat (gourmet) costs around Rs. 300/ per Kg and each adult bird can yield 25 to 30 kg meat, 0.75 meters of body leather, leg leather (used for manufacturing of bags, purses, jackets and protective clothings), 3 to 4 liters of oil (which is used for skin care, cosmetic and for application and medicinal use for massage in cases of rheumatic arthritis, joint pain and for healing of wounds. It has a good market and is sold @ Rs. 2500/ to 3500 / per litre (as per purity grades.). In addition Emu feathers are very attractive and colourful and has a very big market for manufacturing artistic purses and various gift articles.

Management and Health Problems

Emu birds are very docile and sturdy and easy to manage. They do not require large sheds and prefer open barren land to move about. They do not prefer bushes and shady trees and can bear hot and dry atmosphere and can thrive summer temperatures of 52 degree celcius and above without any discomfort. Emu birds prefer standing and wandering for most of the day time and sit during night hours and during dust bathing. A pair of Emu birds requires space of 100 ft x 25 ft and 4 pairs can stay in a open plot of 100 ft x 100 ft. which need to be provided with a wire compound of a type that a bird's head or legs can not get trapped,with about 8 ft height.The fencing should be such that it should be easily seen by the birds, strong enough to withstand birds colliding with it, resilient enough not to injure the birds, free from projections and sharp parts. About 400 sq.ft space is enough for rearing 40 growing young ones.

Farming Systems

In the wild emus are well adapted to the environment in which they have evolved. The process of natural selection favours those that are best adapted to their suitable environment. When exposed to environmental changes, the birds first try to modify themselves to adverse conditions or they leave to look for more suitable places for their needs. Farming alters the natural selection process by providing the birds with food and shelter and by partially or totally restricting their freedom of movement.

There are basically three types of farming system available for the emu production - extensive, semi-intensive and intensive. The choice as to which system to use is essentially governed by availability and price of land, scale of production labour and feed costs.

In the first two systems there is an additional choice whether to use natural or artificial incubation, with intensive system, artificial incubation and hatching of eggs are always employed.

I) Extensive system

This type of system requires a large area of land in excess of 6-7 acre. Apart from cost of birds, land is the major capital requirement. The birds are kept and raised as near as possible to their natural habitat, with minimum interference.

The main advantage of this type is the greatly reduced cost of keeping adult birds in large numbers. Moreover, incubation cost are not incurred if the brids are allowed to hatch their eggs. Thus production cost are extremly low.

Disadvantages

1. No control over breeding conditions can be exercised.
2. Monitoring and identification of the birds and collection of eggs is difficult.

II) Semi-intensive farming system

The area required for this type of system varies from 3 to 4 acre. The birds are kept in relatively small paddocks or territories. They are able to roam freely to a certain extent thus obtaining some of their nutritional requirement from the pasture. Feeding sites should be located near the perimeter fencing to increase the accessibility and reduce the degree of disturbance caused by frequent entry into the paddocks.

Advantages

1. Savings in feed and fencing cost.
2. Freedom provided to birds to choose their mates and hence increase compatibility.

III) Intensive farming system

This system is popular as an emu farming system because of the small land involved half acre. However, it requires high expenditure on feed and buildings (fencing).

Advantages

1. Easy to keep records.
2. Selective breeding of quality birds can be performed.

3.   Full control on breeding programm.

General Considerations

Farm location

Distance from traffic and industrial areas is an important factor to consider.

Land topography

Hilly, mountains, slopping, rocky, or steep ground is not suitable since emus prefer flat open terrian.

Excessive tree covering can be a problem and also attracts wild birds.

Availability of water and Electricity: A clean underground water source or mains water supply is vital because emu drinks plenty of water.

Design of facilities

There are number of designs to choose from. The most widely used is the simple rectangular design with a long serving area running down the centre of the pen.

Fencing

Fencing should be at least 4 ft high for birds upto 3 weeks of age and 6 ft high for birds more than 3 weeks of age and is made of chain link 2" x 4".

Fencing must be

1.   Easily seen by the birds.
2.   Strong enough to withstand birds colliding with it.
3.   resilient enough not to injure the birds.
4.   Free from projections and sharp parts.
5.   of a type that a birds head or legs can not become trapped.

Space requirement

Floor space 2-4 sq. ft. floor space per chick upto 3 weeks will be required.

5 sq. ft. shelter and 25 sq. ft. run/bird.

100 ft. x 25 ft. floor space/ breeding pair is required.

Floor	Chicks	Grower	Breeder
Feeding space	4″	6″	8″
Watering space	1″	2″	2″

Management of Chicks

Emu chicks weigh about 370 to 450 g depending on size of egg. First 48-72 hours emu chicks are restricted to incubactor for quick absorption of the yolk and proper drying. Like chicken emu needs brooding during their early life. Clean and disinfect brooding shed thoroughly well in advance of receiving chicks, spread litter (paddy husk) cover new gunny bags over the litter. Arrange a set of brooder for about 25 to 40 chicks giving 2 to 4 sq. ft. per chick ofr first 3 weeks. Provide brooding temperature of 90°F at first 10 days and 85°F till 3-4 weeks. Provide 24 hours of 40 watt bulb for every 100 sq. ft. area. Chick guard must be 2.5 feet height to avoid jumping and straying of chicks. After 3 weeks of age, slowly extend the brooder area by widening the chick guard circle and later remove it by the time chicks attain 6 weeks. Feed starter mash for the first 14 weeks or till attaining standard body weight of 10 kg. Ensure proper floor space for the birds housed as these birds require run space for their healthy life hence floor space of 40′ x 30′ is required for about 40 chicks if out door space is provided. Floor must be easily drained and free from clampness.

Do's

- Never make over crowd in the pen, first few days provide sanitized water and antistress agents.

- Clean waterers daily otherwise automatic waterers are preferable.

- Monitor birds daily for their comfort, feed intake, water intake, litter condition etc. for making immediate corretion if any.

- Practice all-in-all-out rearing to maintain better biosecurity.

- Ensure proper mineral and vitamins in the feed for healthy growth of chicks and to avoid leg deformities.

- Spraddle condition of legs that are seen commonly can be managed by holding the legs together during first 72 hours of chicks. This can be done particularly in the incubator.

Dont's

- Never handle the birds during hot hours. Birds easily excite, hence calm and quite environment in the pen is required.
- Birds easily grab any item, so avoid certain objects like nails, pebbles, metal pieces etc. in the vicinity of birds.
- Avoid unauthorized persons, mateirals into the farm. Proper biosecurity must be ensured.
- Never keep the birds on smooth surface as the young chicks easily excite, run and break their legs due to slipperiness.

Grower Management

As emu chicks grow they require a bigger size of waterers and feeders and increased floor space. Identify sexes and rear them separately.

Feed the birds on grower mash till birds attain 34 weeks of age or 25 kg body weight. Offer green about 10% of diet particularly different kinds of leaf meals for making the birds eat adopt to fibrous diet.

Provide clean water all the time and offer feed as much as they want. Ensure dry litter conditions throughout the grower stage. If necessary add required quantity of paddy husk to the pen provide 40' x 100 space for 40 birds if out door space is considered.

Do's

- Monitor flock at least once daily for alertness of birds, feeding and watering troughs.
- Notice leg deformities, dripping and isolate birds.
- Never keep in the vicinity of the adult birds:

Dont's

- Never keep the sharp objects, pebbels in the vicinity of the birds. Birds are mischievous and grab anything that comes in their vicinity.
- Never handle or disturb the birds during the hot weather conditions.
- Provide cool and calm water throughout the day.

Breeder Management

Emu birds attain sexual maturity by 15-24 months age. Choose flock or pen mating. Keep sex ratio of male to female 1:1. In case of pen mating the pairing should be done based on the compatibility. During mating, offer floor space about 2500 sft. (100 x 25) per pair.

Trees and shrubs may be provided for the privacy and to induce mating. Offer breeder diet well in advance i.e. 3-4 wks prior to breeding and vitamins to ensure better fertility and hatchability in brids.

First egg is laid around two and half year age. Eggs will be laid during October to February particularly cooler days of the year. The time of egg laying is around 5.30 pm to 7.00 pm. Eggs can be collected twice daily to avoid damage in the pen. Normally the hen lays about 15 eggs during first year cycle, in subsequent years the egg production increases till it can reach about 30-40 eggs. On an average a hen lays 25 eggs per year. Egg weighs abut 475-650 g with an average egg weight of 560 g. Egg appears greenish look like tough marble. The intensity of colour varies from light medium to dark green. The surface varies from rough to smooth. Majority of eggs (42%) are medium green with rough surface.

Feed the breeder ration with the sufficient calcium (2.7%) for ensuring proper calcification of egg with strength. Feeding excess calcium of the breeding bird before laying will upset the egg production and also impairs the male fertility. Provide extra calcium in the form of grit or calcite powder by placing in separate trough.

Incubation and Hatching

Collect eggs frequently from the pen. If eggs are soiled, clean with sand paper and mop up with cotton. Store the egg in a cooler room providing 60°F temperature. Never store eggs for more than 10 days to ensure better hatchability. Eggs stored at room temperature can be set every 3 to 4 days for good hatchability.

Set the fertile eggs after adjusting to room temperature and place in a **horizontal** or in **slant arranged row** wise in a tray. Keep ready egg incubator by cleaning and disinfecting thoroughly well in advance and switch on the machine for setting the correct incubating temp. i.e., dry bulb temperature about 96 to 97°F and wet bulb temperature about 75-80°F (about 30 to 40% RH). Place carefully the egg tray in a setter once the incubator is ready with set temperature and relative humidity and place identification slip for date of set and pedigree if needed.

Fumigate the incubator with 20 g potassium permangnate + 40 ml formaline for every 100 cu. ft. of the incubator space. Turn the eggs every one hour till the 48th day of incubation. From 49th day onwards stop turning, the eggs and watch for pipping, by 52 day incubation period ends.

The chicks need drying. Hold the chicks for at least 24 to 72 hours in the hatcher compartment for (reducing the down) absorption of yolk and to become healthy chicks. Normally hatchability will be 70% or more.

Nutrition (Feeding)

Emu need balanced diet for their proper growth and reproduction. Feed can be prepared by using common poultry feed ingredients. Feed alone accounts for 60 to 70% of the production cost, hence least cost rations will improve the margin of returns over feeding. The feed intake per emu breeding pair per annum varied from 394 to 632 kg with a mean of 527 kg. Cost of feed was Rs. 6.50 and 7.50 during non-breeding and breeding season respectively.

Restraining

Emus are not easiest to catch. To handle the bird it is best to catch it while it goes by, getting behind it and grabbing the two small wings. Once grabbed the two small wings then pull the bird very close to you with the rump of bird held tightly against you and between your thighs.

Health

The birds usually do not have many health problems.The general health of the flock affects egg productivity. If the oviduct is not properly formed, females may ovulate internally. The infundibulum fails to engulf the ovulated ova, which then remain in the abdominal cavity, such females develop a pot bellied appearance and are normally termed as internal layers. Prolapse of oviduct is another condition associated usually with young females in their first season. In addition some females may become egg bound, in that case the bird is unable to deposit or expel the completely formed egg. The egg may not always be palpable in the caudal abdomen.

Encephalomyelitis is the only disease that may poise a problem sometime as it is transmitted from horses but is not communicable to human beings, so due precautions to avoid proximity to horses and other equines be taken as a preventive measure.

Economics of Emu Farm

Initial requirement is that of an open land provided with a strong wire net compound of 8 ft. height, a small shed inside for rest and shelter, and some utensils for food ,water and green vegetables and grasses.It is better to have a concrete tank for water storage and a good bore well for a perennial fresh water supply. A pair of Emu birds can cost about Rs. 12000 to 14000/ as an initial investment as per the size of farm that is anticipated. The female Emu can give about 40 young chickens per year.

Feeding

Usually a readymade commercial feed can be used or the feed can be compounded by crushing grains, maize, oil cakes and wheat or rice bran as we do for poultry. It is advisible to use ready made feeds available as **Starter, Grower, Breeder, Maintenace and Finisher** feeds.

A fully grown one year old adult Emu needs 750 to 1500 grams of maintenance feed per day.

The feeding schedule is as under:

0 to 8 weeks old bird — — —Starter feed — ad lib.

8 weeks to 9 months — — — —Grower feed — — ad lib.

9 months to 18 months — — —Finisher feed— —ad lib.

Breeder Age /Breeding Season— — — Breeder feed ad lib.

Maintenance ration for other times for all adult birds.

Emu Farming is a good subsidiary business for any

agriculturist and once established, needs very little management skills and supervision is required as the Emu birds are very sturdy and except and beyond adequate and fenced open space with a shed inside very few things are required and with a very big life span of over 25 to 30 years, the initial number of 10 or 20 pairs with which a beginning was made, the number of birds may cross 3 to 4 hundred within a span of 10 to 15 years which will mean a very good and profitable investment. The Emu farms are increasing rapidly as a new industry and one who is interested to start, must visit and get adequate practical experience and the know-how before start.

Chapter 16

Goat Farming

Rearing of goats is considered a very lucrative animal husbandry activity and more and more farmers and educated unemployed youths are attracted towards this industry.

The reasons are:

(i) Fast multiplication of their number.

(ii) Comparatively low investment and assured market.

(iii) Relatively less accommodation required and low cost of maintenance.

(iv) Ability of goats to thrive on relatively uncommon vareities of feed and fodder not consumed by cows.

(v) Lesser problems of disease control due to their habits (in small & medium size units).

(vi) High nutritive value and higher content of milk, making its use desirable for growing children, and old and sick persons.

With the above points of view new projects on goat keeping are coming up in suburban and rural areas. Once upon a time goat keeping was considered a big hazard due to their habit of close grazing on tender leaves of grasses disallowing them to grow up for larger ruminants and other animals and thereby creating problems of soil erosion. However, with the advent of new varieties of grasses and shrubs and new farming practices it is now possible to exploit the potentials of milk and meat production from this animal. Promotion and facilities advanced by Government and Banks, this industry is likely to help in solving unemployment problem of youth to some extent and side by helping in enhancement of milk and meat production.

BREEDS OF GOATS

There are several breeds of goats and such as *Jamunapari, Beetal, Barbari, Cutchi, Osmanabadi, Surti, Malberi,* in various parts of India "Pashmina" breed common in Ladakh. Tibet and Kashmir is famous for its fine undercoat used as a natural textile fiber famous for "Shawls". "Angora" goat is an important breed from Turkey and Asia minor and is famous for undercoat used for weaving "Shawls".

However, following two breeds are most common and abundant in India.

(i) **Jamunapari**

A large sized breed with convexface and used as a milch breed. Body is white with chestnut brown and a black patches over body.

(ii) **Barbari**

Is a dwarf wedge shaped breed prevalent inU.P. (Agra, Mathura & Etah). The coat is fine and has a straight face. Body colour white, brown and black patches ove body. Average body weight of adult animal ranges between 75-100 kg and female gives 2 -3 litres milk.

Housing and Management

Housing and feeding are closely related with maintenance of good health of animals. A properly ventilated shed with high thatched roof is ideal under Indian conditions. The size of 20 x 30 shed should normally accomodate about 50 adult goats of medium size (Barbari breed). The flooring should be hard remmed murrom with good slope to prevent water logging and be free from pointed stones which could injure udders. The fence should be about 4 ft. high with adequate number of shady trees around. Separate arrangements are necessary for housing pregnant does, kids and breeding bucks. One breeding buck is enough for breeding 80 - 100 females. Goats do not like rains, moist and watery surroundings. The house should have hay racks and fresh water trought as well should provide shelter from strong hot winds, cold and rains. Goats are allowed grazing normally for 8-9 hours per day if enough grazing pasture

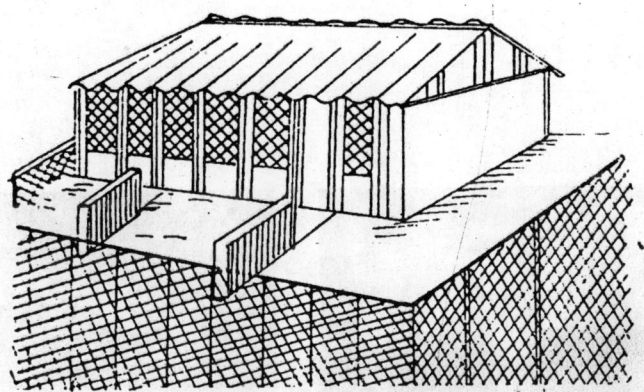

Fig. 15. Ideal House of 20 x 30 size

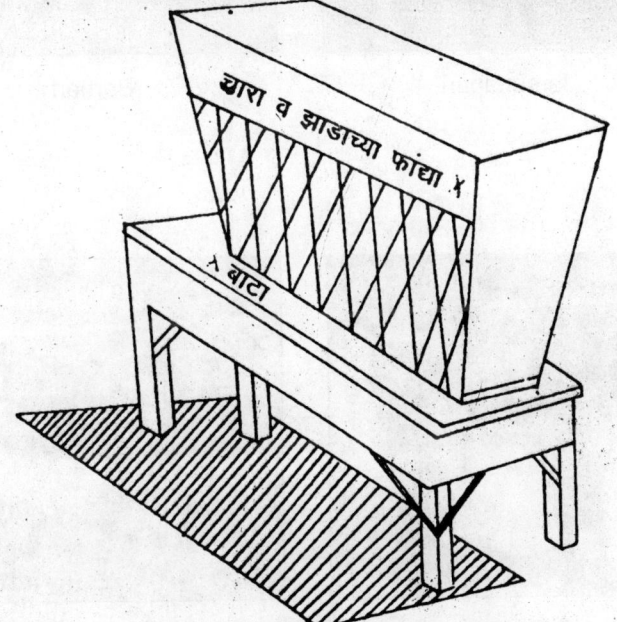

चारा व झाडाच्या फांद्या

बाटा

Fig. 16. Feeding troughs for goats.

land and forest is available. This gives adequate exercise to the animals.

House should have an attached space for the movements of animals and should have trees nearby. Separate rooms be provided for isolation of sick animals, for parturition (*Lambing*) and growing kids.

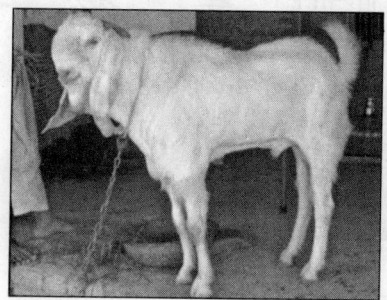

Jamunapari

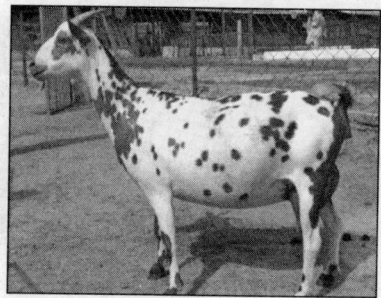

Barbari

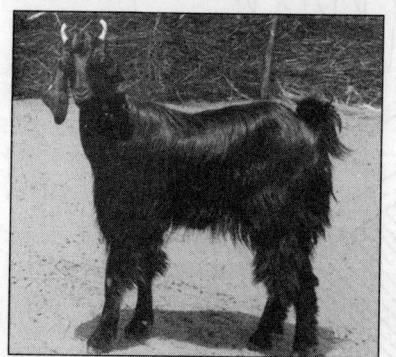

Marwadi

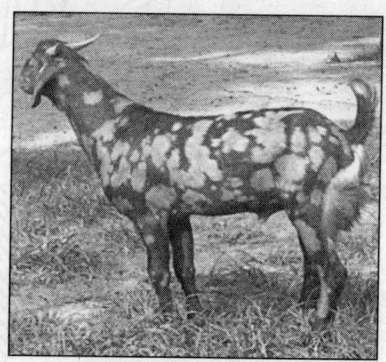

Sirohi

NUTRITION

The nutritive requirements of goats are considerably higher than for cows on account of greater body surface in amount of total digestible nutrients (TDN) over and above their maintenance requirements per kilogram milk produced than do cows (about 20 - 25% additional feed for maintenance and about 10 - 15% more TDN per kilogram of milk produced).

Concentrate mixtures are given to the flock in stall feeding to growing lot, milking lot and breeding animals.

Various concentrate mixtures are given depending upon availability of ingredients.

Following are some examples:

1)	Crushed gram	1 part
	Crushed maize	2 parts
	Linseed or G.N. Cake	2 ½ parts
	Heavy Wheat Bran	2 parts
2)	Wheat Bran	50 parts
	Crushed Maize	15 parts
	Crushed gram	15 parts
	Crushed Linseed or Groundnut cake	20 parts

2 percent mineral of standard quality be added to above concentrate mixture. Rock salt licks be kept in the shed.

Feeding routine should be as under

8-9 A.M.	:	First concentrate meal
6-7 P.M.	:	Second concentrate meal.

Grazing is allowed between 10 A.M. to 5 P.M.

Total quantity of concentrate is given @ 600 - 750 g per adult divided in two meals per day.

About 10 goats will require approximately the same amount of feed as one good average milk yielding cow.

Fodders such as *Napier, Lucerne, Barseem, Cabbage, Cauliflower leaves, leaves of vegetables, leaves of "Subabool" Shevari* or other trees

221

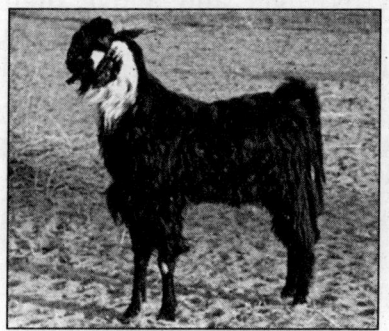

Kachi

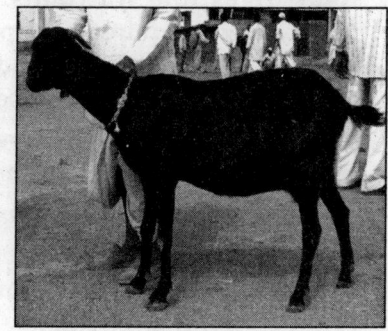

Usmanabadi

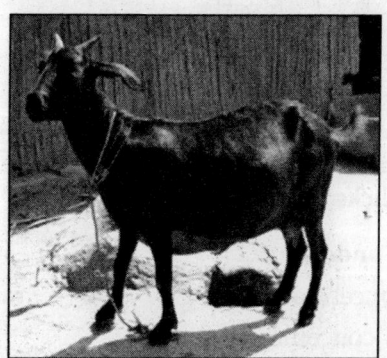

Blackbangal

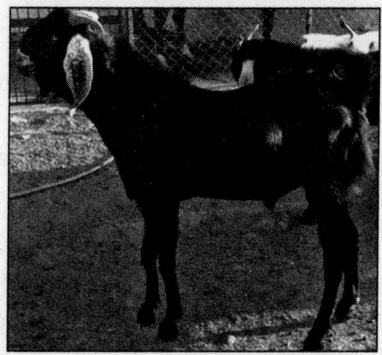

Zakrana

as per availability are given in hay racks or hung up in bundles tied from the roof. The grasses should be perfectly dry and each adult may require about 4 to 5 kg of fodder every day (including grazing).

Goat is considered as "poor man's cow" and good milch breed animal (*Jamunapari*) may yield average of 2-3 litres milk per day which is sufficient for a family. Milk contains about 4 per cent fat in finely emulsified form and hence is easy to digest than cow milk. Goat milk does have some "goaty" flovour or smell but one get used to and start liking the taste. The milk is alkaline in reaction, much more rich in minerals as compared to cow milk. It contains 9 minerals as compared to 5 minerals in cow mik. Goat mik is rich in Iron, Phosphate and Potassium which are deficient in cow milk. This makes the goat milk ideal for sick individuals and young children.

Diseases and Health Problems

Goats, because of their clean habits, and hardy nature are usually naturally more resistant to diseases. However, they do suffer from certain health problems which are mostly due to dietetic errors and bad hygiene. Goats do not relish rains, dampness and moist enviornment. Grasses and leaves should be dry and if moist, this may promote worm infestation.

Indigestion

Usually occurs due to consumption of kitchen wastes, state food, grain engorgement and consumption of toxic or poisonous plants. (*Hiver pods*). This causes impaction and rumenal acidity and sometimes tympanites. If unattended, acute cases may result into death. Treatment consists of correction of rumen pH (*neutralizing acidity or alkalinity*) administration of iv fluids, antihistaminics, carminatives, rumenoteries and B-complex compounds in proper doses as described for cattle Battisa, turpentine in sweet oil, and digestive tonic powders are commonly employed for treatment.

Diarrhoea

Is mostly an indication of intestinal worm infestation or fascioliasis in certain areas. Faecal samples be examined and regular periodical deworming with suitable drugs be given. Antibiotics and antidiarrhoeals for bacterial infection.

Respiratory Tract Infections

Are characterised by fever nasal discharge, cough,adventitious sounds on auscultation of chest and varying degree of dyspnoea. Treatment comprises of heavy dose of broad spectrum **antibiotics** given parenterally and other supportive treatment. Blood examination for TLC/DLC be done for diagnosis of C.C.P.P. and H.S. which are serious life threatening infections.

Other Specific Diseases

Following infections, diseases may occur at the goat farm

Rinderpest

May occur during an epidemic amongst cattle, but rinderpest is almost eradicated. An incidence of Peste-des-petits Ruminants (PPR) has recently been reported at Goat Breeding farm in Orissa where 103 out of 212 goats (53.3%) succumbed with symptoms and lesions very similar to Rinderpest. Mobilivirus was confirmed, AGPT was positive to rinderpest hyperimmune serum. Newly procured animals mostly suffered. Disease was controlled by vaccination of incontact animals with TCRP vaccine and treatment with high doses of tetracycline and vitamin-mineral supplements proved useful. The outbreaks of PPR have since then been reported from Maharashtra and southern States of India at organised goat farms resulting in severe mortality. TCRP vaccination can control outbreaks after it is confirmed.

(ii) **F.M.D.**- Independently or during epidemic amongst cattle.

(iii) **H.S.**-During early monsoon as sporadic cases.

(iv) **C.C.C.P.**- A serious infectious pneumonia of goats causing heavy mortality.

(v) **Goat Pox**- A comparatively severe form of pox and may cause considerabe losses due to mortality.

(vi) **Contagious Ecthyma**- A viral infection common in sheep and goats. Lesions are restricted to lips and mouth.

(vii) Dermatitis and Mange

Could be a serious problem in the flock if neglected and if premises are damp and humid.

Most of the above diseases are preventable by carrying out regular prophylactic vaccinations. Special Tissue Culture vaccines are used for prevention of Rinderpest and F.M.D. if *necessary*. Vaccination against CCPP is a "must" and should be carried out annually. Ear-tip vaccination of 0.2 ml. IV.R.I. vaccine is commonly employed. However, vaccine prepared from locally isolated PPLO strain is always preferable. *Product instructions must be strictly followed before undertaking any vaccination.*

Breeding

Goats breed throughout the year but breeding time can be decided so as to get good nourishment to dams and kids. The gestation period is about 147-150 days. Mating should be arranged in the months of May-June-July so that kids will be born in October, November and December which is usually the healthy season. Does (female goats) as rule, come into oestrus (heat) throughout the year at an interval of 27-28 days and the duration of oestrus is about 20 hours. Usually the does often have two oestrous cycles with the interval of 7 days.

The age at first mating may be 10 -15 months and shall give kids twice in 15-18 months and continue breeding till 12-14 years of age. Does usually gives 2 kids (54%) 1 kid (35%) and 3 kids (3%) at a time.

Training Programmes

Special training programmes are arranged for the interested farmers and youths by State Animal Husbandry Department and the Animal Science Universities. It must however, be remembered that goat farming as a large scale industry will have limitations as it will need ample free grazing land which could not be utilised for other profitable cultivation.

It can, however, be an ideal supporting side business for a family to keep 2- 4 adult goats of Barbari breed (or 1-2 goats of Jamunapari breed for milk) in urban or suburban area where moderate extra space is availble. The goats would yield about 2- 3 litres of milk per day (for about 150 - 250 days lactation period) which would be sufficient for family comsumption and some little quantity could also be sold. Two to 4 goats could be maintained on kitchen waste, greens and some concentrate mixture. Surplus male kids could be sold out as and when possible.A recent survey in U.P. has revealed that 76% persons had small units (1-5goats), 14% has medium size units (6-10 goats) and only 10% has more than 10 goats. Small and medium size had lesser problems of mortality, got regular kidding and milk, the manure (about 1.5 quintal per adult goat) could be utilised for own field or gardens and surplus goats could be sold out. *Barbari* was found suitable.

Chapter 17

Pig Farming

Pig Farming is becoming increasingly popular in areas where marketing pork and bacon to multistar hotels in and around cosmopolitan cities. Normally, there is a limited market for pig meat in selected pockets of India.

Pigs have good ability to convert foroges, damaged feeds by products of meat, milk and grains into nutritious meat.

Pigs are prelific breeders. They grow fast, attain puberty at the age of 6-8 months and breed twice a year. Under able management a sow delivers 10-12 piglets at a time. The carcass return is 65-80% of the live weight. Scientific breeding, good feeding adequate housing and sound health care practices are the key to profitable piggery.

Breeding

Domestic breeds of swine vary in colour pattern, body size conformation and appearance of head and ears. They are small in size with poor feed conversion abilities. Exotic breeds like **Large White York Shire, Middle White York Shire, Landrace, Saddle back, Tam Worth** and **Bark Shire** have been tried in India. Among them large white york shire and landrace are widely used for upgrading the local stock. Cross breeding plays a key role in the development of piggery in India.

Breeds in India

Following 3 breeds are seen in India

1) Large White 2) Middle White and 3) Black Berkshire

Crosses of Middle white and Berkshire have also proved economical. In addition to these breeds, Yorkshire, Hamphsire, Herford and Meriland are some more breeds available in some piggeries in India. One can get complete information about

227

breeds, and their availability at some of the following centres:

(i)   Pig Breeding Farm, *Bastar* (C.G.)

(ii) I.V.R.I., Izatnagar (U.P.)

(iii) Manager, Pig Breeding Station, Hissargatta

(iv) Manager, (Production Bacon Factory, MAFCO, Borivali National Park, *Mumbai-66*

(v)   Jawaharlal Nehru Krishi Vishwa Vidyalaya, *Jabalpur*

Pig farming is now developing in India because:

1)   We get good animal protein as food.

2)   Comparatively low investment cost due to early maturity and faster weight gains.

(3) Excellent food conversion capacity of animals which convert about 2 to 2.5 kg feed into a kg of live weight and the animal can be sent to slaughter house as it attains weight of about 150 kg within the period of 10 months to an year.

4)   Due to the prolific breeding capacity a female gives 8-12 piglets twice a year.

5)   Comparatively low disease problems is due to shorter period of rearing.

Housing

Pig "sties" are provided for different age groups such as Boars, Sows, Piglets and isolation. An adult pig requires about 10-15 sq. feet floor space and a shed of 150 sq. feet can accommodate about 10 pigs. Housing should be such as to give protection from hot sun, rain showers and cold breezes. Houses should be properly ventilated and should provide mangers for feed and troughs for clean water at reasonable height. Pregnant mothers and young piglets should be provided separate accommodation. The floor should be properly levelled and should always be kept clean.

Feeding

Pig is a simple stomach animal. Hence high protein low fibre feed is essential to boost the growth.

Piglets are weaned at the age of 8 weeks. However, creep feeding should start from second or third week. After weaning piglets grow exceedingly well when fed with maize, sorghum, oat and barley. They need 1.2 kg feed/kg weight gain. Starch and fat form the main source of energy. The total digestable nutrient of the feed should be 70%.

The feed compositions vary according to the storage of growth as presented in Table 1.

Table 1. Formulation of Feeds

Ingredients	Composition in present		
	Creep Feed (upto weaning)	Grower ration (20-40 kg body wt.)	Finisher ration (40-90 kg body wt.)
1. Oil cakes chunni	16-18	14-16	13-14
2. Animal portein	8-10	4	2
3. Grains (Maize, Millets)	60-65	50-55	40-45
4. Bran	5	10	20
5. Lucerne meal (if available)	-	5-8	-
6. Mineral mixture	0.5	0.5	0.5
7. Iodized salt	0.5	0.5	0.5
8. Antibiotic (mg/100kg)	40	20	10
Required protein content in feed	18-20	14-15	12-13

Pregnant females must get a good balanced ration, green fodder and good mineral mixture. A pregnant female weighting above 150-200 kg should get total of 3-3.5 kg feed divided in 2-3 instalments. Supplements of Vit. A and D necessary. Care should be taken to provide good mineral mixture containing **Calcium, Phosphorus, Iron** and **Iodine** so that the mother should not suffer from any deficiency.

Iron is a very essential and the suckling piglets as they commonly suffer from Iron deficiency anaemia and this can sometimes create a serious problem and result in mortality, particularly amongst piglets upto 2 weeks age hence there is a practice to paint the teats with 2% solution of Ferrous sulphate daily so that the piglets will get adequate iron during suckling.

1. Calcium, phosphorous, iron and zinc are critical minerals for boosting the growth of pigs. Hence the ration should be fortified with fish or meal/milk by-products or limestone with dicalcium phosphate.

2. As cow's milk is deficient in iron, feeding 0.6-1.2 g Ferrous sulphate /day is beneficial.

Water

Pigs require plenty of water particular in hot weather. Hence, fresh water should always be made avilable. Piglets and dry sows require 5 litre of water during farrowing while boars need 15-20 litres of water per head daily.

Guidelines for Management

Preliminary Care

1. Procure healthy stock from reputed breeding units.
2. Maintain newly purchased animals in isolation for 20 days.
3. Place a foot bath contining 5% phenyl solution at the entrance of the shed.
4. The attendants working in the shed should have good health and should be free from tuberculosis.

Maintenance

1. Group the animals according to their age and size and house them in separate pens. Keep the pens clean and inspect them daily.

2. Segregte the sick animals and treat promptly. Examine their stools regularly and treat if faeces are liquidish. In case of injury, treat the animals with turpentine and boric acid paste.

3. Feed troughs should be cleaned every day, unconsumed food is an indication of either sickness or poor quality food. Avoid feeding damaged grains. If garbage is used, boil before feeding and ensure that it is free from salt, tea leaves, banana rinds, broken glasses and metal pieces.

4. During hot weather, keep the floors, roof and walls wet and reduce the calorific value of feed.

5. Poor growth of animals can be genetic or due to parasites or mucosal viral disease. Such animals should be examined and treated.

Selection for Breeding

1. Selection and culling of animals should be a regular activity. Cases of abortions and still birth should be studied carefully. If these are related to genetic base and diseases, such sows should be culled. Do not maintain weak and anaemic animals, which do not respond to treatments.

2. Weight gained in between two to six months of age is a good baiss for selection. Select a sow having a proven record of giving good litters and tending to them.

3. Cull the repeat breeders and sows furrowing small and dead piglets. Sows which are ferocious, careless or deficient in milk, should also be culled.

Important Diseases

Pigs suffer from common ailments as do other animals. The treatment is carried on the similar lines as in case of other animals.

Swine Fever

Swine Fever or Hog Cholera is an infectious septicaemia. characterized by haemorrhages. The pig is the only susceptible host.

Clinical symptoms

Initially slowness or "Weaving" gait. Anorexia, rise in body temperature upto 41.5°C (108°F), profuse discharge from eyes associated with conjunctivitis, moderate to severe nasal discharge, constipation followed by severe watery diarrhoea. Purplish discolouration of abdomen, snout and ears.

Diagnosis

Gross lesions characterized by enlarged and mottled lymph nodes with haemorrhages. Button ulcers in colon. Leueopenia, AGPT, CFT and HA.

Treatment

Effective treatment of secondary complications can help in saving the affected pigs.

in saving the affected pigs.

Prophylaxis

Freeze dried live vaccine

Primary vaccination

Piglets born to non-immune sows on the seventh day

Piglets born to immune sows: In the absence of any threat of disease, vaccinate at six weeks of age. When there is threat vaccinate at 3-4 weeks of age.

Booster Vaccination

This should be adminstered after 5-6 months and then at an interval of 6-12 months according to local needs.

For piglet intended for breeder stock, booster vaccination is necessary at least one month before puberty (5-6 months of age).

Pregnant sows may be vaccinated in the last two months of pregnancy using tissue culture vaccine but not lapinized live attenuated vaccine.

Dose : 1.0 ml deep im in the neck or thigh muscle.

Foot and Mouth Disease

In pigs, lameness is the first conspicuous symptom to be noticed. The animals suffer from fever and blister appear on the feet and mouth. As in cattle, blister may appear on the dorsum of the tongue, on coronary band, between claws and even on feets of sows. Young pigs may die. Abortion is occasional.

Vaccination Schedule

Disease	Primary	Booster	Repeat
Swine fever	2-3 weeks	5-6 months	6-12 months
FMD	3-4 weeks	30 days	Yearly

Other Common Diseases

Pox

Fever (40°C) cutaneous lesions

PM : Cutaneous lesions

232

Pneumonia

Caused by *Mycoplasma hypopneumoniae, Salmonella bronchiseptica, Pseudorabies virus.*

Clinical Symptoms : Dyspnoea, cough, anorexia, fever, abdominal respiration.

P.M. - Plum red atelectatic lesions with variable intralobulr oorema.

Treatment

Sulpha drugs and or antibiotic.

Salmonellosis

Restlessness; common in piglets, fever (40.5 to 41.6°C), watery yellow faeces, huddling.

P.M. - Catarrhal to haemorrhagic and neocortic enteritis.

Treatment

Furazolidone and/or antibiotic.

Colibacilosis

Mild to severe diarrhoea common in piglets. Vomitting in some cases.

P.M. - Stomach often full; congestion and oedema of intestine.

Treatment - Furazolidone and/or antibiotic.

Erysipelas

Above 3 months to below 3 years. Fever (40-42°C) chill, stiff gait, diarrhoea, cutaneous lesions.

P.M. - Diffuse lutaneous hematasis in the skin of snout, ears.

Treatment - Antibiotic therapy.

Prophylaxis - Killed vaccines are used as prophylactic agents.

Pasturellosis

Pasturellosis

Dyspnoea, thumping. All age groups but most common in adults. Dry non-productive cough, fever, depression, anorexia.

P.M : Purulent bronchopneumonic lessions with fibrinous pleuritis.

Treatment - Sulpha and/or antibiotic

Prophylaxis - Autogenous bacterians

Bordetellosis

Affected piglets snuffle, sneeze particularly in piglets and snort with serous and mucopurulent nasal discharge.

P.M. - Catarrhal rhinitis and variable amount of turbinate hypoplasia

Treatment - Sulpha and/or antibiotic therapy.

Parasitic infections can be a problem if the premises are unhygienic and insanitary. Routine faecal examination be followed by administration of broad spectrum dewormer if faecal examination reveals worm infection. Regular deworming be carried out with broad spectrum **dewormer** such as **Albomar** or **Panacur** every 6 months.

Iron deficiency anaemia should be prevented in time and suckling piglets should be looked for signs of this ailment. Injectable iron preparations are available and should be used if situation demands.

Chapter 18

Common Poisonings

Poisoning is usually accidental and very rarely malacious. Detailed enquiry and circumstantial considerations are important. Must rule out a specific infectious disease of peracute nature, electric shock and snake bite in case of history of *sudden death*.

Some of the important considerations are as under:

1. No. of animals show symptoms of varying intensity simultaneously if the toxicity is of food origin.
2. Enquire about history of recent spraying of some insecticide or pesticide, painting of sheds, access to industrial waste water etc. Consider the possibility of residual insecticide toxicity in fodders also.
3. Accidental over-dosing with some poisonous drug.
4. History of access to jowar or linseed field (HCN poisoning).
5. Use of rat poisons, skin application in case of pets.

General Symptoms of Poisoning

1. Usually afebrile (*exception is chlorinated hydrocarbons*) Temp. is usually subnormal depending on the stage.
2. Pupilar responses either absent or weak. Pupils usually dilated. (*Exception-organophosphorous poisoning*).
3. Respiration and heart beats arrhythmic.
4. Convulsions, spasms, tremors, paddling, champing of jaw and such other uncontrolled movements. *Rule out Rabies.*
5. Bloating, frothing of mouth, regurgitation, diarrhoea.
6. Vomiting very common in dogs.
7. Depressed consciousness and coma.

235

General Prinicples of Treatment:

1. Stop further ingestion/absorption of poison, in detected or suspected. *Stop giving suspected feed.*

2. Removal of residual poison from alimentary tract/skin (By giving emetics where indicated, gastric lavage, purgatives, washing of skin with plenty of water) For Dogs : 5 ml Hydrogen peroxide or one teaspoonful salt in little luke warm water given orally induces vomiting. Inj. Apomorphine 20 microgram/1b iv. Preserve vomitus for detection of poison).

3. Neutralization of residual poison

   Oxidizing Agents- Tannic acid which precipitates alkaloids.

   Milk Eggs. In irritant and corrosive poisons.

   Chemical Antidotes - which render poison insoluble or harmless.

   Calcium -In most poisonings as universal antidote.

   Activated Charcoal - Adsorbs the poison in stomach. (5 teaspoonsul in 100 ml water as a slurry given by stomach tube followed by 20 g Sod. sulph after one hour. In ruminants emetics are of no use and hence ativated charcoal @ 1-3 g/kg body wt. (300 -500 g as aveage dose) should be administered and repeated if necessary. It adsorbs hydrocarbons, organophosphorous, compound, mycotoxins, plant alkaloids. This should be followed by a saline or oily purgative after about an hour.

4. Supportive Therapy - Fluids in dehydration, demulscents in gastroenteritis, sedatives in excitement, stimulants in CNS depression.

Steps for Confirmation of Poison:

Conduct post mortem examination whenever possible and make a detailed note of gross abnormalities.

Collect- Stomach contents, (ruminal and abomasal contents spearately in ruminants); *Liver* (about 500 g). *Kidney* (one) and intestine (*about 12" long piece*) ligate at both ends. Pack separately in sterile airtight containers. Send preferably on ice or use *saturated salt solution* as a preservative. In suspected HCN or Nitrate poisoning send about 500 g rumen contents preserved with about 5 ml chloroform in airtight container. Send a piece of long bone in suspected arsenic poisoning. Also send blood and muslces on ice. One per cent solution of mercuric chloride is very ideal for preserving viscera in case of suspected HCN poisioning. Also send feed and fodder sample. (*Mention the preservative used in all cases.*). *Forensic labs accept material only from medicolegal cases.*

Common Poisonings and their Treatment

Lead

Ruminants are commonly affected. Poisoning through licking oil paints, lubricants, ingestion of metallic lead (*car-batteries, lead shots*).

Clinical Symptoms

Staggering, spasms, bellowing, convulsions, pupils dilated, blindness, mania, hyperaesthesia, initally ruminal atony and constipation, later diarrhoea and signs of acute colic.

Treatment

Mag. sulph. orally. **Calcium Versante (Ca EDTA)** 70 mg/kg as 12.5% sol. iv in two divided doses along with dextorse. **For dogs:** @ 25 mg/kg subcutaneously in repeated doses for 4-5 days. Sedation with Largactil or Siquil to control hyperaesthesia and excitement.

Arsenic

Poisoning through dipping and spraying of animals for ectoparasite-control, arsenic weed killer, insect-killers, over dose of arsenical drugs etc.

Clinical Symptoms

Severe gastro-enteritis manifested by acute abdominal colic, grinding of teeth. Vomiting even in cattle, foetid diarrhoea. In dogs vomitus has a *garlic-like odour,* Cynosis, weak pulse, shock and collapse.

Treatment

Sodium Thisoluphate 15-30 mg in 200 ml iv followed by oral doses of 30-60 g BAL (2.3 dimercaptopropanol) 2-3 mg/kg im (BAL- Inj. 100 mg. available (*Boots*).

For Dogs: 3 mg/lb im three times unitll recovery. Intensive supportive therapy.

Hydrocyanic Acid (HCN)

Common in ruminants due to ingestion of jowar (*Sorghum*) plants at certain stage. New sprouts which appear after untimely rains in recently harvested field of jowar are commonly a cause of poisoning when animals graze in such fields. Linseed and certain other cyanogenic plants (*Hiwar pods*) can also cause poisoning.

Clinical Symptoms- Always acute and death occurring within 1-2 hours. Severe dyspnoea, restlessness, bloat, convulsions and opisthotonus, pupils dilated, m.m. bright red. Blood is *bright red*. Rumen contents have a bitter-almond smell. the rumen contents can be tested by an easy *picrate paper test*. Mix 0.5 gm. picric acid and 5 gm. Sod. carbonate in 100 ml. water. Filter paper strips are dipped in this soln. and air dried in dark place. A drop of rumen fluid is placed on this test paper. A red discoloration is a positive test for free HCN acid.

Treatment

Sod. Nitrite.	3 g
Sod. Thiosulphate..	5 g
Dist. water.	200 ml

Inject by iv route. Repeat after one hour if necesary. Feed Sod. Thiosulphate 30-60 gm. orally at hourly inteval 4-5 times. Inj. Calcium borogluconate, dextrose saline and antihistaminics as intensive supportive therapy.

Nitrate and Nitrite

Plants grown on soils heavily fertilized with nitrates. Accidental ingestion of Amm. Nitrate and used as fertilizer, water from deep wells etc. are the causes.

238

Clinical Symptoms

Salivation, abdominal pain and anoxia, muscle tremors, stagging, subnormal temperature. Acute gastroenteritis on p.m. *Blood dark red or coffee brown coloured.*

Strychnine

Once upon a time Strychnine was the most commonly used poison for killing stray dogs by municipal authorities. Dogs are highly susceptible for strychnine. Poisoning not common in farm animals.

Accidental poisoning is possible in dogs

Clinical Symptoms

Dyspnoea, cyanosis, severe tonic and spasms with opisthotonus, death due to respiratory paralysis

Treatment

Evacuation of stomach contents by giving emetics (*Apomorphine* 20 microgram iv). Anaesthetise the patient by Pentbarbital or iv **Intraval sodium** (*Rhone P.*) 0.5 g in 20 ml.distilled weter. @ 30 mg/kg bwt Gastric lavage after anaesthetization. (*Do not use caffeine, opiate and synthetic narotics.*)

Zinc Phosphide

It is a common *rat poison* and a common accidental poison to dogs.

Clinical Symptoms

Vomiting and diarrhoea. Acute dyspnoea, pulmonary oedema, tonic convulsions.

Treatment

Gastric lavage with potassium permaganate solution 1: 2000, Oxygen, dextrose iv unless pulmonary oedema has developed. Caffeine sod. benzoate 0.05 g im.

Chlorinated Hydrocarbons

(D.D.T. Gammexane (BHC), Aldrein, Endrine)

Commonly used insecticides and pesticides in agricultural operations usuallly absorbed through skin and by ingestion of sprayed grass.

Clinical Symptoms

Initially stimulatioin of CNS, excitement, muscle tremors, tetany, grinding of teeth, dyspnoea, inco-ordination of movements and *fever*.

Treatment

Wash the skin thoroughly with soap water Emetics and gastric lavage in dogs if possibility of ingestin. *No specific antidote,* sedation with Pentobarbital iv calborol 200 ml of cattle. *Calcium Sandoz* 5-10 ml iv for dogs. Nikethamide for supporting circulation. Reduce body temperature by cold water packs.

Organophosphorus Compounds

(Malathion, Sumithion, Neguvan)

Commonly used insecticides and pesticides. Also used for spraying over animal body in sheds for ectoparasitic control.

Clinical Symptoms

Salivation,dyspnoea, diarrhoea, muscle stiffness and staggering. *Constriction of pupils,* tremors of head, bloat, collapse and death. They inactivate enzyme cholinesterase and cause increase in acetylcholine in the tissues.

Treatment

Atropine sulphate 0.25 mg/kg body wt for cattle and 1.0 mg/kg for sheep. (Available as 0.6 mg ampules and 10 mg. vial. Average total dose for cattle is 50 mg Half of should be given by slow iv route and half by im route). Repeat at 4-5 hourly interval. Calborol 200 ml iv.

For Dogs: 0.02 mg/lb (av. dose 1ml). Atropine sulphate given by iv route and repeated by subcutaneous route if necessary. *Calcium Sandoz 5-10 ml iv Sedation with barbiturates if excessive excitement and convulsions. Dextrose saline iv.*

Urea

Urea is the most common fertilizer extensively used by farmers. Accidental ingestion by cattle due to carelessness is one possibility. Urea is also used as a cheap source of protein in the cattle feed. If urea is to be fed as a protein supplement, it must be given in very small amout commencing from 0.5% increased to maximum 2 % *gradually*. Adequate proportion of carbohydrates like maize, molasses etc. must be available in the feed if urea is to be added. Sudden addition and overdose usually results in poisoning. 100 Gm. of urea can be poisonous for average size cattle if the animals are not accustomed.

Clinical Symptoms

Severe colicy pain. Incoordination, tremors, bloat, dyspnoea, violent struggling and bellowing. The animal may die within 3 -4 hours. There is a *strong smell of ammonia to the breath* and death is due to respiratory arrest.

Treatment

Not likely to be successful. Oral administration of weak acids (5% acetic, acid, 3 -4 lit) may be effective in very early stage. Evacuation of rumen contents by quick rumenotomy. Large volume of intravenous dextrose saline will help recovery.

Fluorine

Is a **chronic** condition due to continuous consumption of fluorine through water or feed. Some areas are found to have high fluorine content in soil and water (*area around Ramtek in Nagpur district parts of Chandrapur, district for example.*) Some industrial waste waters containing residual fluorides can contaminate the grazing land and deep soil waters in the adjacent areas. Rock phosphates used in mineral supplements contain high conc. of fluorine.

Fluorine is deposited in bones and teeth. It fixed the tissue calcium by forming calcium fluoride. The rumen miroflora is disturbed and chronic indigestion results. Mottling and pigmentation of incisor teeth which show spots and horizontal bands; teeth become brittle, get eroded and are *painful*, animals become lame due to osteofluorosis, joints and bones are enlarged and painful, easily get fractured.

Diagnosis

By estimation of fluorine levels in blood and urine. Soil and water samples must be also be analysed. There is considerable increase in serum alkaline phosphatase.

Treatment

Is not practicable in case where large animal population in involved. Calcium injections to replace the precipitated calcium, glucose, injections, and other supportive therapy is the only possible treatment. Aluminum sulphate @ 30 g daily may be tired as it reduces toxic effects of fluorine. Addition of slaked lime to water @ 500-1000 mg/kg and water allowed to settle for 6 days. This requires large storage tanks.

Oxalate

This poisoning has attracted attention recently. Oxalates in the form of potassium oxalate are present in some plants and grasses. Some fungi like *Aspergillus niger (black fungus)* are capable of producing oxalates and the stored fodders infected with fungus due to humidity, act as potential source of oxalates to animals. There is a fairly high level of tolerance in cattle but continous feeding on fungus-infected fodder over a prolonged period can cause oxalate poisoning under field conditions. Sudden ingestion of highly infected fodder, however can produce acute poisoning in cattle who are not a accustomed to consumption of oxalates in low doses.

Mode of Action : Oxalates themselves cause gastrointestinal irritation. In rumen the oxalates combine with calcium and form calcium oxlate which is insoluble and is immobilised. In blood, the oxalates chelate the blood calcium and produce *hypocalcaemia.* The acute syndrome is therefore like *severe, hypocalcaemia,* continuous ingestion of soluble oxalates cause renal damage due to oxalate crystals in the renal tubules, and injure blood vessels (*causing oedematous swellings at perineal region*).

Symptoms

Acute poisoning- Muscular tremors, staggering, recumbency and coma.

Subacute Poisoning- Muscular weakness, ruminal atony, bloat, incoordination of gait, hematuria, oedematous swelling on perineum and around the genitals.

Confirmation

Suspected fodder or grasses should be analysed for oxalate contents.

Treatment- Inj. Calcium borogluconate 25% sol iv in the dose of 200-300 ml.

or Inj. Calcium levulinate (*Rickelvit- J.P.*) 30 ml. im.

Feeding lime water along with feed, dextrose soln. for energy. The fungus infested fodder should be sun-dried and treated with lime water before feeding.

Aflatoxicosis

Is a type of fungal toxicosis due to some strain of *Aspergillus flavus* which produce a potent hepatotoxin (*Aflatoxin-B$_1$*). The fungus grows on grains, groundnut, maize, jowar, Grains become mouldy due to humid conditions of storage. Actue poisoning may cause death in young calves. The symptoms appear slowly if the toxic feed is consumed in small quantities over a long period. Affected animals suffer a chronic indigestion, nervous signs like inco-ordination, blindness, grinding of teeth and diarrhoea. Milk production is decreased and causes considerable economic losses. Aflatoxicosis may occur in other animals like poultry and rabbits.

Diagnosis

By analysis of suspected feed for presence of aflatoxin-B1 (levels above 100 mg/kg. feed are considered poisonous for cattle).

Treatment

Not specific. Evacuation of rumen in case of obstinate rumen indigestion, intravenous dextrose, calcium and liver tonics may help in some cases. Careful and vigilant observation of feed ingredients and proper storage can prevent the conditoins.

Snake Bite

Clinical Symptoms

Depend on the type and species of snake. Look for the bite marks on lower extremities, head and muzzle. Local swelling and pain, excitement, salivation, hyperaesthesia, tetany, recumbency and paralysis. Death due to asphyxia in 1-10 hrs. in dogs upto 48 hours in cattle and horses.

Treatment

Tourniquet above the bite, give a deep incision at the site of bite to drain blood for some time. Polyvalent antiserum available at Haffkin Institute (Freeeze dried)s. Give 2 ampoules iv as intial dose and repeat till clinical recovery. *Polyvalent serum should always be stocked in dispensary.*

Chapter 19

Care of a Pet Dog

Pet dog is not only the best and loyal friend but a family member. Dog. owners usually possess good information about managemnt by experience, through reading literature and by discussion amongst the other dog lovers. However, there are some misconceptions and incomplete knowledge about scientific facts. It is essential that the veterinary physician should have good information about various breeds of dogs, their normal habits, instincts, food requirements etc. in addition to sound knowledge about treatment and prevention of diseases.

Which Breed is Good?

Selection of a breed is a matter of individual liking and need. Some dog lovers have a special fancy for pure bred dogs and insist on having a dog registered with kennel club because pups born to such registered pure breed parents fetch an attractive price. Pure bred dogs do have appearance and confirmation of the particular breed but continuous inbreeding can result in loss of vigor and appearance of congenital defects and deformities in the progeny.

Common Breeds of Dog

There may be about 250 different breeds of dogs all over the world but all may not be available in India as recognised breeds, it is an individual fancy and the purpose for which the dog is required. The dog is may be kept any of the following purposes:

1. **Purely as a Domestic House Dog for Guarding the Premises, and for Companionship**

   A real liking and affection is needed for this purpose.

2. **For Detection of Crimes (in Police Dog squads)**

   A specialized training is require.

3. **To Detect Narcotics and Explosives by Police Squads**

   A very special type of training is needed.

4. **Participation in Exhibitions and Dog Shows.**

   Proper training of obedience and performance is necessary.

5. **For Making Business of Selling Pedigree Dogs.**

   Good amount of experience of maintenance of dogs is necesary.

It is quite expensive to rear and maintain good dogs in a house. The house members should have liking for dogs, should devote enough time to look after them and have patience to train your dog for obedience and good habits and also for nursing the dog during illness. Yours dog will repay you in terms of loyalty, faithfulness and high degree of devotion. The dog will ignore your status, financial position, education and will only expect love and affection from you.

The breeds are classified according to the utility-watch dogs, hunter dogs, domestic pet as per size of breeds as under-

1) Large breeds-Dogs with height at withers of 55-60 centimeters and above.

2) Medium breeds-Dogs with height between 40-55 cms.

3) Small breeds-Dogs with height between 20-40 cms.

4) Miniature or toy breeds-Very small dogs with height below 20 cemtimeters and body weight ranging from 1 to 5 kilograms. These dogs can be accommodated in a pocket of overcoat while going out for shopping or a walk. Such toy breeds are quite popular in Western countries.

Every breed has his standards prescribed by International Kennel Clubs to be called as "pure breed". These breed characteristics are maintained over generations unless altered due to cross breeding. These decriptions are with Kennel clubs and judges who are recognised for appointment in dog shows.

The brief description of a some common breeds and pictures of dogs is given below to help the dog lover to select his pet dog.

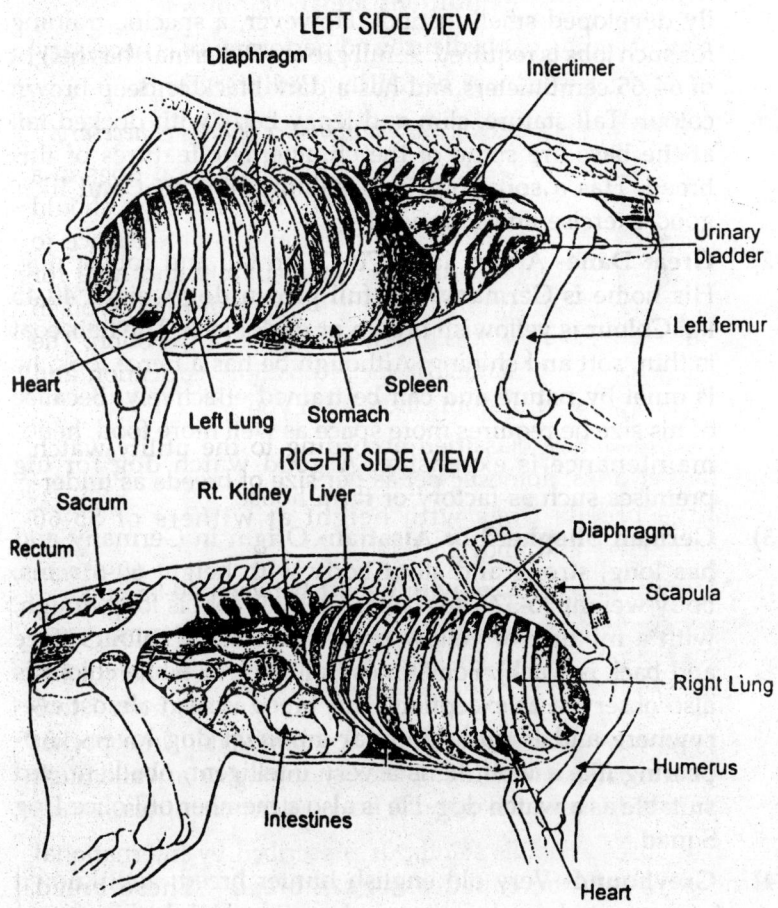

LEFT SIDE VIEW

Diaphragm

Intertimer

Urinary bladder

Left femur

Heart

Left Lung

Stomach

Spleen

RIGHT SIDE VIEW

Sacrum

Rt. Kidney

Liver

Rectum

Diaphragm

Scapula

Right Lung

Humerus

Intestines

Heart

Fig. 17. Regional Anatomy of a Dog.

Large Breeds

1) **Doberman Pincher**-A very intelligent breed with tall and slender body. Origin in Germany. Invariabley a member of Police Dog Squad, utilised for tracking thieves, locating stocks of narcotics and explosives due to his extraordinarily developed smell instinct. However, a specific training for such jobs is required. A full grown Doberman has height of 64-65 cemtimeters and has a dark black or deep brown colour. Tall stature, slim and leggy body with docked tail at the base are some of the chracteristic features of this breed. Has a soft, short and shining hair coat and likes good exercise and long walks.

2) **Great Dane-** A very large 70-72 cm tall and robust dog. His home is Germany and full grown dog weighs 40-45 kg. Colour is yellowish brown or dark black. The hair coat is thin, soft and shining. Although he has a fierce look, he is quiet by nature and can be trained effectively. Because of his size he requires more space as well more food, hence maintenance is expensive. A good watch dog for big premises such as factory or farm house.

3) **German Shepherd or Alsatian-** Origin in Germany and has long, strong and stout body with height 60-61 cms, body weight 35-37 kilograms. The hair coat is long, rough, with a mixture of yellow brown and black colours (face and back is black). Sometimes full black or white colour is also observed as exception. This breed is seen almost everywhere and is quite popular amongst dog lovers. Appearing like a wolf, he is a very intelligent, obedient and suitable as a watch dog. He is also a member of Police Dog Squad.

4) **Greyhound-** Very old english hunter breed, well known and reputed for hunting and racing. Height 55-60 cm, strong body, small ears and long tail. Hair small and has a mxiture of brown hair. Good understanding and co-operative nature.

5) **Blood Hound-** Origin in England, height 66 cms, long loose and hanging skin around eyes and face, ears very long and pendulous. Hair coat short and long tail. Weight 30-

Large Breeds of Dog

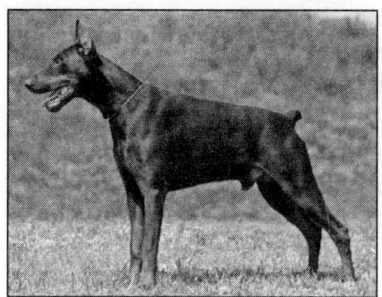

Doberman

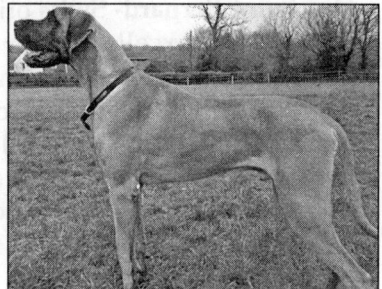

Greatdane

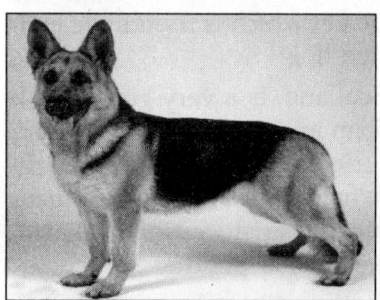

German Shepherd
(Alsatian)

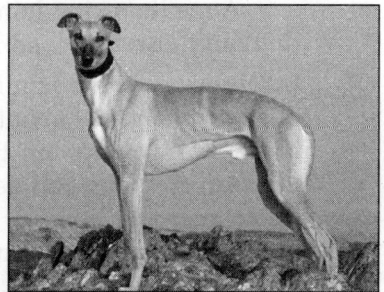

Greyhound

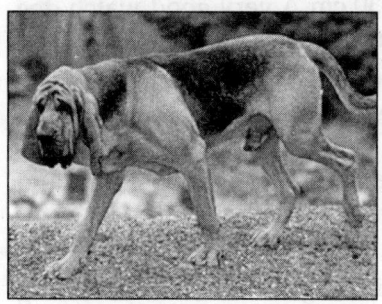

Bloodhound

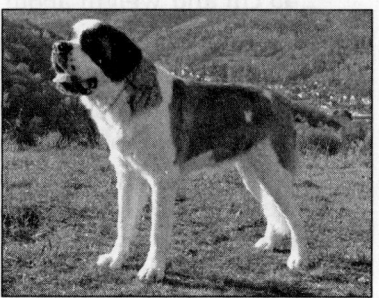

Saint Bernard

40 kg. A vey good hunter dog with strong instinct of smell. Colour-red and black.

6) **Saint Bernard-** Swiss origin and known as old watch dog. Proved excellent path finder to search lost travellers trapped under snow. This is a powerful, strong and muscular dog. Height 71-72cm, 50-60 kg with medium length of coat with a bushy tail. Ears are of medium size. Colour is a combination of red and white patches and tail white. Character is quiet, friendly and reliable.

Medium Breeds

1) **Dalmatian-** Home country is Dalmatia state of Ugoslavia. Also bred in England. This breed is found in several countries. Black or brown coloured round patches over white coat is the identity of this breed. Hair coat is small and soft. A medium size domestic pet which is friendly to children and also is a good watch dog.

2) **Collie-** Dog with origin in Scotland. Is a very good watch dog with height of about 55 cm and weight 40-45 kg Red, brown. and white are the tricolour patches with fairly medium size long and dense hair. Ears small and pointed, snout long and pointed. Nature is aristocratic, is reliable, honest and intelligent and very good pet dog.

3) **Boxer-** German dog trustworthy to his owner, energetic and with a stout stature of body. Face is black and with nose tip pointing upwards and has an angry look. Colour is brownish red and tail usually docked. Height about 40-45 cm and weight about 25-30 cm A very good watch dog which is friendly to children.

4) **Golden Retriever-** A domestic dog with peaceful and quiet nature. Coat colour is golden-brown, ears long and hanging and hair soft and short. Good to participate in exhibitions due to his co-operative nature. Height 35-40 cm and weight 25-30 kg Included in Police dog squad after training.

5) **Labrador-Retriever-** A very intelligent and affectionate dog with brown or dark black colour. Ears long and pendu-

Medium Breeds of Dog

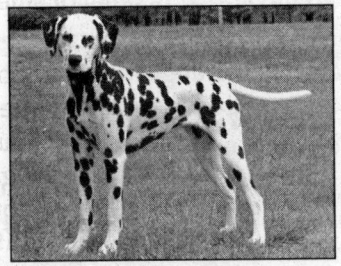

Dalmatian

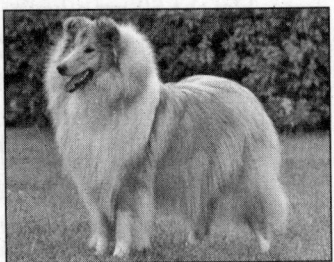

Collie, Rough

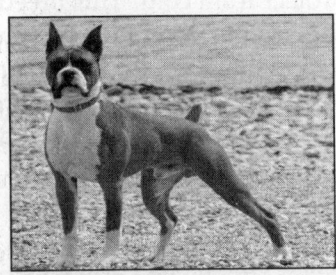

Boxer

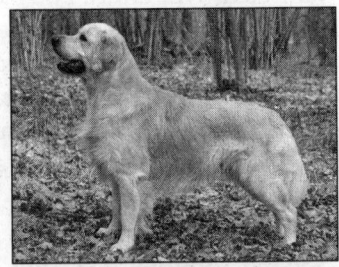

Golden Retriever

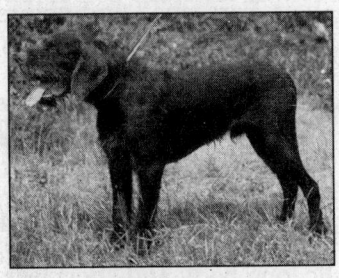

Poodle Pointer

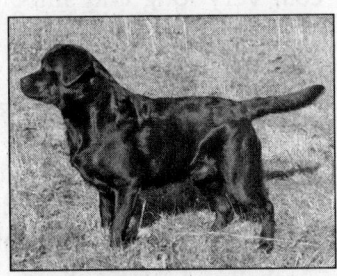

Labrador Retriever

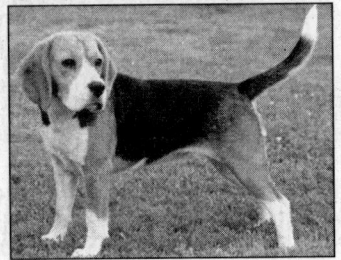

Beagle

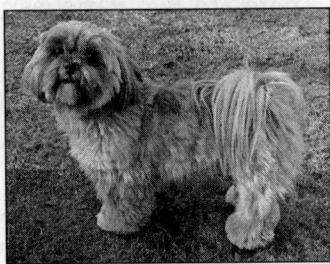

Lhasa Apso

251

lous. Height 50 cm weight 25-30 kg. Good dogs for Police squad after proper training due to his extraordinary strong smell instinct. A very good natured pet dog.

6) **Poodle Pointer-** German dog with 45-55 cm height, medium stature, clever hunter dog. Tail usually docked.

7) **Beagle-** A very good pet dog with good nature. Used in experiments in laboratories. Available in any colour. Hair small and dense. Height 35 cm and weight 16-20 kg.

8) **Lhasa Apsos-** Country of origin is tibet and has long, dense hair coat over entire body to protect from cold. This breed is adopted by many families and seen in good numbers in exhibitions. Extra care is required to maintain the long hair and keeping the ectoparasite away. Colour is usually golden black or snow white. Height 30-35 cm and hairy tail turned on his back. Always alert and energetic.

Small Breeds

1) **Cocker Spaniel-** Very old English breed. Very intelligent and with a mild nature. Ears are long and pendulous. Hair coat very long and smooth. Seen in different colour but black or brown and white are very common. Tail usually docked. A very good pet dog.

2) **Samoyed-** Home is the Samoyed state in Russia. White colour with long hair is very common. Appearance is closely similar to Pomeranian and Spitz but height is more than the above two breeds. His nature has sportsman spirit and is an energetic and intelligent dog.

3) **Dachshund-** Has a characteristic long body and short legs. The snout is pointed and ears are long and pendulous. There are two varieties i.e., long haired and with very short, soft and glistening coat. (See two pictures). Colour is black or brown. The tail is long. Height is between 20-30 cm and body weight about 10 to 18 kg. Nature is usually quiet but is unpredictable. A good house pet who can act as watch dog also.

4) **Spitz-** This breed has close similarity with Samoyed and Pomeranian. Has long hair coat like Lhasa apsos. Basically

Small Breeds of Dog

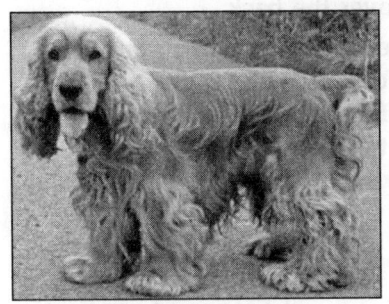

Cocker Spaniel

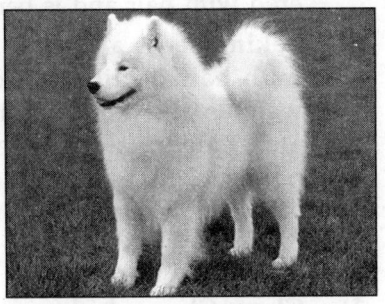

Samoyed

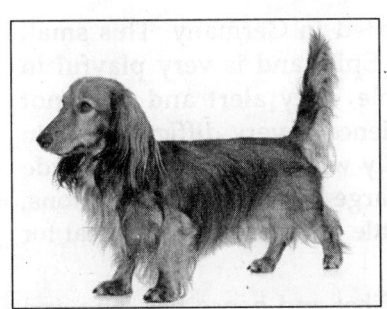

Dachshund (Long-haired)

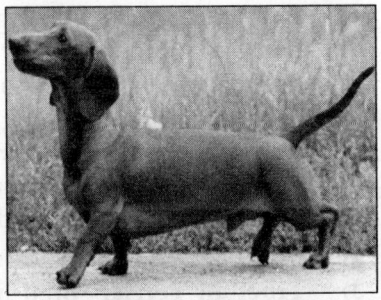

Dachshund (Short-haired)

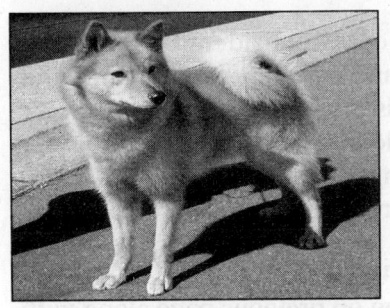

Spitz

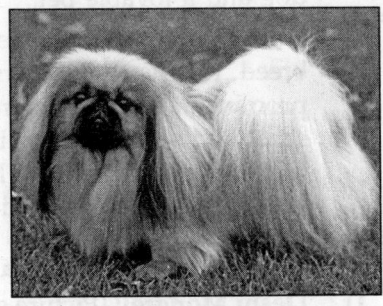

Pekingese

white colour is common but golden and brown shade is also seen. Height varies between 30 to 35 cm Tail is covered with hair and is bent over the back.

5) **Pekingese-** Is a Chinese breed. the body is fully covered with hair of different colour. Hight 20 cm and body weights about 3-5 kg The face is black and proportionately larger as compared to body. Legs are small and pointed. This is a small toy breed known for it's aristocracy and boldness.

Small Miniature Breeds

1) **Chow Chow-** A chinese breed and is very obstinate by nature and attitude is fearless. Has long, thick and soft hair and has red, brown or white colour. Height about 40 cm with a bent tail.

2) **Pomeranian-** Breed originated in Germany. This small hairy dog looks similar to Spitz and is very playful in nature. He is very unstable, very alert and does not concentrate on anything. Hence is very difficult to train him properly. Hair is usually white or has golden shade or black colours. Seen in large numbers in exhibitions. Requires small space and little food hence economical for playing with children.

3) **Tibetian Terrier-** Bred in Tibet and hence has long and soft hair which covers the entire body. Tail is bent and curved on the top of his body. Height 30-35 cm Colour is white, brown, black or golden. Intelligent and good watch dog and a lovable pet.

4) **Chihauhua-** Bred in Mexico. Is considered as smallest breed. Face is round, ears and eyes are very big and and prominent. Body structure is rather long but legs are very short and small and tail is long. Hair is short and glistening. Some varieties have longer hair. Body weight is 1 to 3 kg. Very intelligent, bold and considerate by nature.

Deshi Breeds (With photographs)

1) **Deshi Mongrel:** (Picture seen on previous page along with small breeds)

Small & Deshi Breeds of Dog

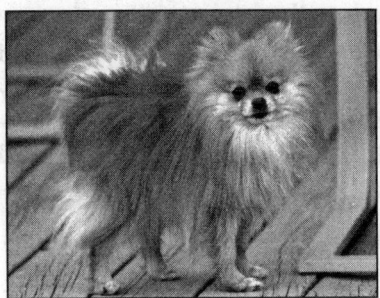

Pomeranian

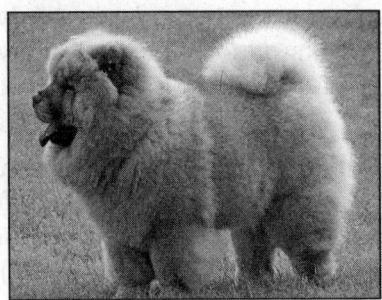

Chow Chow

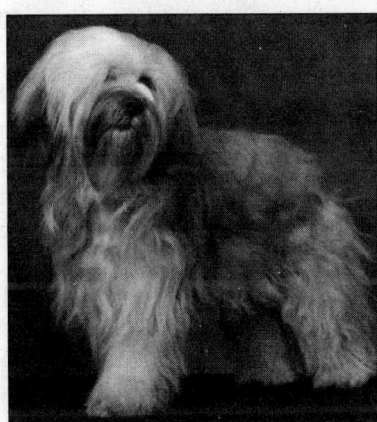

Tibetan Terrier

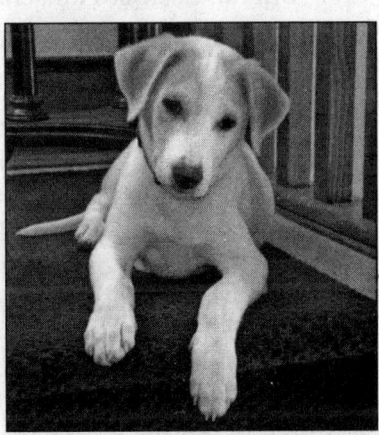

Desi Mongrael

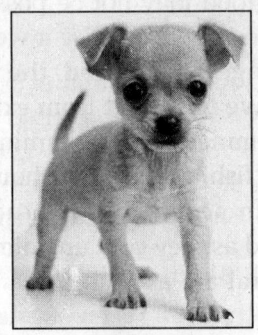

Chihuahua

255

The Deshi breed dogs are seen in different colours of hair coat and are seen all over India. These are essentially cross bred progeny and are sturdy and as they have no particular background, sometimes are very erratic and unpredictable by nature.

2) **Gaddi-** Seen in Himachal Pradesh.

3) **Banjara-** Seen in Maharashtra. This breed is reputed to be hunter type and dogs fearless and of attacking nature. Usually seen with Banjara people (nomadic tribe moving with big herds of Sheep). Seen all over India.

4) **Rampur Hound-** Seen in Madhya Pradesh.

5) **Bhotia-** Seen in Himachal Pradesh.

6) **Rajapalyam-** Seen in Tamilnadu.

7) **Himalayan Sheep dog-** Seen in Himachal Pradesh.

All these are Indian breeds although not recognised by International Kennel Clubs, are very popular with poor farmers who can not maintain pedigree dogs. If these dogs are offered same management, care and feeding and disease protection, these will also turn out to be good pet dogs.

Feeding of Dogs

The opinion and experience of dog lovers may vary considerably as regards feeding practices. In nature, dogs are carnivores and the most natural food for them is the raw meat, bones and occasionally some vegetables. If in a pure vegetarian family regular meat food may not be possible, occasional meat and long bone if given once or twice a week may be desirable. In case of pure vegetarian food the essential nutritive requirements will have to be met from extra supplements such as more milk, eggs, minerals and vitamins etc. Small pieces of bones from poultry, fish, rabbits etc. should never be given as they might cause an accidental obstructoin of throat. Dog biscuits, are also good as they contain animal proteins. The food requirments in general are as under:

Small & Deshi Breeds of Dog

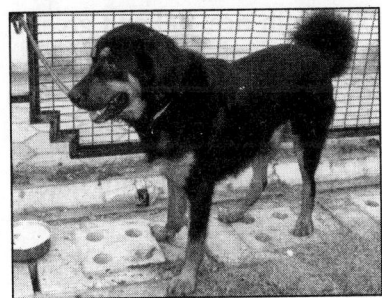
Gaddi

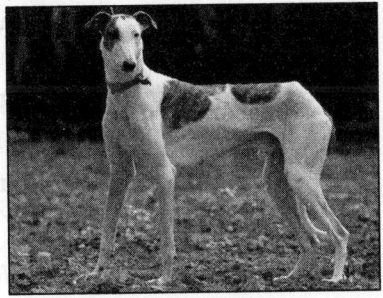
Rampur Hound

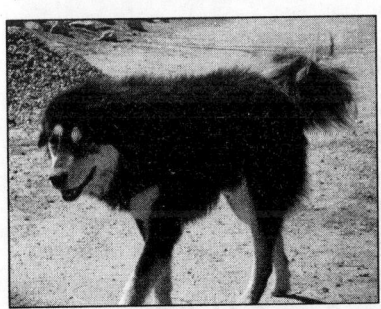
Bhutia

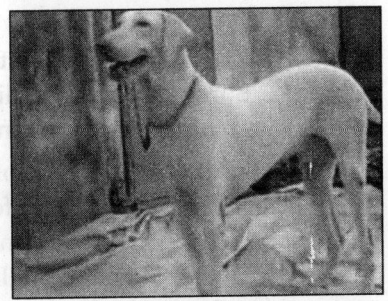
Rajapalyam

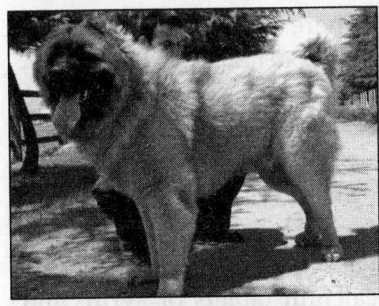
Himalayan Sheep Dog

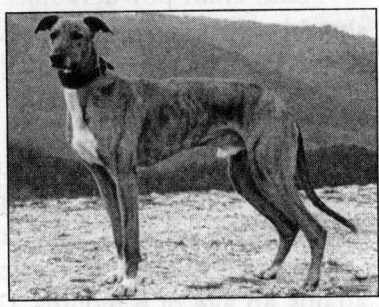
Banjara

257

1) **After Weaning till 10 Weeks Age:**

   Morning: Scrambled or boiled egg and 100-200 ml milk.

   1.00 pm: Raw or boiled meat 50 g with rice, dal and green vegetables.

   6.00 pm. : Rice, dal and green vegetable.

   10.00 pm. : Bread or roti 100 g with milk

   Total bulk about 120 g for small breed and 400 g for large breed.

2) **Ten Weeks to Sixteen Weeks:**

   Quantities to be increased, basic ingredients remaining the same. Daily requirement of bulk is approximately 250 g for small breeds 800g for large breeds.

Above16 Weeks

   Give 2 feeds a day one at 8.00 or 10.00 A.M. and other at 8.00 P.M. Some advocate feeding only once but this is unkind and dog remains unsatified and hungry.

   Total daily requirement of bulk should be about 500 g for small breeds and upto 1500 g for large breeds. Complete bodily development occurs by 9 months age. Milk, egg, biscuits, rice and dal, vegetables etc. should be given in the morning and roti prepared out of wheat or jowar flour, (with little, urad dal or soyabean added) along with boiled vegetables, dal and milk or meat in the evening.

   Salt, chilli powder, spices as well as too much of sweets should not be given in the food. There can be various other combinations made according to the food habits of the family.

Food Supplements

   A growing pup needs minerals and vitamins for optimum growth. If the food is appropriately balanced, these requirements are met with from food. However, to avoid any risk, it is advisable to give calcium and vit. A and D till the dog attains an age of 6 months. Ostocalcium tablets or syrup and multivitamin drops and preparation like **Bonyvet** *(Kosmorex)* or

Vimeral (*Virbac*) if given regularly, serves the purposes. This will ensure growth and prevent rickets which is avery common condition in young growing pups. Several nutritional supplements are now available as feed additives and **anyone of the following** may be given regularly.

These supplements when regularly made available, the nutritional inadequacies and presence of trace elements are taken care of in the feed and although it might add a little to the feed cost, are beneficial in the long run.

1) **NUTRIPET** (*Pectcare*) given 4 teaspoon powder twice daily in food or milk as food supplement.

2) **PROMIX-Y** (*Alembic*) tablets 2 to 4 tablets twice daily given regularly with food.

3) **NUTRIBIX** (*Petcare*) and Probix dog biscuits containing animals proteins and vitamins can be given regularly.

4) **VISORBEN** (*SKF*) Liquid feed supplements as growth promoter and coat conditioner.

5) **NUTRILIV**-Fote (*petcare*) Liquid 4-5 ml twice daily as oral tonic and conditioner.

6) **SILFUR** (*Serum Inst.*) 10-15 g daily 2-3 times with milk.

7) **VETRIL** (*Vestas*) Liquid 1-2 tsp twice daily.

8) **VITAPET** (*Agrivet-Glaxo*) as food supplement.

9) **ZIGUP** syrup (*Ind. Herbs*) as health tonic.

10) **CHOLYMBI** (*Lyka*)-for lustrous hair and shiny skin.

11) **PROCOFUR** H.P. (*Life laboratories*) 1 tsp in milk twice a day.

12) **YEA-SACC** powder (*Petcare*) 1/2 tsp in milk twice a day.

Housing and Management

Dog should be kept leashed (unchained) as far as possible. The pup when young should be provided with box of suitable size with bedding and kept at well protected place. Top of the box should be open and whenever necessary half of 3/4 of the top could be covered to protect during cold and rainy weather.

For adult and grown ups a similar arrangement or a cage house located in an attached enclosed verandah or in the front portion of house so that the dog can watch the vistors. Food and water utensils should be kept scrupously clean by washing with boiling water. *Phenyl or carbolic acid should never be used.*

Training and Exercise

It is possible to train the dog for good habits and obedience if a pup is reared from early life.

Food should be offered at fixed tmes but water should be availble at all times. The pup can be trained or defaecation and urination habits after it is about 2 months old. The dog should be taken to the place which he is supposed to use this purpose. If the dog defaecates or urinates at other places in the house, he should be punished for that and express that you have not liked his behaviour. If he obeys your instructions, he should be patted with love in appreciation. Dogs can be trained for obedience in the similar manner. This requires a little patience but will soon pick up good habits and will always try to please the owner.

Regular exercise is a must. A good morning/evening walk will do a considerable good to the dog and will have minimum digestive disturbances in general.

Prevention of Disease and Immunization Programme

Digestive upsets, gastritis with vomiting and diarrhoea are the common ailments. Switching over to cow milk after weaning should be done gradually. Proper boiling of milk cleaning utensils of food, milk and water are very essential, periodical administration of gripe water as we do for children, prevents flatulence and other digestive disturbances, persistent vomiting and diarrhoea should not be neglected as they might produce serious dehydration and hence need timely attention.

The pup needs to be protected from cold weather, and on rainy days. Long haired breed need special care to keep them clean and dry. Frequent bathing of long haired breeds might prepitate an attack of colds.

The young puppies should not be brought in contact with other dogs till all its immunization programmes are completed. Taking an unprotected pup to the hospital is not free from risk.

Never neglect a dog bite. Dog bite is never free from risk. The wound should be flushed with a running tap water using any alkaline soap *immediately within 20 minutes of the bite.* This reduce the changes the rabies infection and is more important than trying in control a little bleeding.

Following diseases can be communicated to man from dogs:

(i)   Rabies

(ii) Leptospirosis

(iii) Herpes virus

(iv) Round worm infection

(v)   Tapeworm infection (*Hydatidosis*)

(vi) Ringworm

(vii) Scabies

(viii) Toxoplasmosis (*rarely*)

(ix) Allergy to dandruff and hair.

It is therefore necessary that the owner be informed about taking adequate care to protect himself from getting diseases from his pet. The pet should not be allowed entrance in the kitchen and dining room or in the bed.

Immunization Programme

The pup must be in excellent healthy condition at the time of immunization. It is advisable to give deworming dose one week prior to immunization. This is necessary for better immunization response.

(1) Distemper Vaccination

Distemper is the most important killer disease of young pups. Appropriate age for vaccination is 12 weeks. If the mother was vaccinated or had recovered from distemper. The pup is most likely to have received maternal antibodies through colostrum. These maternal antibodies will protect the pup for about 10 to 12 weeks. These antibodies also interfere with development of immunity by vaccination and therefore, vaccination is not usually done untill these maternal antibodies disappear by 10-12 wks. age. This creates two possibilities.

(i) The assumption that the pup has received maternal antibodies may not be actually true (*It is not so easy to measue this*) and in this case the pup is at a risk of getting distemper in a very severe form, if not vaccinated before 12 weeks age.

(ii) Vaccination done before 12 weeks. age may not produce protective immunity because of the neutralizing effect of maternal antibodies.

Hence, if you do not wish to take any risk, do the first vaccination at 4 to 6 weeks age. At the most this might be wasteful but there is no harm. (*For this you can use monovalent distemper vaccine alone which is cheaper*) second or a booster dose must be given at 12 weeks as usual.

This double vaccination may be little more expensive but you avoid any risk. Subsequently annual revaccination is advised atleast for 3 more years.

Distemper vaccine is available as polyvalent in combination with hepatitis, Leprospirosis, parvovirus and Rabies antigens.

The vaccine is a live attenuated tissue culture vaccine of distemper virus.

Following different vaccines are available:

(i) *Distemper Vaccine*-(single antigen)-I.V.R.I Izatnagar

(ii) *Distemper + Hepatitis* - **BIVIROVAX** (*Iffa*)-

(iii) *Distemper Hepatitis & Leptospirosis*

Caniffa-IFFA (*Serium Institute*)

NOBI-VAC-DHL (*Intervet*)

CANLEP-DHL (*Virbac*)

CANDUR DHPPI +L (*Intervet*)

(iv) *Distemper, Hepatitis, Leptospirosis & Rabies-*

Canadivac-DHLR (*Behring*)

Pentadog (*IFFA*)- (*Serium Instt.*)

(v) *Distemper, Hepatitis, Parainfluenza, Adenovirus (CAV-2) Leptospirosis and Parvovirus* **(multicomponent)**

Adenomune-7 *(Vestas)*

Galaxy-6 *(Tech. America)*

Duramune *(Fort Dodge)*

Vanguard -S/L seven way vaccine.

Magavac-6 multicomponent canine vaccine *(Ind.Immunol)*

(Note: The above multicomponent vaccines do not contain rabies vaccine).

The combined vaccines are mostly imported at present and marketed by distrubutors in India. However, these vaccines are manufactured in India by Indian Immunological for example and there is a continuous progress of technoology in India. The vaccines may not be regularly available in the Pharmacy. The vaccines are to be transported on ice and stored in the freeze at 4 degree C. The availability may be enquired with some of the following dealers.

(i)   Modern Agencies-Gandhibag, NAGPUR.

(ii) Mahal Medical Stores-Fawara, Chowk, NGP.

(iii) Akbarallys-Fort, MUMBAI.

(iv) Bhagat Traders- Matunga, MUMBAI.

(v)   Intervet Pharma- Pragati Bhawan, NEW DELHI.

(vi) Veterinary Service Centre-E-20, Defence N Colony NEW DELHI-24.

(vii) Serum Institute of India. Hadapsar, PUNE-28.

(viii)"VESTAS' A-21, Rajouri Garden, NEW DELHI.

(ix) B.C.Animal Hlth Product,Dhenu mrkt, INDORE.

In big cities these vaccines are available at all times. it is advisable to deworm the pup atleast a week before distemper immunization. It should not have any other illness and should be in best health. This is necessary for production of good immune response.

Beyond a mild febrile reaction, the vaccination is quite safe.

(2)   Antirabies vaccination: *(Pre-bite or Prophylactic)*

Antibrabies vaccination is a *must*. Different vaccines are available. First dose of vaccine is to be given at 3 months age. It is better to use a proper, potent and safe antirabies vaccine preferably as a single antigen.

Age at first vaccination – 3 months, **Immunity**- 3 years.

Inactivated Vaccines (*Single rabies antigen*)

(*Inactivated rabies virus grown on cell culture*)

(i)   **NOBIVAC -R** (*Intervet*)

(ii) **DURARAB** (*Vestas*)

(iii) **RABIGEN** (*Virbac-Vestas*)

(iv) **ANUMMUNE** (*Fort-Dodge*)

(v)   **RAKSHARAB** (*Ind. Immunological*)

(vi) **IMRAB** (*Rhoe Merieux*)N)OVI-VAC

(ix) **IMRAB** (*Rhone Merieux*)

(x)   **CANDUR-R-VET** (*Hoechst*)

* *Flurry-LEP strain grown on chicken fuibroblast cellculture and inactivated.*

Dose : (For all above) : 1 ml sc or Intramuscular.

Primary vaccination : At 10-12 weeks age.

Booster dose on 28 th day after primary.

Annual revaccination thereafter.

Immunity: One to 2 years. However, annual vaccination recommended in India.

Inactivated Vaccines (*Combined with rabies*)

(i) **LEPOTRAB** (*Iffa*) a combined Leptospirosis and Rabies vaccine

(ii) **CANDUVAC-DHLR** (*Behring*)- A combined vaccine against Distemper Hepatitis, Leptospirosis and Rabies.

Immunity : 1 to 2 years (Annual vaccination recommended)

(3) **Vaccination against Infectious Hepatitis and Leptospirosis**

When combined vaccines are used the protection against these disease is taken care of.

(4) Vaccination against Parvovirus Infection

This is a newly identified disease causing hemorrhagic gastroenteritis with heavy mortality. Vaccine is now available (**Candur-P**) and **Parvocine** (*Serum Institute*) Annual vaccination should be done. *Galaxy-6* **and** *Adenomune-7* are polyvalent vaccines from U.S. and contain Parvovirus antigen

Parvovirus vaccine (*Modified live virus* of feline cell line origin) of *FROM laboratories Inc. Graffon. Wiscouncin (U.S.A.)* is also available.

"Commander" Parvovirus type D2 modified live virus vaccine by "Blocor' is also introduced.

"VANGUARD-CPV Parvo vaccine is also available.

(5) Canine corona virus infection

Disease similar to Parvo virus infection, prophylactic vaccination at 6 wks age is recommended.

Periodical Deworming

Roundworms

Roundworms (*Toxocara-spp*) and Hookworms (*Ancylostoma-spp.*) are the most common worms causing menace. Every dog gets one or the other worm infection at some stage. Periodical faecal examination is necessary to keep the worm infections under control. Round worm infection is very common in young pups who may receive the infection *even before their birth, from mother through the placental barrier.* Diarrhoea, vomiting, fits and pot belly are the common symptoms.

Piparazine compounds (*Piparazine liquid, Antepar, Wormex, Piparex etc.*) are very useful against round worms of Toxocara species. Human products such as Nemocid can as well be used and the dose rate is as per body wt.

Blood in the faeces, black coloured stools, dysentery, anaemia, itching, loss of condition are the signs of hookworm disease. Get the faeces examined. Hookworm infection must be treated in time. Inj. **Ancylol** (as per body wt.) two injections given 21 days apart are very effective. Other drugs given orally such as *Pantelmin, Mintazole, Mebex, Eizol, Wormin, Eben etc. are* *the human products* containing *"Mebendazole"* or allied compound given @ 100 mg B.D. for 3 days have been found quite effective as broad spectrum dewormer in canine practice.

Albendazole has been found highly effective against hookworms @ 5 mg/ per kg body wt. (**Albomar**-*Virbac*).

Pyrantel pamoate (**Nemocid**) or **Thalmax** (BPL) tablets or syrup @ 10 mg/kg. *as single dose repeated after 21 days is also effective.*

All these drugs are slightly toxic and hence the general care and precautions are very essential. A detailed check up of a dog and close observation during treatment is necessary. *Self medication by dog owners should be discouraged.*

Tapeworms

Rubbing of anus on the ground, restlessness, general debility etc. are the symptoms of tapeworm infestation. Segments of tapeworm look like cucumber seeds or boiled rice grains and are seen in the stool and sticking around the anus. *Stool examination be done for confirmation.*

Any of the following drugs are prescribed.

DRONCIT (*Praziquintel-Bayer*) or **PRAZI-PLUS** (*Vetcare*) - A new drug very effective against tapeworm

Tablets : (50 mg) @ 5 mg/kg as single dose followed by a laxative

NICLOSAN (*Niclosamide*) tablets. @ 500 mg/ 3 kg b.wt. twice a day for 2 days.

Maintenance of general cleanliness and hygiene are very essential for preventing worm infestations. Always remember that the worms in dogs could be source for *human infection for the members of family.* It is therefore necessary to examine faecal sample regularly and given regular treatment.

Ectoparasite Control

Ticks, mites and lice are the important problems. ticks suck blood, cause anaemia and also transmit certain diseases. Mites burrow in skin and produce "Mange" or "Scabies". Lice cause restlessness and constant itching resulting in loss of hair.

Application of gammexine dust 5% combined with hand picking of ticks regularly is the safest method. Other drugs like **malathion, Sumithion, Asuntol** etc. are deadly poisons. Very dilute solutions like 0.2 % are used applying on body by a small spray pump and about 2 % soln. is used for spraying by dog house and the places where dog is housed. Great care is necessary while using these drugs. Absorption through cuts, tick-bite injuries can lead to absorption to poison through skin. Immediate antidotal treatment **(Inj. Atropine)**must be employed in case symptoms of poisoning are observed.

NOTIX scrub (*Petcare*) containing 10@ *Carbaryl* in shampoo base is found very effective. To be used once in a month and followed by NOTIX talc for regular use while brushing.

BUTOX (*Deltamethrin*) is a new generation ectoparasiticide highly effective against ticks and lice. A solution of 1 ml. in a litre of water useful for spraying over body. Use the drug with great care and avoid eyes, mouth parts, of dog and keep food and water utensils away. Wash hands with plenty of water.

EKTODEX (dip solution *Amitraz 5%-Petcare*) Dilute @ 6 ml. per litre water. First give a bath with warm soap water and dry up with towel. Apply the dip solution liberally all over body using a sponge specially over the lesions. Allow it to dry. Do not wash. Repeat once a week.

TAKTIC (*Intervet*) is a new product introduced.

Mites are very small microscopic parasites which burrow in the skin and produce **"Scabies"** or **"Mange"**. There are three types of mites namely **Sarcoptis, Psoroptis** and **Demodex,** out of which first two mites are easily controlled but demodex is very difficult to eradicates and cure completely. **Demodecosis** is usually seen in young age and lesions commence on face, around eyes and also spread on other parts of the body. There is no itching and lesions appear as pustules and hairless patches. Mites comes out with pus when the pustules are pressed. Thse mites proliferate when the general vitality and resistance of the patient is lowered due to malnutrition or any other cause. Inj. **Ivermectin** along with **Levamisole** have been found effective. The skin scrapings must be examined for confirming the type of mites infection.

The Sacroptic and Psoropic mites cause intense itching, rednes of skin, loss of hair on affected parts of body. Scrapings have to be examined for diagnosis. The affected part must be cleaned by shaving hair, washed thoroughly and dried before application of medications.**Ascabiol, Petmosol** lotion or **Himax** ointment etc. are quite useful. Sulphur Ointment, Golden Lotion are equally effective. Pestoban and Laurell *(Ind. Herbs)* are Ayurvedic herbal compounds found effective and safe very applying over the body after diluting 3- 4 times with water. **IVOMAC** (*Ivermectin*) an injectiable drug (**M.D. Agvet**) is highly effective against all types of mite infections.

Dose: 200-400 mcg/kg sc as a single dose treatment, repeated after one week if necessary.

Regular grooming is necessary in long haired breeds. Bath may be given once a week or fortnight depending on weather and season. Never use carbolic soap like **Lifebuoy** for a dog. **Petmosol, Sulphur** or **Neep soap** should be used. **SII Shampoo** (*Serum Inst.*) **Canifur** (*Cadila*) **Blaze Shampoo** (Ind. Herbs) are used for improving shining of coat and keeping it clean. **Flematic skin oil** *(TTK)* is useful mild ectoparasitic infestation.

For **lice** infection the gammexine dust or **Dalf** dust **Licil** or **Crotorax** lotion etc. along with brushing and combing is usually enough. Regular brushing and hygiene alone can control lice infection.

Flea Infestation

Fleas are common on dogs and cats. They may become a nuave in long haired breeds. Fleas cause continuous irritation due to release of salivary secretions in the skin. They also cause allergy (flea-bite dermatitis) characterised by rash which occurs repeatedly. Flea faeces contain blood and make the skin dirty.

Control- By regular brushing, use of shampoo and ectoparasitic sprays. Flea repellent belts may be tried but have limited use if infection is heavy.

Some Important Infectious Diseases of Dogs

Canine Distemper

This is another viral disease more commonly affecting young pups below 6 months age. Newborn pups usually get protective antibodies through mother's colostrum (*first milk after whelping*). This protection lasts only for a few weeks and then they can get the infection from other sick dogs. Disease is widely prevalent and infection from other spread like influenza through infective droplets. High fever is an early sign. The fever appears to have come to normal for a day or two and then again there is a relapse with signs of bronchitis, pneumonia, yellow pustules with symptoms like rash on abdomen, diarrhoea and weakness. The animal may suffer trembling and convulsions because nervous system is affected. The majority of pups do not survive but those who survive suffer from polyneuritis- There is a continuous and involuntary contraction and relaxation of muscles of legs, face, ears(similar to Parkinson's disease in human beings).

This is known as *"Chorea"* or *'St.vitus dance"*. The condition is incurable. Animal cannot stand or walk or eat properly, ultimately the dog lingers for a long time and becomes miserable. Though it is a disease of young pups, occasionally the adult dog may also suffer if they did not develop immunity. This disease is not *communicable to man*.

Diagnosis of the disease is easy from symptoms.

Treatment- Mainly symptomatic Antibiotic cover, intravenous fluids and nutrients, high doses of vit. C etc.

Rabies

Rabies is the oldest known and *fatal disease* of dogs caused by a virus and **communicable to all warm blooled animals including man** through bite of the infected animal. Dog is the chief source and is highly susceptible. Disease is important because of the close association of pet dog with all the family members at home.

How Does the Disease Spread?

The virus of rabies is present in the *saliva* of the *infected dog*. So any bite wound from such a dog or its saliva coming in contact with existing wounds, abrasions on the body of healthy dog or man can be dangerous.

The virus enters the body through the wound and within 15-20 minutes it attaches itself to the nerve cells and then starts traveling towards brain. Higher the nerve supply at a part (*i.e., more sensitive part like finger tips & tender skin have rich supply of nerve fibres*) and nearer the bitten part from brain, more will be the risk. Once the virus gets attached to nerve fibres, it is difficult to neutralise it. The virus ultimately reaches the brain and from there the *virus migrates to salivary glands*. Hence the time required to symptoms of disease after the day of bite will be variable and depend on the nature of bite (whether deep or superficial, whether *directly on the skin* or the bitten part was covered by cloth) sensitivity of the part and the distance from brain.

How to Know that Your Dog could be Rabied?

The symptoms are seen when the virus reaches brain and produces encephalitis.

The first symptom is the change in behaviour. The dog may become *unusually docile or furious*. The *vision appears defective with a typical "vacant look"*. He does not behave as usual. There is disorientation, does not identify the members of family and does not obey the usual commands of his master; may become irritable, excited or hide himself in corners or under the table and bed. The voice appears changed to hoarseness and frothy salivation surrounds the lips. Dog may become uncontrollable and may bite anybody *without provocation*, may run long distances, attack any moving object, eat anything like stones, bite any object and get teeth and gums injured. Dog is *unable to eat or drink* and becomes weak, exhausted and *ultimately paralysed*. Death usually occurs within 5-6 days after appearance of symptoms. Maximum period could be 14 days.

What should a Dog Owner Do?

Get alert as soon as you find any *change in behaviour* of your dog. Isolate the dog and tie it securely in a protected room.

Do not handle the mouth parts. Don't allow children to play with him. Give food and water from a distance and observe carefully. *Consult the veterinarian.* Check up if he has bitten any member of family, or licked anybody's skin. Handling such a dog is not free from risk either for the owner or for the doctor. Once the doctor is satisfied that it is rabies (after taking into consideration several factors and after observation of the dog) the dog will have to be put to sleep preferably by shooting. *There is no treatment for rabies.* Confirmation of rabies can be done by histopathological exam. of brain after death. Post mortem is to be performed very carefully by qualified veterinarian. Brain is removed and a portion is sent for virus detection test in 50% glycerine saline to the laboratory where facility exists. A portion of brain (*hippocampus*) is sent in 10% formalin for detection of "*negri bodies*". Presence of negri bodies confirms the disease but their absence does not rule out rabies.

The carcass has to be disposed off by deep burial with salt after thorough disinfection. If anybody who handled the rabied dog is bitten or has injuries on fingers or hand, he must consult the family physician and get antirabies vaccination as per his advise.

Regular annual vaccination against rabies and preventing contact of your pet with stray dogs is the best and safest way to keep yourself free from rabies. Never handle the mouth parts of dogs while founding and playing. Wash your hands and bite injuries immediately within 15-20 minutes with plenty of soap and water. This will wash out and neutralise the virus in the wound and thus the chances of infection will be considerably reduced. After doing this first aid you should consult your family physician about further treatment of wound and antirabies vaccination etc.

Infectious Canine Hepatitis (ICH) (Rubarth's Disease)

Also know as canine adenovirus (CAV) infection. Is a specific viral disease of canines and *not communicable to human beings.* There are two stains of virus CAV-1 and CAV-2.

The CAV-1 strain cause more severe and generalised disease, damages vascular endothelium and liver cells. Young pups are more severely affected. Recovered dogs excrete virus in faeces and urine for several months. CAV-2 strain produces a mild disease.

Clinical Symptoms- Fever which fluctuates, without returning to normal, jaundice, loss of appetite, thirst, painful and distended abdomen due to liver enlargement. There may be swelling (*oedema*) on head, face and under the skin.

Pin point haemorrhages, *delayed clotting time* and corneal opacity are some of the signs.

Treatment- Is mainly paliative because there is no specific remedy against virus, continued nursing, rest, antibiotic cover and nourishment by way of intravenous glucose, liver tonics, may save the dog if there are no complications. *Corticostroids* should not be used, as far as possible as it might lead to opacity of cornea.

Prevention- Is easily possibly by regular periodical vaccination every year, *after getting a thorough health check up.*

Haemorrhagec Gastroenteritis
(*Canine Parvo-Virus infection*)

The virus of this disease is closely similar to *feline panleukopenia* virus of cats. The virus is very resistant and spread very rapidly. *Disease not communicable to man.*

Dogs of all ages are affected but young pups and imported breeds suffer more heavily.

Clinical Symptoms- High fever followed by enteritis and severe diarrhoea with sometimes frank blood in the stool. There is also vomiting. The dog becomes very much exhausted due to loss of blood and dehydration. In young pups the virus causes damage to the heart muscle and resultant respiratory distress.

Diagnosis- Mainly from symptoms and some blood tests and tests on faecal matter (if specific facilities are available in laboratory).

Treatment- Mainly a supportive symptomatic treatment.

Antibiotic cover to prevent complications, lot of intravenous fluids. It is desirable to make blood estimation for *Sodium*, *Potassium* and *Chlorides* and select the most appropriate intravenous therapy. **Inj. Vitamin C** in high doses, **Inj. Straden, Coagulin** may control bleeding. Homeopathic drug "Ipicac" cotrols vomiting. Vit-K. Perinorm, Buscopan etc. are useful as supportive therapies.

Leptospirosis

Is a bacterial disease caused by spiral shaped organism. There are several species of this organism but *L. canicola* and *L. icterohemorrhagica* are the the most common organisms affecting dogs. The organism localise in kidneys and are excreted in urine. Infection of other dogs occurs due to contamination of food and water with urine of a sick dog and due to unclean habits and close contact with pets in case of human beings.

Diagnosis- From symptoms, examination of urine by special methods, serological test, *(agglutination test)* conducted in some laboratories.

Treatment- Successful treatment is possible. With the use of antibiotics given in time and at proper doses for adequate period. Late treatment when kidneys and liver are extensively damaged, may not be successful.

Prevention- Vaccine is available and usually in combination with distemper and hepatitis. Regular annual vaccination is recommended. The contamination with dog urine must be avoided scrupulously.

Toxoplasmosis

A coccidia-like protozoan *infection mainly of cats* and occasionally in dogs and communicable to man. Transmission from dogs to man is very rare. Symptoms in dogs, are not very characteristic. The intermediate stages (*tachyzoites*) of the protozoan may be localised in internal organs like liver, muscles, brain of dog.

Diagnosis- By special serological test (Sabin-Feldman dye test). Faeces of cats is more important source of infection to dogs and man. Hence adequate hygienic care must be taken.

Treatment- Sulpha drugs are effective.

Prevention- No vaccine available.

Common Worm Infections of Dogs

Round worms and tapeworms are quite common infections in dogs. Worms are present in the intestines where they not only cause irritation, but also utilize the nutrients in the food for their own growth. Some worms attach themselves to the intestinal mucosa and suck nutrients and blood thereby causing considerably blood loss. The dog with worm infectin has therefore digestive upsets, pain in the bowels and remain weak and anaemic. The pups do not grow well. The skin and haircoat becomes dull lustreless. Some worm larvae penetrate through skin and thereby cause continuous itching and losses of hair making the appearance dirty. Dogs can obtain roundworms from ingesting the ova. Toxocara canis is often obtained transplectelly from the mother. Tissue migration by immature forms can result in hepatic Fibrosis and significant pulmonary lesions.

Some worms may produce bronchitis,pneumonia and liver disease. In case of some tapeworms. (Taenia multiceps, Echnioceccus glanulosus) can produce big cysts in the acts as an intermediate host due to accidental ingestional of infected flea carrying a cysticeroid (*Hydatidosis*).

Important round worms are :

Toxocara canis

These round worms of intestines are about 7-15 cm Long and cause diarrhoea, vomiting and growth retardation. The larval stages may cause bronchitis and allergic breathing difficulty. This worm can infect man if eggs of worm enter through food/water contamination.

Diagnosis- By examination of stools which contain eggs or worms. Sometimes in severe infections adult worms are seen in stool. The larvae of worms can cross the uterus of pregnant bitch and infect the puppies before birth.

Treatment- Drugs like Piprazine is quite effective and should be used every 15 days till the pup achieves age of 3 months periodical deworming. Pregnant bitch should be deowormed.

Ancyclostoma canicum (Hookworm)

These are small worms (less than 2 cm.) of intestines and are blood sucking worms. They attack themselves with their special fangs-like mouth parts to the intestinal wall and such blood. The worms pass eggs the stools. The eggs hatch into larvae which penetrate other dogs through skin, and reach intestines to becomes mature. The infection can reach puppies in the uterus of a pregnant bitch. So, the pups before birth may also have an infection if the bitch has worms. Human infection is possible with any ancylostoma species.

Diagnosis- Symptoms of black faeces, itching of skin, Confirm by faecal examination for eggs of worms.

Treatment- Check up faeces. Inj. **Ancylol** 0.2 ml/kg b.wt. sc, or Inj. **Ivermectin** 0.5 ml sc for 25 kg bwt Tablets of **Mebendazole, Pyrental pamoate** etc.are claimed to be effective drugs which may be used for periodical deworming. Treatment for anaemia and for general improvement of health is also necessary.

Tapeworms

Dipylidium caninum

Is the long worm having small segments. The worm attaches itself to the wall of intestine with its head (*scolex*) which has spikes. Number of worms can block the intestine and cause chronic indigestion, diarrhoea and colicy pain. The segments of worm are passed in the faeces and look like cucumber seed. They contain egg capsules. This worm needs an intermediate host (*flea*) in which infective stages develop. Man may get infection (*through the accidental ingestion of infected flea*) as a very rare chance.

Diagnosis- By faecal examination and observing segments of worm in faeces. The dog rubs his anus on the ground which is a typical observation. and when the owner reports tapeworms segments like rice grains in the faeces or sticking on the perineal region.

Treatment- Praziguiantel (**Droncit or Prazip-plus**) is effective drug which should be given after computation of dose as per body weight and general condition of health.

Other medication for tapeworms e.g., **Niclosamide, Bunamide** are not as effective and may be more dangerous.

Prevention of tapeworm- Involves controlling the intermediate hosts i.e., flea and lice.

VECTOR BORNE DISEASES
(Diseases Transmitted through the Insect Bites)

Babesiosis

This disease caused by protozoa *B. canis* and *B. gibsoni* are the two common species out of which the latter one cause a more serious disease. The parasites are transmitted from a sick dog to the healthy dog by the ticks which come from other dogs by contact. The parasites invade the red blood cells and destroy them in large numbers. The affected dog has *high fever, anaemia and jaundice.* Acute infection is usually fatal if not treated in early stage. Diagnosis by blood smear examination for intraerythrocytic parasites.

Treatment- Berenil in appropriate dose as intramuscular injection, antibiotics to control secondary infections and treatment for anaemia and jaundice. Intensive supportive treatment and nursing is necessary under veterinarian's supervision. Control of tick infection is the only way of prevention.

Tryanosomiasis

This is an another protozoan infection transmitted by ticks from other dogs, cats and bovines. *T. evansi* is the parasite which is long flagellated organism outside the red blood cells. The pararasites invade vital internal organs like spleen, liver and cerebrospinal fluid causing generalised illness with high fever, congestion and pin point haemorrhages, nervous signs, and corneal opacity.

Diagnosis- By examination of blood smears for parasites.

Treatment- **Berenil** in appropriate doses (0.25-0.5 g in distilled water im) is effective. Treatment may have to be repeated if necessary.

Breeding and Whelping

Dogs are seasonal breeders. Females come into heat twice in a year. A female might show signs of first heat at about 5 months of age depending on the season. Although bodily development is complete by the age of 9 months it is advisable to allow some more time to have full development and maturity. Breed the female at about 15 months of age.

When the female is in heat, she becomes restless, anxious to meet males, has a swelling on vulval lips and has bloody discharge, males will be trying to be after such a female in heat period. It is very difficult to keep the female restrained inside the house. The heat period lasts for about 14 days. Best time to breed the female is around 10th day onwards of the heat period. Take care that male and female are healthy, free from any worm or ectoparasitic infections and veneral granuloma.

Preventing Conception

Conception due to accidental mating with unwanted male can be prevented if an injection of **Vetoestrol** (*Stilbesterol*) 0.5 mg/kg (*max. dose not exceed 25 mg.*) or **Estradiol benzoate** 1-3 mg or Inj. **Mixogen** 2 ml. is given soon after mating and within 48 hours.

Breeding of females or males can be permanently ceased by surgical operations similar to those which are done in human side. Removal of uterus together with ovaries is the operation called **"Spaying"** and can be done at any stage to prevent conception. In males, vasectomy or castration is done. Hormonal contraceptives can also be used.

Inj. of **progesterone** given one month prior to the expected period of heat. This will prevent the bitch coming into heat and the injection can be continued throughout life every time during the season.

Osterone (*Lyka*), **Proluton depot** (*German Rem.*) are the progesterone containing injectable preparations. Dose to be computed in individual animal.

Tablets of **Perlutex** 5 mg or **Permolut** can be given daily during heat period to avoid conception likely to be due to accidental mating.

These ways of hormonal contraception are preferred to spaying operation by many people, but these are not very much dependable.

Care During Pregnancy and Whelping

Gestation period is 60-62 days. Signs of pregnancy are clearly visible as enlargement and rounding of abdomen, enlargement of mammary glands and the foetal palpation is possible at about 30 days gestation. Pregnancy diagnosis is a matter of experience in **abdominal palpation and auscultation of foetal heart sounds** developed by an individual veterinarian. Heart sounds can be audible at about 23-25 days of gestation. There are no validated assay procedures for diagnosis of pregnancy in bitches. Placental hormones have not been demonstrated in the urine of bitches. Pregnant female should be properly looked after and fed well with balanced diet. Moderate exercise of walking is necessary. Drugs containing *corticosteroides must never be given during pregnancy.*

As the day of whelping approaches the female becomes dull, silent and seeks isolated place. She should be provided with a spacious box with good bed.

During first stage of labour, the uterine contractions occur every 5-6 minutes and are mild. This may continue for 20-24 hrs. Bitch may remain restless and off feed.

During second stage of labour the cervix is fully dialated. Bitch will lie on one side start straining. A watery or *greenish discharge* is seen followed by a pup. Let the mother have it infront of her.

The pups are delivered at different interval along with the placenta covering attached to each foetus. The mother usually cleans up the foetus. If she allows to handle, the nose and mouth of newborn pup should be cleaned and the cord should be cut and disinfected with tincture iodine or betadine.

If there is unusual delay in expulsion of pups due to uterine inertia, contractions can be stimulated by administration of oxytocin (*Post Pitutary extract*) providied it is dialated and foetal presentation is normal. Inj. **Epidosin** *(TTK)* 5 ml also helps in dilation of cervix and stimulates uterine contractions. Homeopathic drug **Cauliophyllum** 200 C be given once a day during last week of pregnancy. This will ensure safe delivery. (whelping).

Imminent bitch should not be disturbed as far as possible. It is most essential to provide warmth to newborn pups particularly in winter and rainy season. Hypothermia and trampling are the common causes of pup losses within first week. Pups should be allowed to suckle liberally so that they get enough colostrum through which they receive maternal antibodies. In case of primipara, mother needs to be helped for suckling, keep a close watch on mother. She might get an attack of Eclampsia i.e., hypocalcaemia which is characterised by spams, trembling, fits, stiffness etc. She will need immediate attention and calcium therapy. Withold suckling for 24 hours in such a case. Pups will open eyes in about 8-10 days time.

Give enough of milk, calcium, liver soup and vitamins to the mother. Do not give heavy food. Let her be with the pups as much time as she prefers.

Training the Dog for a Show

A dog show gives you an opportunity to learn new information and get in contact with other dog lovers. A well maintained and trained dog is a matter of pride. Dog is a very intelligent animal and can be trained for special purposes. His wonderful sense of smell and eye sight makes him a highly efficient assistant in the investigation of crimes, detection of explosives, narcotics etc.

Any average dog irrespective of his breed, can be trained for obedience and performance as under. The dog usually obeys commands of one particular person and it requires good deal of patience to make your dog learn, the lessons with perfection. Training should be started at the age of 3-4 months.

	Obedience		Commands
1)	Sit	:	to sit on his legs.
2)	Down	:	to lie down on the floor.
3)	Get up	:	from any of the above positions.
4)	Stay	:	to stay in each of the above positions.
5)	Heel	:	to walk on the left side and with the speed of the handler.
6)	Come	:	to approach the handler, sit in front to the left side and sit.
7)	Go	:	to go in the specific direction.
8)	Hold-Drop	:	to hold suitable things in his mouth and drop in the handler's hand.
9)	Pick-up	:	Any suitable things lying on the floor.
10)	Fetch	:	to retrieve any suitable things thrown by the handler.
11)	Fetch	:	specific handkerchief from 4-5 non smelling handkerchiefs.
12)	Fetch	:	to retrieve a thing over 3 feet hurdles.

Owner must have mouth patience and should pat the dog with love and affection when he complies your orders.

	Performance		Commands
1)	Shake hand	:	only with the right paw.
2)	Bow	:	one kind of namaste.
3)	Beg	:	second kind of namaste.
4)	Jump	:	to jump over 3 feet height hurdle.
5)	Jump	:	to jump through rings.
6)	Jump	:	to jump through burning rings.
7)	Speak	:	to bark on order of the handler.
8)	Watch	:	to guard owner's property.
9)	Attack	:	to attack a stranger.
10)	No	:	to refuse food given by a stranger.
11)	Find	:	to track out a hidden person.

Common Querris of the Dog Owners

What is Rickets ? and How can it be Prevented ?

Rickets is disease of young pups, which one growing. Slight deformity or bending of limbs, pain on bone and joints are early signs. Once bony deformity occurs it is permanent unless it is treated in time. Rickets occurs due to deficiency of vitamin D_3 and calcium. Normally in the country like India where sunlight is available in plenty the deficiency of vitamin D occurs rarely unless the animals are housed totally indoors.

For prevention of rickets 1 tablet of **Ostocalcium** (*Sandoz*) or **Rejucalcium** (*Indo. French*) be given twice a day till dog is 4 months old.

or **METACAL –D** (*Almet*)

or **OSTOPET Liq.** (*Virbac*)

or **VIMERAL (liq)** (*Virbac*)

or **ASCAL** (*Alembic*)

or **REJUCALCIUM** (*Indo-French*)

or **VETKRAL-B$_{12}$** (*Sarabhai*)

One teaspoon of any one of the above syrups be given twice daily in milk till 4 month of age. Multivitamin drops till 6 months age.

Inj-**Vit-D$_3$** usch as **Arachitol**,Inj **Adecelin** (*Virbac*), **Macalvit** (*Sandoz*) or **Caldee-12** (*Wockhardt*)1 ml. twice a week be given as soon as symptoms of deficiency are suspected.

If the growth rate is not satisfactory the protein sparing and tissue building preparations such as **Orabolin** (*Organon*) or **Dinabol** (*Ciba*) may be tried in suitable dose with due care.

Balanced diet, Calcium-Vitamin supplementation, regular exercise and exposure to sunlight are the essential prerequisites for preventing rickets in a young puppy.

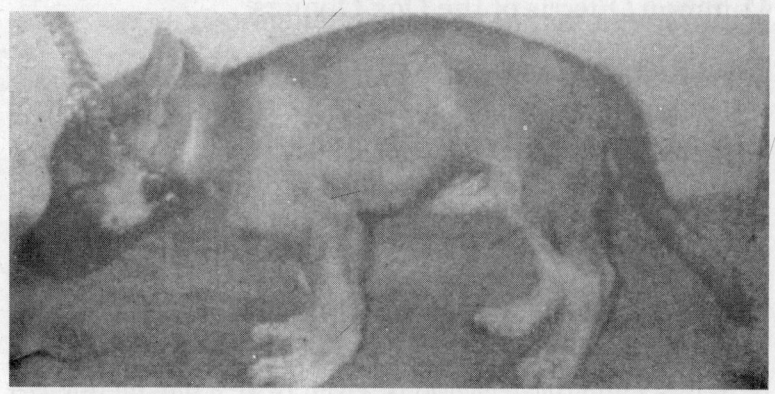

Fig. 18. Rickets - Note the deforming & bending of vertebral column legs.

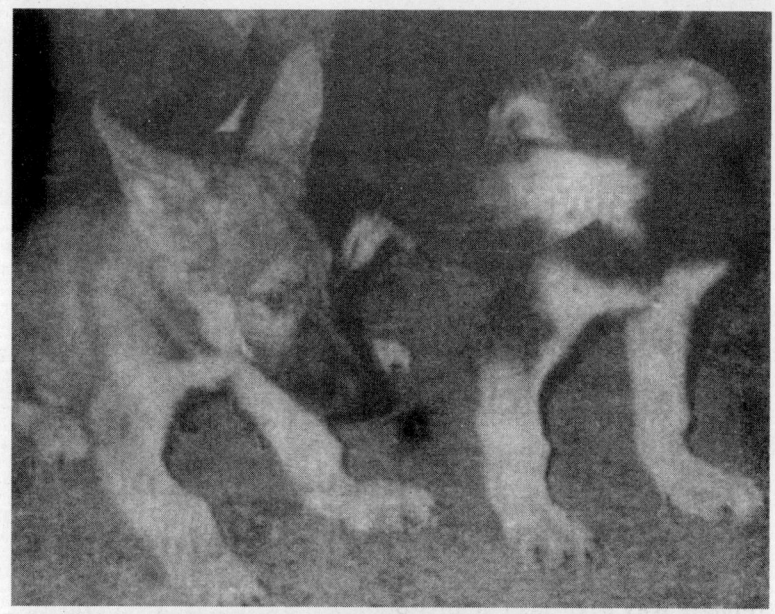

Fig. 19. Rickets - Note the deformed forelegs with bending & swelling of joints.

Q. Should we treat a case of Rabies ?

No. Once rabies is confirmed by symptoms and history of a previous dog bite it is no use treating rabies. On the contrary it is risky for owner as well as the doctor. Dog should be isolated and observed. After it dies the brain exam. may be done for confirmation. If the dog is suspected for rabies it can be killed by shot of a gun, The Negri bodies may not be seen in the brain in such a case.

Q. If " Negri bodies" are not seen in brain, should we presume that it was not rabies?

This is not true. If a dog dies early or is killed, then *"Negri bodies"* may not develop. For confirmation of rabies, mouse inoculation and virological studies are essential. *Presence of Negri bodies confirms rabies but their obsence does not rule out rabies.*

Q. Should an antirabic vaccination course be taken even if a healthy dog bites man or another dog ?

Dog bite is *never* totally free from risk. A healthy looking dog or a dog in *incubation stage* might be having rabies virus in his saliva. To prove or disprove the presence of rabies virus in the saliva is not an easy procedure. Although the possibility of getting rabies from the bite of known healthy looking dog are very less, still *take no chance* with a dog bite. Recommend a complete course of post bite anti rabies vaccination. Washing the dog bite wound with plenty of soap water immediately within *20 minutes* minimises risk considerably.

Q. If a dog is regularly vaccinated against rabies is it that he is completely protected and shall never trasmit rabies if he bites anybody ?

Regular prophylactic vaccination against rabies is quite a reliable way to protect against rabies. If the dog is never allowed to go stray and is carefully looked after, not allowed contact with other dogs, then the fear is still minimised. However, although there are improved and better vaccines available, it is not easy to ascertain that each vaccinated dog has developed satisfactory immunity. It is only an assumption and it might prove to be wrong in a particular case although such a case may be 1 in 1000. Hence the decision is to be taken by the person concerned with full responsibility. To give a complete foolproof advice, it is better to undergo a course of antirabies vaccination. Now safe and effective vaccines are available for human use. Regular prophylactic vaccination for dog owners and high risk group like vets is advisable.

Q. When can we get the female spayed? Is the operation risky?

Spaying can be done at any stage after 6 months age even in case the female has never given any pups. However, it is desirable to get her spayed after taking crop once. Operation is done under *general anaesthesia* and beyond the normal risk of anaesthesia, the operation is quite safe if performed by qualified graduate veterinarian.

Q. Can a dog get reaction to injection of penicillin as in human beings ?

Fatal reaction to Penicillin in animals are comparatively less common. However, in some cases reactions may be recorded not only with penicillin, but also with other antibiotics, Vit. B-complex, liver extract, thiamine, Berenil and other chemotherapeutic agents like Ancylol. It is necessary to have antihistamine drugs and adrenaline always at hand and the dog should be observed at least for 15 minutes after *any* injection.

Q. Are the medicines used for human treatment useful for a dog ?

Most of the antibiotics, vitamin preparations, tonics, analgesics, tranquilizers used in human practice can be used in treating a dog. Doses are also more or less similar. *Self medication should be avoided by owners* because there are certain contraindications which a qualified veterinarian alone can decide.

Q. What is false pregnancy and how to deal with it?

This is also called *Pseudopregnancy or hyperluteoilism*. This is observed quite repeatedly in some bitches. The noraml changes during *metestrus* are intensified and prolonged. Metestrus is the stage after termination of estrus (*heat*) when the *corpus luteum* is formed in place of ruptured graffian follicle, from which ovum is expelled. Corpus luteum persists during pregnancy and secretes hormone progesterone which prevents maturation of other graffian follicles and prevents estrus. This is called as *"Pregnancy Corpus luteum"*.

In case there is no conception the corpus luteum regresses in about 4 weeks time.

In exceptional cases the corpus luteum grows and persists even when the female has not conceived. This secretes hormone *Progesterone* and as a result, secondary signs of pregnancy are seen even though there is no foetus growing in the uterus. This is **false pregnancy.**

The signs may be mild or severe and become evident about 45-60 days after estrus. There are psychological changes, nervousness, restless, desire to adopt pups etc. The mammary glands get enlarged and lactation appears.

Diagnosis- Pregnancy diagnosis must be done with confidence. This requires good experience. Non gravid uterus can be confirmed by palpation, X-ray exam. or Sonography.

Treatment- The secondary signs of lactation can be controlled by daily administration of 01 to 1.0 mg diethylstilbestrol until signs of false pregnancy disappear. Alternatively, testosterone proprionate 10-15 mg im may be given daily. Combination of Oestradiol and Testosterone available as Inj. **Mixogen** can be given 1-2 ml twice a week, may be given for 2-3 weeks. Oral testosterone preparations are also useful. Doses of hormones and duration of treatment should be judiciously worked out in individual cases.

The mammary glands should be covered with *many tailed light pressure bandage* to prevent milk secretion.

Ovariectomy is recommended in case of habitual incidence of pseudopregnancy. However, this operation must be performed during anestrus period and not when lactation of false pregnancy is continued.

(7) Why do some dogs shed lots of hair?

Shedding of hair or loss in hair (*alopecia*) leading sometimes to patches of baldness is seen in some dogs. Shedding of hair is particular problem in long haired breeds who need special care. There are several reasons for loss of hair.

The bitches normally shed lots of hair after whelping particularly due to heavy lactation if the number of pups is more, if diet is inadequate or not properly balanced in respect of proteins, minerals and vitamins. Protein rich diet such as egg. meat, milk etc. with vitamin supplement usually has beneficial effect.

Infectation of lice, ticks and skin diseases like scabies cause continuous irritation and leads to scratching and biting. This causes injuries to hair follicles and as a result there is a hair loss. The skin disease must be treated first. General hygienic care, use of Seledruff shampoo and regular brushing may be tried. For correct diagnosis and its confirmation it is necessary to get the skin scrapings examined in the laboratory, so that proper treatment could be adopted. For effective treatment the hair must be clipped close so that medicament will come in contact of skin. Superficial application of skin ointments and lotions in long haired dogs will not cure skin disease until and *unless hair is clipped.*

Medicines that will improve circulation and nutrition of skin and stimulate hair follicles are indicated. Arsenical preparations and vit. A are useful. Arsenical preparations must be used very cautiously and under proper supervision, otherwise may lead to undesireable effect and toxicity.

In addition to above causes there is one type called *hormonal alopecia.* This usually occurs in animals between 6 to 9 years age group.

Hypothyroidism results in generalised dryness, dullness and thining of hair coat. Skin looks full of scales and crusts. Dog gains weight very fast and looks dull and fatty. Serum cholesterol values may be as high as 500 mg. per 100 ml. After a thorough checkup and ruling out other complicating conditions associated with age, treatment with **Thyromixe** @ 6 to 10 per kg. b. wt may prove useful. Dose to be regulated under proper supervision. (*Eltroxin-100 mcg. tabs*).

High levels of estrogens also inhibit hair growth both in males as well as females. Gonadal hormones such as testosterone in properly regulated doses are useful. Androgen as well as estrogen may be indicated in some patients.

Operations for removal of ovaries and castration may prove useful but there is guarantee of expected results in all cases.

(10) Do the dogs suffer from Heart dieases like man?

YES! Dogs do suffer from various types of heart problems such as Congestive Cardiac Failure (CCF) myocardial dilatation (Dilated Cardiomyopathy-DCM), MyocardialIschemia (MI) and congenital abnormalities such as Persistant opening between ventricles and valcular insuffiency etc. Surey conducted at Veterinary Colleges indicated about 20% dogs suffering from some or the other kind of cardiac dysfunctions, evidenced by elctrocardiographic. (ECG) abnormalities. Most dysfunctions are observed in dogs more than 10 years of ago and have relationship with dietary abnormalities. Increase in levels of cholesterol (HDL), triglycerides is also recorded. These abnormalities can be reversed by dietary corrections and regular exercise in the intial stages. Control of obesity, regular exercise, maintaining adequate protein in the diet, restricting fats and sodium in the diet, supplementation of amino acid "taurine" vitamin B_3, correcting potassium levels etc. are very important preventive measures. Loss of body weight and loss of lean body mass (*Cochexia*) in congestive heart failure is mostly due to chronic anorexia, fatigue and dyspnoea due to right sided heart failured and dilatation of heart.

The only thing necessary is to conduct specific studies and evaluate the ECG findings and blood biochemical profile for proper assesment of Cardiac disorders.

(11) Do the dogs suffer from food allergies and resultant also rashes as in human beings?

YES! Very commonly some dogs do not tolerate foods particularly some readymade common foods. Many times change in food brings about remarkable relief in case of allergic skin rashes and pruritus. Some dogs have allergic to beef, chicken meat, fish or even milk.

One has to obseve the allergen by process of trial of elimination. Sometimes the allergies are drug induced also. Hence it is better to consider these possibilities while dealing with skin infections and cases of breathlessness (dysponoea).

Common Health Problems

It is necessary for the dog lover to know something about common problems of the pet who is like a family member.

How to Know When Your Pet is not Well:

If you are very well attached to your pet in the house, you know his normal habits of food, likes and dislikes as well as his normal response. In such a case if you find any change it is easily noticeable and you can start looking for a sign of illness. Aversion for food, milk or water is a very common sign that is observed in almost sign that is observed in almost every illness. It is important to differentiate between the illness accompanied with *fever* and *without fever*. Similarly one should be able to judge the extent of rise in temperature by moving your hand on the inner side of thighs. It is easy to record rectal temperature for any literate person and a good quality thermometer should always ke kept handy for use. The normal range of rectal temperature is 38° to 39°C. (100.5° to 101.5°F). The range of rectal temperature is recorded when the dog is quiet and unexcited. Little excitement and exercise like running and chasing may raise the temp. by one or two degrees but this is transient and comes down as soon as the animal is at rest.

Similarly, while temperature recording in hot day of summer we should not overlook the influence of atmospheric temp. which causes the mercury to go up immediately while you are reading the thermometer. The thermometer should be dipped in cold water in such a hot weather. The bulb of thermometer should be lubricated with vaseline or oil before inserting inside the rectum. It should be inserted about an inch length inside slowly with rotating movements or supported with a lubricated finger while the pet is pacified and petted with affection or is well restrained with a tape muzzle to prevent biting. Allow the mercury bulb of thermometer to remain in contact with the inner mucous membrane for about 2 minutes. Withdraw gently and clean the inserted part with a wet cotton swab and record the temperature. Temperature above 41°C (106°F) should be considered as alarming and immediate help of Vet is advised. Till the time Veterinary aid is received administer. Paracetamol syrup and keep cold compresses on head.

(A) Illness not Accompanied with Fever

Most of the illnesses that are not accompanied with fever are some kinds of digestive upsets, which are very common. The usual complaints are as under:

(1) **Constipation-** The faeces are scanty and hard. Animal strains while passing faeces. The appetite is reduced and the animal is dull and lethargic.

Treatment- Mild purgatives or laxatives are indicated in such condition. The medicines used in human practices are safely used such as:

Milk of magneis or Liquid Paraffin	1--2 teaspoonful daily in evening for 2-3 days

Castor oil 1 teaspoonful or tablets of *Vaculax, Dulcolax, Purgolax, Glaxenna, Laxecon or Cellubrill* etc. could also be used. Vitamin B-complex syrup or tablets. Liv-52 drops or tablets should be given for about a week so as to restore the normal digestion and appetite. Glycerine suppositories are inserted in the rectum if the stool is very hard to the extent of causing bleeding while straining. Animal should be given good exercise regularly.

(2) **Diarrhoea-** The animal passes liquid faeces in varying quantities depending upon the severity. The blood may contain

blood and mucous if it is dysentery. Simple diarrhoea may be caused due to irritant foodstuffs and is a natural response to get rid of the same. Passing loose motions twice or thrice is not a matter to be worried. If the diarrhoea is persistent also accompanied with vomiting, it may lead to dehydration and should be attended to early. Chronic diarrhoea is also caused due to intestinal worms. Blood and mucus in the stool is also a symptom of hookworm infection which is very common. Viral gastroenteritis is quite a severe condition and is characterised by shooting diarrhoea with lots of blood into the faeces.

Treatment- Depends on severity. A simple diarrhoea due to food irregularity can be controlled with a few tablets of *Perinorm or Intestopon* which regulates the bowel movements and reduce the spasm. Faecal examination is needed for diagnosing worm infection which can be treated with effective drugs. The bacterial or viral gastroenteritis needs intensive treatment and fluid-electroyte therapy. Diarrhoea is sometimes accompanied with gripping pain and the animal shows intermittant spasms of colic. In such a case antispasmodic like **Piptal** or **Carmicide** paediatric drops (2 to 6 drops depending on age and size of dog) can be given for relief. **Normet** (*iMetronidazole* and *Norflaxacin*) is a very good antidiarrhoeal suspension given @ 1 TSF B.I.D. **Azitral-100-, Econorm** sachets containing essential intestinal flora given twice a day in addition to oral rehydration therapy like Electral/Peditral are also useful.

(3) Vomiting- Vomiting is a very common symptom observed in several conditions as the vomiting reflex is very much developed in dogs. It is of two types:

(a) Projectile vomition means a sort of overflow when the dog overeats or eats very fast and thereby a mild gastric irritation is produced. The dogs induce vomiting by eating little grass. This type of vomiting is without much of retching action and occurs once a while. This should not cause and worry.

(b) True vomition is as a result of gastric irritation and is accompanied with retching and spasm. Its frequency and persistence depends on severity of gastric irritaion. True vomiting is accompanied with diarrhoea in gastroenteritis caused due to bacterial or viral infection. This causes rapid dehydration and shock and the animal needs immediate attention.

Treatment- Gastric irritation is reduced by antacids and demulcent like Gelusil, Digene, Milk of magnesia, Pectocap, Spectol-M and preparations containing Kaolin and Pectin. etc. If milk and water is also not retained, then it is better to maintain animal on intravenous glucose, electrolyte and fluids. Oral feeding should be avoided till gastric irritation is reduced. Antiemetics which act centrally are employed to control persistent vomiting and gastric spams. Inj. Siquil, Anicalm, Largactil or Stemetil are employed for this purpose in properly calculated doses. Appropriate electrolyte solutions such as Lactate Ringer's soln. Isolyte M, E, G etc. are employed depending upon the requirements to correct acidosis or alkalosis as the case may be Plasma extenders like Dextrans of various molecular wt. are also indicated in certain instances. The degree of dehydration is judged by examining the elasticity of skin fold and also by packed Cell volume exam. PCV about 60 mm, percent is considered as critical stage of dehydration. Estimation of Na^+, K^+ bicarbonates and chorides in blood gives very useful guidelines for treatment.

The fluid and electrolyte therapy is to be combined with specific treatment like broad spectrum antibiotics to control the bacterial infections. Blood transfusions may be necessary in case of severe blood loss. The convalescence period is very long and the normal feeding should be restored gradually within a period of 2-3 days after control of vomiting.

(4) Chronic indigestion and Malabsorption Syndrome

This is the type of digestive disorder associated defective or impaired functions of digestion and absorption. The animal has either normal or reduced appetite and gradually loses condition, body wt. and general lusture of body coat. The parasitic diseases should be ruled out. Malabsorption is difficulty in digestion and in absorption of nutrients of food. The pet does not gain weight or continues to lose weight and suffers from chronic indigestion or diarrhoea. This is because of deficiency of exocrine digestive enzymes of pancreas responsible for digestion and assimilation of carbohydrates, fats and proteins

291

or the endocrine secretion of insulin which in necessary for regulation of glucose level in the body system. The exocrine secretary deficiency is characterised by undigested pasty/ unformed faeces. Presence of endoparasites may worsen the problem. The specific tests such as *Liver function tests*, *Pancreatic function tests* are necessary for accurate diagnosis and appropriate treatment. Enzyme preparations and liver stimulants are recommended after completing the investigations. PANCREOFLAT (*Duphar*) tablets. FESTAL (*Hoechst*) tablets are the pancreatic extract enzyme preparation. Diet should be well balanced and rich in enzymes and probiotics.

(5) Ulcerative Stomatitis

Is a very common condition in dogs, due to deficiency of Vit-B6 (*Pyridoxine*). The mucous membrane of gums, cheek and tongue is ulcerated, with dirty saliva and foul smell. Animal cannot eat any food. Tab. BENADON 40 mg. B.D. or Inj. **Beplex-forte** iv or im will cure in 3-4 days. Give Vit. C in addition to above in high dose.

(B) ILLNESS ACCOMPANIED WITH FEVER

General Considerations

Except hyperthermia or pyrexia which means rise in body temperature due to high atmospheric temperature causing failure of heart regulating mechanism. (*Sunstroke or Heat stroke*), fever which is accompanied with malaise is usually a result of some kind of infection. The infection may be caused by bacteria or virus and may be generalised type or localised in any organ or system of body. The degree of rise in fever is in proportion to the severity of infection. Fever is the manifestation of normal defence reaction by body to fight the invading infection and is an index of activity of body defence mechanism. Fever therefore, is a desirable response on the part of body and unless the rise in temperature is abnormally high as to cause damage to brain, there should be no hasty attempts to bring down the fever rapidly.

Symptoms of Fever- In addition to rise in body temperature the animal is dull, respiration rate increased, eyes become red

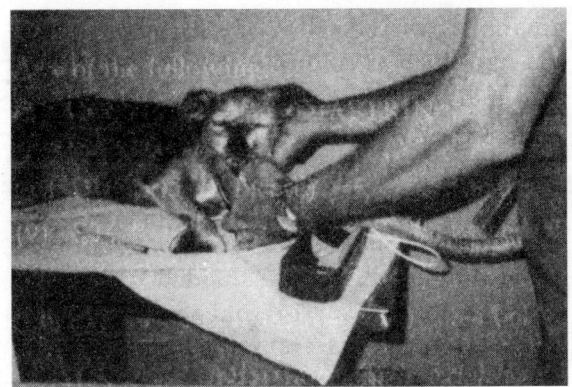

Fig. 20. A case of squamous cell carcinoma.

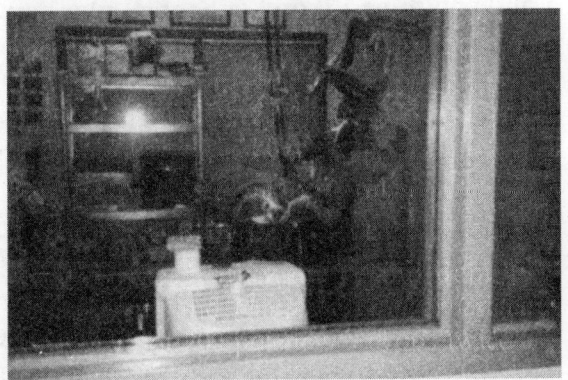

Fig. 21. Chemotherapy for Cancer Patient.

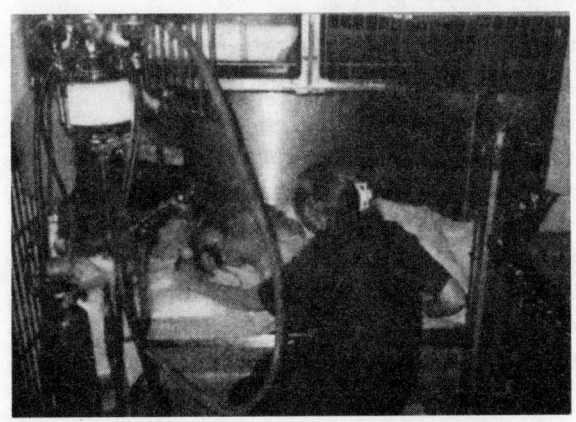

Fig. 22. Intensive Care Unit for Dog.

and there is lacrymation, nose becomes dry. Urine output is scanty, concentrated and deep in colour.

If respiratory system is involved as in case of distemper, bronchitis and pneumonia the breathing becomes difficult, there is nasal discharge and adventitious respiratory sounds are audible.

Treatment- The patient should be kept in a well ventilated room; but, direct wind draught should be avoided. High fever can be controlled by keeping ice bag or cold water packs on forehead and administration of **Paracetamol, (Crocin)** or **Nice** syrup 1 teaspoon at every 2-3 hourly interval. In case of respiratory distress use preparations containing antihistamine and ephidrine **Vikoryl** or **Seumol-plus** syrup, are more suited. The animal should always have plenty of fresh water available for drinking.

Blood examination must be done in every case of fever to rule out the specific bacterial or haemoprotozoan infection and also to know the leucocytic picture.

Suitable antibiotics, fluid and other supportive therapy will be necessary as per specific requirements under the expert supervision.

Dog owners should be advised to get their pets regularly protected against specific diseases like Distemper, Hepatitis, Leptospirosis, Parvovirus and Parainfluenza against which effective vaccines are available.

CARE OF SKIN AND EAR INFECTIONS

Skin infections (*scabies, ectoparasites, fungal infections etc.*) and allergic dermatitis or rashes are very common problems of pets that bother owners quite a lot. Frequent bath and use of inferior quality soaps, carbolic soaps and detergents are not desirable. They make the hair coat rough. weekly bath with some good quality herbal shampoo and daily grooming will keep the hair coat bright and shining. Proper nutrition and diet containing proteins, minerals and vitamins is the basic need to keep the skin healthy and bright. **Flemetic** skin oil (*TTK*) is useful in improving skin lustre and control of ectoparasites as well.

Ear infections (*otorrhoea*) come to notice when they get will established. The pet lovers must therefore be very watchful about skin and ear infections. A regular and careful examination by the master is necessary. Skin and ear infections infact can be prevented if the standards of hygience are excellent. Regular grooming, particularly of long haired breeds is absolutely necessary. Periodical insecticide spraying of the room, preventing contacts with other stray dogs, immediate steps to get rid of ticks and lice as soon as noticed are some of the rules of hygiene. the ear cavities should be examined during the bath and inside of ears cleaned with a soft cloth. Johnson's Ear buds can be used carefully to clean the canal of ear or remove the oily secretions which cause irritation if allowed to accumulate.

It should always be remembered that a healthy, clean and a well cared pet with disciplined habits is loved by all.

Biochemial Values of Healthy dog

Parameter	Adult Dog
Serum Urea Nitrogen(mg/dl)	8-23
" Glucose (mg dl)	71-115
" Total Bilirubin (mg/dl)	0.1-0.6
" Total Protein (g/dl)	5.2-7.0
" Albumin (g/dl)	2.7-3.8
" Alkaline Phosphate (IU/I)	10-82
" Calcium (mg/dl)	9.8-11.4
" Inorganic Phosphorus (mg/dl)	2.8-5.1
" LDH (IU/L)	8-89
" AST or SGOT (Trans Act units/Litre)	13-93
" ALT or SGPT (IU L)	15-70
" Total CO_2 (mEq/L)	18-25
" Ceatinine (mg/dl)	0.5-0.81
" Uric Acid (mg/dl)	82-282d
" Triglycerides (mg/dl)	10-42
" CPK(IU/L)	12-84
" Sodium (mEq/L)	143-151
" Potassium (mEq/L)	4.1-5.7
" Magnesium (mEq/L)	1.4-2-4
" Chloride (mEq/L)	103-115
Plasma Bicarbonate (mEq/L)	17-24
" T_4 (RIA) µg/dl	1.52-3.60
" T_3 (RIA) mg/dl	48-154

Blood constituents are liable to show marketly different values depending upon methodology employed.

PHYSICOLOGICAL NORMS IN DOG

Rectal Temperature	100-101.6°F (37-38°C)
Pulse Rate (per min).	70-120
Respiratory Rate (per min.)	15-30
Blood pressure	140/100 Hg
Gastation Period (duration)	62-64 days
Oestrus (Heat Period) (duration)	10-12 days

HEMATOLOGICAL VALUES IN HEALTHY DOG

		Average
Total RBC Count (million)	5.5-9.5 c mm	(6.0)
ErythrocyteSedimentation Rate (ESR-mm/hr)	5-20	(10)
Packed Cell Volume (PCV) %	37-55%	(45%)
Hemoglobin (Hb) gm/dl	10-16	(12)
TotalLeucocyteCount (Thousand)	8-14	(10)
Differential Leucocyte Count (DLC)	-	-
Neutrophil	60-70%	(65) %
Lymphocyte	12-30%	(25) %
Monocyte	3-10%	(5) %
Eosinophil	3-10%	(4) %
Basophil	1-2%	(0-1)%

SOME CONTACT ADDRESSES FOR PEDIGREE DOGS

1) **Mohd. Rasheed**
   C/o. Crystal Kennels
   C-52/A Balanger, **Hyderabad**-500 037.
   PH; 3772615 (O). 3813412 (Kennel)

2) **Jayashri Sharma**
   C/o. Kalpana Kennels
   109, Rajiv Nagar, Behind, A.G. Colony,
   Erragadda, Hyderabad-500 045,
   Ph : 3813412

3) **Mrs Chandra Malik**
   18/26, R.K. Puram Officers Colony,
   Secunderabad -500 056
   Ph : 040-7741042

4) **Rametaav Kennels**
   Mrs Meher Mathrani
   Goolshirain, 13/14, Uday Bang,
   Madapur I. E. P.O. Pune -13.

5) **Nariman M. Shakeebai**
   6-3-577/1, Aryanoushi's Khairtabad.
   Hyderbad-4.

6) **Bhogadi Kennel,**
   Hyderabad.

7) **Y.V. Ramane Reddy**
   B-2-1, Karamanghat,
   Hyderabad-74.

8) **Naab Nazeer Yar Jung**
   The Penta House, Dhruvastara,
   6-3-652, Samajignda, Hyderabad- 500 082
   Ph : 040-3310615.

9) **Ahmed Alam Khan**
   1-7-140, Musheerbad, Hyderabad-500 048
   Ph: 76167, 7616658.

10) **B.J. Thomson**
    1-7-18 D/3 , Bakaram, Mursheeradbad,
    Hyderabad,
    Ph: 7732305.

11) **Nawab Yousefuddin Khan**
    3-5-786/22, Shergatre,
    King Kothi, Hyderabad,
    Ph : 240410.

12) **Lt. Col. Sukhjeet Singh**
    C-15, Sainkinkpuri, Secunderabad,
    Ph : 7117838.

13) **Mr Roshan Vijay & Mr. Vijay Ramaskrishna**
    10-3-28, East Morredpally, Secunderabad,
    Ph. : 7732305.

14) **G.P. Veerbhadram**
   30, SBI Officers, Colony,
   Bagh, Amberpet, Hyderabad - 500 013.

15) **Mr Ramesh Chabbara**
   11-1-776/14, Beside Amara, Ralkies
   Chikalgnda, Secunderabad,
   Ph. : 76459013.

16) **Mr Azeen Farooqui**
   60, Rastha Peth, Nilkanth Apartment,
   Pune-11.

17) **Mr. M. Balraj**
   1-7-827, Gemini Colony, Zamisthapur

18) **Mrs Ajita Vijayan**
   C/o, Col. K.K. Murthi
   E-11, Sainkipuri, Secunderabad-500 094.
   Ph. : 711 1140.

Table 2. Differential Diagnosis of Common Conditions & Lab. Diagnostic Tests (for Dog)

Predominant Symptom	Age Group	Typical Symptoms	Possible Diagnosis	Laboratory Tests Recommended
FEVER (Above 103°F)	Pups below 6 months	* Cough and Colds with Nasal) Discharge and severe dullness	Distemper (if not protected) Respiratory distress Bronchitis/Pneumonia	Blood for TLC (initial Leucopenia) and DLC (Lymphopenia) and later stage shows fever and Neutraphilia
		* Jaundice & tenderness on liver site	Infections Canine Hepatitis (if not protected)	Blood for TLC (initial Leukopenia) and DLC (Lymphonehnia). Blood Clotting Time (increased) & Liver function tests (abnormal)
		* Diarrhoea & Vomiting	Parvo-viral gastro enteritis (if not protected)	Blood for TLC (initial Leukopanis) and DLC (Secondary Leukocytosis) Serum Sodium, Potassium & Chlorides, E.C.G., Elisa test if possible
	Above with 6 months	* Jaundice abortion in females	Leptospirosis (if not protected)	Blood for TLC (Leukocytosis) and DLC (Neutrophila) Serum of agglutination test

Predominant Symptom	Age Group	Typical Symptoms	Possible Diagnosis	Laboratory Tests Recommended
		* Jaundice and severe anaemia. Ticks on the body	Babesiosis and Trypanosomiasis	Blood smear for parasities. Blood for Haemoglobin & Liver Function Tests. Repeated smear exam. necessary
		* Nervous Signs, Epilepsy, convulsions, tremors	Meningitis or Encephalitis, Clorea as after effect of Distemper. Rule out Rabies	Blood for TLC (Leukocytosis) and DLC (Neutrophilla) CSF for culture
		* Foul smelling uterine discharge (in females associated with whelping)	Metritis or Pyometra if with fever, consider Renal and urinary infection	TLC (Leucocytosis) DLC (Neutrophilia), uterine swab for culture and sensitivity test, Kidney funtion tests may be considered
		Summer	Sunstroke	High Rise in PCV (increased in severe dehydration), serum Na., K
DIARRHOEA and occassional vomiting	Pups below 6 months	Severe diarrhoea with yellow/white watery stools	Bacillary Diarrhoea	PCV (increases in dehydration) faeces for bact. culture, Serum Na, K and Chlorides

Predominant Symptom	Age Group	Typical Symptoms	Possible Diagnosis	Laboratory Tests Recommended
		Black & reddish faeces with occasional mucus and body itching with alopecia	Hookworm infection	Faeces for Parasitic Ova, Blood for Hb. check for dehydration
	Above with 6 months	Persistant, non responding to routine treatment. Presence of fats & undigested food particles.	Maldigestion or Malabsorption Syndrome	Special tests for Amylase, Lipase and Pancreatic enzymes, Liver Function Tests
		Persistant diarrhoea with inflammation & swelling of rectum	inflammation of rectal glands	Examination of Rectal glands and their gentle squeezing with sterile mop. TLC/DLC for infection
		Black stool, itching of skin & warting	Hookworm infection and other worms	Stool exam for parasitic ova and routine Haematological tests

Chapter 20

Care of Crossbred Heifer

Expected resuls of early maturity and optimum production are possible only if the heifer-calf is brought up on the following lines.

(1) Give enough of colostrum (at least 2 kg) within *first 12 hours of* life. Allow enough milk @ 10% of body weight till at least 3 months age. Gradually replace milk with the starter ration containing about 20% proteins.

Feeding Schedule

Although it is ideal to provide whole milk upto an age of 3-4 months wherever possible. there is practical difficulty because of poor milk-yield of dams as well on economical considerations. Hence the whole milk can be replaced by a following calf starter ration containing about 22% proteins.

Maize yellow (*crushed*) 55 parts		3-5 g of **TT-50** (Pf*izer*) & 2-4 ml of Vimeral (Virbac) should be added per head up to 2 months of age
G.N. cake powder	35 parts	
Wheat bran	8 parts	
Mineral Mixture	2 parts	

Calf should be allowed a little quantity of good hay after an age of 15-20 days and gradually increased to eat lib. at 3-4 months age. Whole milk can be replaced by skimmed milk. the above calf starter should be given from 15 days age starting from 10 g/day gradually incrased to 1 kg. of 2 months and 2 kg at 6 months.

(2) Give mineral supplements like **AIRES formula-100"** @ 1 kg in 6.5 tonnes feed or 1 teaspoonful daily.

(3) Deworming-for round worms once a month (*see under parasitic diseases*). Get the faeces examined for coccidiosis in case of diarrhoea.

(4) Give any broad spectrum anthelminitic (*See under parasitic disease on relavent page*).

(5) Get FMD vaccination (*Intervet, or Indian Imunologicals*) first at 3 months age, booster dose at 6 months and then twice a year regularly. In case of outbreak in nearby locality, younger calves can also be vaccinated.

(6) H.S. and B.Q. vaccination in *June every year.*

(7) Take rectal temperature twice a day as a routine if possible and take immediate steps as soon as high fever is noticed. *Examine body for presence of ticks.*

(8) Keep the shed clean and get it sprayed periodically with either 5% DDT or 2% *Malathion or Butox* for prevention of tick infection.

(9) Examine conjunctivae for detection of anaemia and watch if there is any enlargement of lymph nodes. (*Pre-femoral and Pre-scapular*). These are the symptoms of Theiloeriosis which is a common ticborne disease of cross bred and exotic cattle. Get blood smears examined in case of slightest doubt. Also get haemoglobin estimated.

Vaccination against *Theileriasis* is now possible with **"Rakshavac-T"** (*Ind. Immunol*) and can be undertaken regularly if advised by the Vet.

(10) Adequate exercise, prevention of adiposity, adequate nutritious diet with minerals are essential for early maturity and reproductive efficiency.

(11) The crosss bred animals need to be protected from high atmospheric temp.in summer. Provide a cool shed with thatched roof and good cross-ventilation. If money is no consideration provide khus tatties,room cooler etc.so as to prevent room temp.rising above 37°-38°C.

(13) Watch the growth as per following expected schudule:

Month

Age	at birth	1	-2	-3	-4	5	-6	-8	-10
Expected body wt.(kg)	20.5	34	-57	-73	-88	-101	-116	-164	-192

If growth rate is proper the heifer should have girth measure of 150 cm which indicates her body wt. of 190-200 kg If this is not attained, check up feeding schedule. **Laurabolin** (*Organon*) or **Dinabol** (*Ciba*) have protein-sparing and tissue building properties and can be used in suitable doses with due care.

(13) Get the hiefer examined at 8-9 months age by an experienced Gyanecologist to ensure that everything is normal.

Chapter 21

Ethnoveterinary Medicine (Alternate Medicine)

There has been a worldwide rethinking over past decade about animal health care. There are certain managemental practices, indigenous methods and remedieswhich if practiced can keep the emergencies away and can keep the dairy farm in its optimum level of production. Certain management practices such as prompt feeding of colostrum after birth toanewborn calf; adoptiong proper milk in practices, sanitary measures to prevent udder and uterine infections, periodical vaccinations, deworming, feeding balance diet and providing mineral-vitamin supplements etc. have no alternative.

However, there are occasions when animal needs attention for its health problem and expert veterinary aid is not always available harmless but well tried and authenticated alternative remedies are very much needed by our poor farmer. This has given rise to the concept of *alternate medicine or Ethnoveterinary Medicine (EVM)*. These remedies are practiced in every village by tradition and are known by keeping their remedies as more or less a professional secret. They mostly use the herbs available locally and are identified by them. Efforts are being made to know their remedies and find out how far their medicinal utility can be scientifically authenticated or validated.

In addition to the herbal products, there are homeopathic drugs which have been tried in certain diseases for which effective allopathic treatment is either not available or is extremely cost involving. The examples are viral disease like foot and mouth disease. Mastitis Gynaecological disroders like prolapse of uterus with tenesmus, opthalmological problems like corneal opacity, treatment of septic wounds. etc. Several

305

scientic studies have been carried out by qualified vets, unqualified livestock owners and common persons but there is very little authentication and publication in research journals. Homeopathic remedies are generally considered by harmless but objections are raised over the issue for authority for using them. This issue needs to be tackled at proper authoritative forums to find solutions. Research findings presented at All India Homeopathic Association have been widely appreciated and the homeopathic medicines are widely used in day to day practice for treatment of animals. There are many books dealint with homeopathic practice by authoritative persons published and findings of scientific trails are also published in journals, and presented at national and international conferences. (*Recently two international conferences on Ethnoveterinary Medicine were organised at Pune (Maharashtra) between 4- 6 Nov 97 and other at Calicut (Kerala) between 4-6 Feb. 99 and about 100-150 delegates from outside India participated*).

Based on discussions in the seminar following general suggestions can be made:

1. Neonatal diarrhoea, infections and calf losses could be prevented by feeding colostrum during early hours after birth of a calf and adopting sanitary measures and avoiding overcrowding. Withholding milk, giving sterile water containing little salt and sugar to avoid dehydration administration of astringent powders like **Neblon, Diaroak, Chalk-Catachu** mixtures are quite effective in diarrhoea but antibiotics are needed in fever and respiratory symptoms (*colisepticemia*).

2. Digestive tonic powders, containing substances like **ginger, gentian, asafoetida, black salt, caraway seeds, black pepper, ajwain** or commercially available powders like **Battisa** followed by Liver stimulant powders containing Tefrosia and other herbal constituents are usually beneficial as a first aid in simple afebrile digestive disorders which are very common. Normally, ordinary digestive upsets get cured within 2 to 3 days and those which do not show improvement could be because of change in rumen pH, consumption of some traumatic or non traumatic

undigestable foreign bodies or vagal indigestion and need a thorough chck up by a qualified vet. Frequent and sudden change in the feed must be avoided as a general rule.

3. In case of retained placental or even after a normal delivery the cow/buffalo should be given a cleaning dose containing ext. ergot and mag. sulph or herbal preparations like **Replanta, Hormotone** for a day or two. Intrauterine antibiotic pesseries must be inserted at least for 2 to 3 days by a Vet.

4. Prolapse of uterus or vagina are common after calving and can be treated by homeopathic drug **Arnica, Pulsatilla** and **Podophyllum** after the prolapsed mass is reduced in position after thorough cleaning with disinfectant containing cold water. You can take help of an experienced veterinary technician for reducing the prolapsed mass by gentle manoeuvering. Homeopathic drugs are found to reduce straining and recurrence of prolapse. Sometimes a rope truss can be applied to prevet recurrence. However, antibiotics are necessary for 2 to 3 days.

5. Subclinical mastitis and blood tinge in milk can be successfully treated with homeopathic drug **Phytolacca** and **Ipicac**.

6. Further research on clinical cases of mastitis with homeopathic remedies is essential as it is difficult to make a generalisation because the causes of mastitis are multifarious and experiences of clinicians are different.

7. Fresh wounds, injuries and septic wounds can be effectively treated with combination of homeopathic mother tincture of **Calendula** and **Glycerine** mixed in equal parts. It is necessary to keep the wound clean by thorough washing and necrotic tissue by local application of mag. sulph. powder initially for a day or two. Ayurvedic and herbal preparations such as **Himax** lotion and ointment. **Wisprec, Charmil** are also effective. Fly repellents like **Lorexane,** Maggocide creams are also useful.

8. Sprains of muscles and tendons can be effectively treated by use of rubifacinet liniments used for massage only after ruling out fracture. Homeopathic drugs **Arnica** and **Rhus** tox are also useful.

9. Problems of reduction in milk yield and difficulty in letting down can be dealt with herbal galactogogue preparations containing **Leptadena, Ashwagandha** and other ingredients available commercially as **Leptaden, Morolac** tablets, **Galog, Gwala, Lactovet, Payapro** powders in addition to providing balanced ration and mineral supplements.

10. Breeding problems of cows/buffaloes such as anoestrus condition, infertility due to various causes repeat breeding and abortions are widely prevalent and several herbal and hormonal remedies are available in the market which make high claims of success. However, all cases cannot be alike and there may be a different causative factor for each individual animal. Normally it is better to get the problem animal examined by a qualified Gynaecologist before spending time and money on treatment. Nutritional and deficiency conditions must be ruled out as the first step. **Prajana, Sajani, Janova, Aloes compound, Hitali** are some of the non hormonal herbal compounds. and claim reasonably good response in non specific problems and may be tried for some time. Research is necessary in the field of homeopathy although claims are made by some clinicians.

Foot and mouth disease can be prevented and rapidly cured without complications by use of Homeopathic remedies **Cantheris, Merc. Sol.** and also by use of the propritary mixtures marketed in the name of **"Khurenol".**

There are several types of skin diseases and various types of ointments and lotions recommended for getting relief ,but here again the treatment is not likely to be the same for all situations. On human side Dermatology is a separate independent branch and it is the general experience that the skin diseases need a prolonged treatment.

It will thus be recommended that a holistic approach and use of different alternate medicines is the need of the day and the research scientists and the universities should direct the research to validate claims of such non conventional medicinal prepations with open mind.

Chapter 22

Diseases of Wild Animals
in Captivity

Veterinarian are occasionally required to attend and treat zoo animals in captivity either in zoological parks or circus and are required to advise on health matters in respect of wild animals in national parks or project tiger etc.

Dealing with zoo animals and their health problems is in fact a specialised branch and some big zoos and National parks have their own Veterinarian employed exclusively for this purpose. They gain valuable experience by virtue of long association and observation of wild animals. Advice of such experienced persons is valuable and should be sought for whenever possible.

In this chapter attempt is therefore made to give some guideline which may be useful while dealing with health problems of zoo animals.

Need to Know about Normal Habits and Behaviour of Wild Animals

It is very essential for a Veterinarian to have some information with regard to the normal habits, behaviours and health norms of the common zoo animals. This information should be obtained by visiting zoo and observing the animals as frequently as possible and by discussion with the persons concerned with day to day work at zoo.

Need of Proper Facilities for Restraint

Proper restraint of the animal in question is the most important need while dealing with zoo animals and without this proper clinical examination, diagnosis and treatment becomes difficult or even impossible. Isolation cages and squeeze cages are very useful and essential for this purpose. particularly the wild feline species (*tiger, lion, Leopard etc.*) Most of the zoos have such cages and if not they should be advised to have the same. The animals can be persuaded by familiar attendants or by offering attractive food such as fowl so that wild felines can be taken inside the squeeze cage. Elephants respond to command of their keeper (*mahouts*).

In certain cases the animal is captured and immobilised by strong ropes and poles with the help of attendants who are used to handle the animal (*manual restraint*). However, the *behaviour of animals cannot be predictable* and there is a certain amount of risk in this procedure. Catching the animal by chasing in respect of deers, antelopes and other animal creates a tremendous stress and animals just collapse and die due to shock and fear. Use of nets may be sometimes made (*for rodents, small felines*).

It is possible to give some sedative and tranqulilizers to avoid stress and shock. Oral administration is not dependable because the dose cannot be correctly assessed and ingestion of medicine cannot be assured. Special types of injection guns (*remote injection system*) are devised and have a range of 20 to 60 meters. They are fitted with suitable size syringse and needle with automatic ejection system. These tranquilization equipments and drugs are availble with "HELPRO Health Products & Services" at *D-53, Shopping Complex, INDORE 8,* who are the sole distributors. Anaesthetic stage can be produced by use of drugs like **Ketamine HCL** (Inj. **Ketalar -PD**) @ 10 mg./ kg.body wt. by remote injectable method followed by intravenous barbiturate (*Intraval sodium*) in appropriate dose for surgical work. Doses of these drugs have to be adjusted in individual animals and there can be great variations in response. **Rompun** (*Bayer*) and **"M-99** (*Reckitt*) are the other drugs.

General Precautions and Prophylactic Measures for Zoo Animals in Captivity

Visitors and particularly those with sadistic habits are the greatest enemies of zoological parks. Irritating the animals by throwing stones, sticks etc. may make the animal ferocious.

Throwing food material may give rise to digestive upsets and sometimes even food poisoning. So while investigating the disease problem specific enquiries should be made. Foot and mouth disease outbreaks have been reported among deers and other cloven footed animals due to throwing grass while the FMD outbreak was prevailing amongst cattle in the nearby locality. Such incidents are very common in deer parks located in the crowded parts of cities.

Non Human Primates

(**Apes and Monkeys**) These are the most frequently handled patients and since they are more closely related to human beings, there is high degree of susceptibility to human diseases like *tuberculosis, salmonellosis, amoebiasis, helminthiasis, poliomyelitis, small pox* (Monkey pox is more closely related to human pox — variola and vaccinia and less closely to cowpox). Other health problems like nutritional deficiencies, anaemia, rickets, nervous, disorders (*psychological problems like frustration, vicious biting self injury, refusal to food etc.*) cataract etc. are similar to human beings. The general principles and treatment are same as for human beings and study of human medicine and consultation with human practitioners will be useful.

The physiological norms are given below

Diarrhoea due to *salmonella infections* is quite common. Sick

Species	Normal Body temp.	Gestation (Days)	Life (Years)
Chimpanzee	37.2 °C	216-261	over 50
Orangutan	37.0 °C	275	over 35
Gorilla	37.2 °C	251-289	about 40

animal should be isolated as far as possible because the infections spread quite fast and young population is at high risk. Cleanliness, fly control, control of mice and cockroaches in the animal house are some important measures which prevent entry as well as spread of infections. Easily digestible food such as rice or barely water, vegetable soup with little salt are ideal.

Astingent mixtures, oral electrolytes in water (*Electral,*

Peditral etc.) are indicated. Hyperperistalsis and intestinal spasms causing pain can be controlled by spasmolytics such as *Buscopan or Antrenyl or Bellodenal* 1-2 tablets twice a day should be given with food or water. Antibiotics for infection control are *Chloramphenicol, (Chlorostrep Syrup), Dependal M suspension, Kaltin with Neomycin, Pesulin-O* suspension. They should be given in appropriate doses and for atleast 3 to 4 days. Vitamin supplements such as Vimeral or Winstress liquid. Vit. B-complex syrups and probiotics form excellent supportive therapy.

Tuberculosis is another imporatant disease causing heavy losses in primates. Tuberculin testing (*Intrademopapabral test with PPD*) should be carried out and those which are negative should be vaccinated with BCG (single dose 0.05 to 0.1 ml. intradermally in the delotoid region). Animals with known tuberculosis should be destroyed. Isolation and treatment with Isoniazid and Streptomycin may be done in the case of valuable and irreplaceable animals. Source of tuberculosis infection should be searched in attendants and bovines in the premises.

Infection with pox viruses (*monkey pox*) which is closely related to human pox are reported in monkeys. Cases of chicken pox due to human infection are also reported. *Measles* and *Poliomyelitis* are also reported. Fungal skin infections due to *Microsporum canis* are seen in orangutan and chimpanzee. The sites affected commonly are toes, finger, dorsal part of hand and head. The lesions are round or oval and with constant itching. The lesions spred to other animals and also to attendants. Topical antimyotics such as *Multifungin or Microgel ointment, Tinanderm with oral griseofulvin* preparations should be used (*Grisovin, Identifulvin, Grisaction etc.*).

Endoparasites

Regular periodical deworming with any broad spectrum anthelmintics should be a routine practice. *Thiabendazole, Tetramisole, Mebendazole* @ 10-20 mg./kg. body wt.for 2 to 3 days and repeated after ever 4-6 months. Periodical faecal examination be carried out.

Large Felines (*Felidae*)

(*Tigers, Lions, Leopard, Cheetah-Panthers*)

Physiological Norms

Species	Normal Body Temp.	Gestation (Days)	Life Span (Years)
Lion	38-39°C	110-112	30
Tiger	"	103-110	25
Leopard	"	93-105	21
Cheetah	"	91-95	15

Round worms (Toxacara leona, T. Cati), Hookworms (Ancylostoma spp.) and tapeworm (Taenia spp.) are common problems.

Regular periodical deworming with broad spectrum anthelmintic drugs (*Thiabendazole Mebendazole, Tetramisol etc.*) in appropriate doses is one of the routine programmes that must be followed at every zoo. Periodical faecal examination must be carried out to assess the efficacy of deworming programme. If this is satisfactorily carried out, the problem of gastrointestinal helminths is usually taken care of. For tapeworms **Niclosamide** and **Droncit** are the drugs which may be used.

Individual cases of *coccidiosis* may be encountered. Diarrhoea with dynsentery and anaemia are the clinical symptoms. After confirmation by faecal examination the animal can be treated with *Amprolium or Furazolidone or Sulpha drug* preparations be employed for 4 to 5 days.

Haemoprotozoan infection like *Babesiosis* is likely to be suspected. Anemia, icterus and haemoglobinuria are the symptoms which should arose suspicion. Confirmation by blood smear examination. In endemic area infection with *Trypanosomiasis* is also likey and can be diagnosed by blood smear examination. **Inj. Berenil** in appropriate dose may be effective.

Amongst *Bacterial diseases, tuberculosis* is suspected in case of symtpoms like cough, reduced food intake, loss of weight and low range fever are seen over a long time and particularly if no response is seen after treatment. Confirmation is not easy in large felines and tuberculin test is not very reliable. Animal should be isolated and throat swab or sputum for microbiological exam. should be collected by use of squeeze cage and anaesthesia. Animal may be treated in early stage.

313

Salmonella infections may become a serious problem in young cubs and occasionally in adults. Faecal culture confirms the disease. Treatment comprises of *Chloramphenicol, Sulphadrugs, or nitrofurans* along with astringent preparations for diarrhoea and fluids in case of dehydration.

Amongst *Viral diseases, infectious panleucopenia* (IPL) *also known as feline distemper* is an important disease caused by a DNA virus which is very resistant to disinfectants can remain infective for over on year. The disease may be peracute, acute or subactue. The important clinical symptoms are initial fever followed by gastroenteritis (*Vomition and diarrhoea*) with blood in faeces, rapid dehydration and exhaustion. During febrile stage TLC may drop to 1000 and below. This leucopenia with relative lymphocytosis is characteristic of this disease. Many animals may be simutaneously affected *by food and water contamination.*

Treatment: Symptomatic-Rule out parasitic infections or bacterial diarrhoea (*Salmonella*). Isolate the animal. Fluids and electroytes to combat dehydration, antibiotics, (*chloramyphenicol, nitrofurans, ampicillin etc.*) to control bacterial complications, *Vit. C, haemostatic* and *gammaglobulins* (*if available).*

Prophylactic vaccinations may be done by use of *Feline panleukopenia vaccine available* from (VESTAS Aero Industries, A 21, Rajouri Garden, New Delhi-110 027) on request.

In addition, Feline Infectious Rhinotracheitis and Infectious peritonitis, Meningo encephalitis and Rabies are the other viral infections which may be occasionally seen.

Skin Diseases

Mange or Scabies (*Sarcoptic and Notoderes*) and Ringworm (Microsporum and Trichophyton) are the common skin problems. Their importance should be remembered, confirmation be done by exam. of skin scrapings. Treatment of scabies comprises of isolation, application of sulphur lotion or ointments. Utility and safety of Inj. **Ivermectin** needs to be established.

Ringworm can be treated by oral administration of Griseofulvin tablets (dose 20 -40 mg/kg) for 4-5 weeks (doses to be regulated in individual cases).

Nutritional Deficiency Problems

Deficiency of Vit. B1 (*Thiamine*) cases neuromuscular symptoms such as *ataxia, star gazing, circling,convulsions, head pressing etc.* Diarrhoea may be present, postmortem lesions are cerebral oedema and supportive meningitis. Treatment is easy and rewarding (*Inj.Tribivet, or Neurobion, Neuroxin-12 etc*). Vit. A deficiency causes lacrymation, vision problems, stillbirths and breeding problems. Feed supplements be given when deficiency is suspected. Rickets is common if Ca : P ratio is disturbed. Mineral-Vitamin supplements like **ALVITE-M** (*Alembic*), **VIMERAL** (*Glaxo*) may be beneficial to prevent rickets and osteodystrophy.

BEARS

Normal Rectal temp. : 37.5°C -38°C

Gestation Period : 155 to 245 days.

(Vairable depending upon time of implanation)

Longevity : 20-30 yrs.

Parasites

Ascaris infection is common and Piparazine compound @ 50 mg/kg body weigt given for 3 days are effective. For tapeworms Niclosamide @ 10 mg/kg x 2 days. For hookworm and other round worms. Thiabendazole or similar broad spectrum anthelminitics @ 25-50 mg/kg body wt.

ELEPHANTS

Body temp : 36.4°C

Gestation Period : 21-22 months (upto 2 years)

Longevity : 40-45 years

Oral medication is done by mixing with jaggery or honey and placed on the tongue. It can also be given in bananas. Subcutaneous injection is most convenient and given at a site behind the upper third of the ear fold or skin behind elbow or infront of thigh, *Intramuscular inj. may cause swelling and abscess formation.* Deep intramuscular Inj. can be given on the gluteal site of shoulder muscles. I/v injections can be given in ear veins at the back of the ear after pressing the ear forward when the veins at the back become prominent. (*Elephants and their diseases. Supdt. Govt. Printing and Staty. Union of Burma Rangoon 1961 by Evan.s G.H.*)

Restraint: Chloralhydrate @ 4 g/50 kg given iv can produce anaesthesia effect. If preanesthetic is given then dose of chloral hydras can be reduced to 2.5 gm/50 kg Various pre anaesthetics such as chlorpomazine are suitable or minor purpose the animal is usually controlled by mahavats.

Parasitic and Protozoan diseases

Fascioliasis (*Liver fluke disease*) is common and the animals show symptoms of anaemia, diarrhoea with foul smell and oedema. Faecal sample examination should confirm this. Stronglyles are also commonly encountered. Chr. diarrhoea and colic may be seen. *Thiabendazole* @ 30 -55 mg/kg body wt. or *Albendazole* may be employed.

Trypanosomiasis is the important disease, Intermittent fever (38.5°C and above). fatigue, emaciation, anaemia and oedema are the symptoms that arouse suspicion. Treatment and any trypanocidal drug may be effective. Periodical checking of blood smear should be done.

Bacterial Disease

Tuberculosis with pulmonary involvement is reported and can be fatal. *Anthrax* and *Pasteurellosis* occur sporadically and cause sudden deaths. *Salmonella* infections are also quite common cause of diarrhoea and death in young lot. Antibiotics and sulphonamides are useful if given well in time. Tetanus is also reported. Symptoms of locked jaw (*Trismus*) and tetanic spasms are seen.

Viral Diseases

Pox disease is seen in countries where it is prevalent in human beings. Human pox vaccine virus (*vaccine virus*) can cause disease in elephants. Typical pox lesions are observed. (*Freshly vaccinated persons can spread the disease to unvaccinated elephant*). Foot and mouth disease may also occur in elephants and through the contact with cloven footed animals. Lameness, salivation due to formation of typical blisters are the symptoms Sometimes horn of the sole (food pad) falls off. The ulcers and wounds may get complicated by pus forming bacteria. Treatment consists of antibiotics and antiseptic dressing.

Amongst other diseases are constipation which is sometimes very severe. Occurs due to ingestion of sand, stones and such other foreign bodies. It cause tympany , obstruction and colic. Drugs to stimulate and regulate peristalsis, (Metaclopromide, Neostigmine, Arecoline, Carbachol etc.) may be used if there is no obstruction. Homeopathic drug **Opium** may be tried. Antispasmodic like Inj. Novalgin or Oxalgin if colicy symptoms are present. Warm water enema using a garden hosepipe to evacuate hard faeces may be attempted.

Abscesses and Wound

Are common problems. Draining the pus by incising the absess followed by dressing and Parenteral antibiotics are the measures generally adopted.

ZEBRA (*Equidae*)

Body Temp: 37-38°C

Gestation Period About : 330 - 365 days

Longevity : 25-28 years

These belong to horse family and the general principles of disease management are on the same lines as for horses. The diseases are also more or less the same as observed in horses.

DEER (*Cervidae*)

Body temp. 38°C

Gestation period-About: 200 days (variable with species)

Longevity : About 15-18 yrs. (varaible with species)

These animals are so nervous and excited that capture and chasing can cause lot of stress and shock resulting into sudden deaths. The temperature may be so varaible that it cannot be interpreted. Inj. **Rompun** (*Xylazine*) @ 1-2 mg/kg administered by shot gun is widely employed for immobilization and restraint. General considerations about diseases are more or less same as for bovines. Most of the parasitic infections are controlled by use of *Thiabendazole, Mebendozole or Albendazole* compounds in appropriate doses orally. **Claustridial infections** (B.Q.) and **Pasteurellosis** (*H.S.*) are common fatal bacterial. diseases. *Rinderpest ,Foot and Mouth Disease* (FMD) *Mucosal disease* are the important viral diseases. Vaccinations against F.M.D. by use of gun could be possible. F.M.D. can cause considerable losses particularly when there is proximity of cattle which frequently experience the FMD outbreaks in India. Homeopathic remedies like Merc. Sol. and **Cantheris.**

Food toxicoses are also reported when strict measures of preventing visitors and public from throwing edible food materials are not followed in deer parks and zoos. Homeopathic remedies given in drinking water seem to be a promising method in wild animals and needs to explored.

Chapter 23

Rabbit Farming

abbit meat is considered as a most delicious dish in multistar hotels and metropolis hotel and restaurants now a days. Although rabbit is the most delicate attractive animal which is liked by young children to play with, its economic importance as a meat animal has attracted attention of meat lovers due to following reasons:

1) Meat is ready in short time, is less expensive. Rabbit meat of excellent quality is available at about 11 to 12 weeks/age.

2) Rabbit meat requires only 1/4 th energy as compared to goat meat.

3) There are no religious superstitions and rabbit does not compete with human food and can thrive on Kitchen waste of vegetables.

4) Rabbit grows fast like poultry and the quality meat is comparable with chicken meat.

5) Meat contains higher proteins and mineral percentage as compared to other meat and has low levels of fats.

6) Body weight gives more per cent of flesh than bones and rabbit has a better feed conversion efficiency.

7) Rabbits can grow in any climate and is a prolific breeder throughout the year and we can market meat at our choice in any seasons of the year.

8) Rabbits can grow well on dried green fodder like barseem/Lucern and disease problems are comparatively less.

9) Rabbit is easy to handle and rabbit farming on modern lines can be good and profit earning business.

10) The beautiful hairy skin has very good market demand

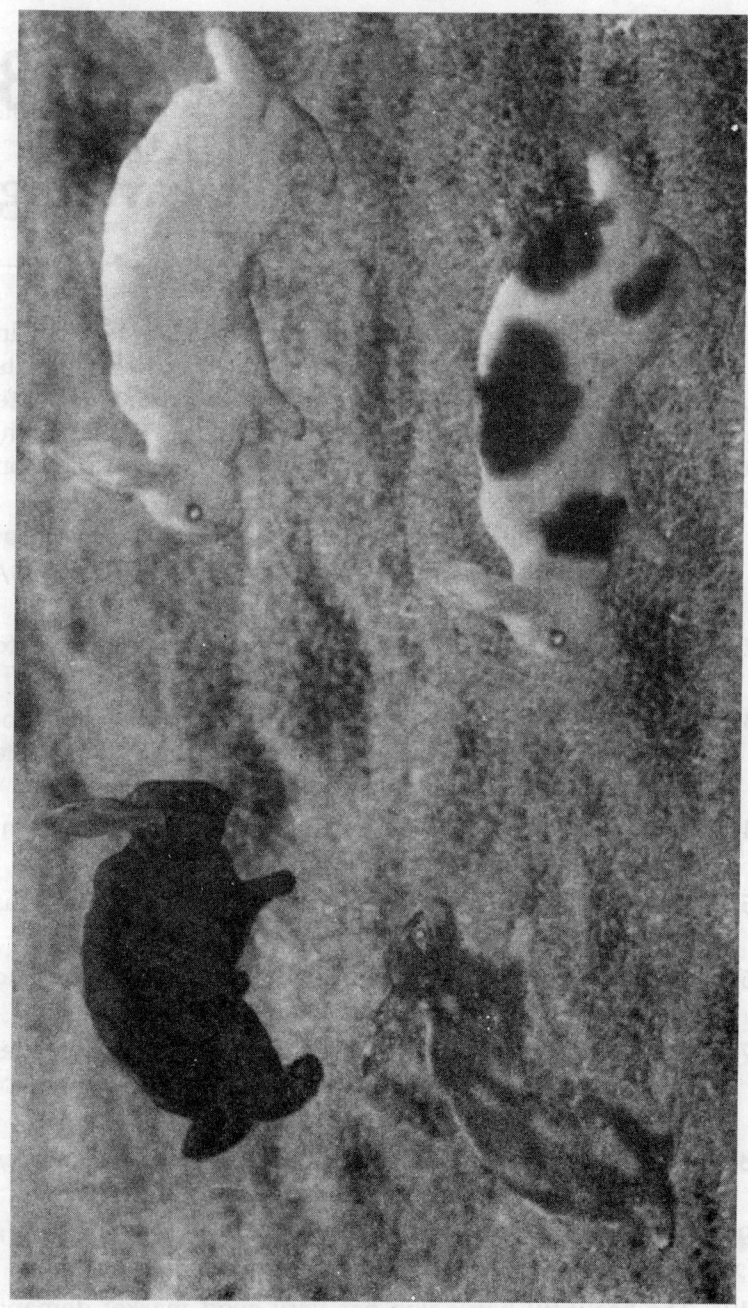

for manufacture of jackets, hand gloves, caps,purses and many other articles. Some breeds are famous for soft wool and as pet animals.

To Start a Rabbit Farm

One must get adequate and 'full' information about the rabbit keeping and must have adequate land with plenty of water and the necessary finance. One must get a good practical experience of working on any rabbit farm so that he get idea of routine working and possible hazards.

This business can be done by an unemployed youth or a housewife and any lady for that matter provided they get the proper training.

Breeds of Rabbits available in India
1) **For wool-** Angora
2) **For Meat and Skin-**
    (i) White giant,
    (ii) Grey giant
    (iii) Newzeland white
    (iv) Soviet chinchilla

The above breeds can be available from following sources-The central sheep and Wool Research Centre-**Avikanagar** (*Rajasthan*) taking one unit (2 males + 8 feamles) and the cages, small rabbit houses and other utensils which would cost about Rs. 5 to 6 thousand.

Usually each rabbit unit would annually require 1 quintal balance feed, 500 kg. greens. These contingent expenses and medicines etc.would cost about 4-5 thousand rupees.

Each unit would give about 180-190 kits and by the time they are ready for sale at 3 to 4 months approximately 130-140 rabbits would be available after allowing some 30% mortality.

The receipts would have to be worked out on existing market rates and one can expect a reasonable profit of Rs. 1500-2000 per unit in 3-4 months time.

One can calculate his earnings as per his investing and managing capacity. It is always better to begin from a small

321

scale so that one an get good experience.

Rabbit Feed

Balanced feed can be prepared as under:

Barseem or Lucern (dried)	40 parts
Maize (crushed)	20 parts
Wheat bran	20 parts
Groundnut cake/soyaben	20parts

To these ingredients 2% mineral and vitamins (like Vimeral) must be added.

When dried grass (*Lucern or Barseem*) is not available we have to increase proportion of other ingredients

The feed requirements are as under

Ist month	@ 20 -30 g per head
2nd month	@ 50-60 g per head
3rd month	@ 80-90 g per head

Above 3 months they should be given feed @ 100 g per day. Green grass/kitchen waste vegetable whenever available should be given over and above the concentrate mixture. Adult rabbits require 150 g feed to 50 g per day.

Rabbits like green grasses very much and hence we must try to give lucern or beseem as far as available and grow these grasses if you have a piece of land and irrigation, or else buy green vegetables in season when theyare available in plenty and use kitchen waste of vegetables in other seaons. Rabbits do well if each one gets about 30-40 grams of greens per day.

The concentrate mixture be mixed with greens so that wastage is avoided, because rabbits usually make lots of wastage while browsing with feed. It is better to use pelleted feeds if available.

Diseases and Health Problems

Rabbits lose appetite when sick and become dull and drowsy and sit in corners. Body temperature also increases which we can feel when we handle them. In respiratory diseases laboured and accelerated breathing, sneezing and nasal discharge are seen. Digestive upsets are usually diarrhoea, dysentery and loss of body weight are the usual symptoms. Diseases can be classified as Bacterial, Viral, Parasitic, Toxic and others.

Bacterial Diseases

1) **Pasteurellosis-** A very common disease for which rabbit is highly susceptible. This is characterised by snuffles (nasal discharge, sneezing and fever), Pneumonia (respiratory distress and high fever) conjunctivitis (swelling around the eyes and severe congestion). Torticollis (The bent neck with stiffness).

The treatment of pasteurellosis is immediate use of broad spectrum antibiotics and commonly effective antibiotics are Tetracyclines which could be given as a injectible (Inj. Terramycin 1-2 ml) or in drinking water (Hostacycline W.S. powder) on large scale in a herd. The feed utensils be sterilized by boiling water and there should be proper ventilation and freedom from dust and fungus in the house.

2) **Tuberculosis-**Rarely occurs, but, if present,can be a health hazard for man.

3) **Abscesses-**Are common in unhygienic premises and if rabbit cages are dirty and not cleaned properly.

Viral diseases are not very common.

Parasitic Diseases

The common diseases are Ear mange caused by *Psoroptes* and *Sacroptes cuniculis* mites. The mange spreads arounds the ears on face and eyes.There is purulent discharge from ears, due to bacterial infection. This causes uneasiness and loss of body weight and ugly appearance. Infection of internal ear can lead to stiff neck and death.

Coccidiosis-Cause diarrhoea with presence of blood and mucus resulting in dehydration and anaemia. The parasites also affect the liver (*Eimeria stidae* infection). Treatment is possible with coccidiostats like **Codrinol** and **Sulpha drugs.** Spread should be prevented by isolating sick animals and hygiene otherwise there can be some mortality. Cleanliness is very important.

Chapter 24

Veterolegal Procedures

POSTMORTEM EXAMINATION

Technique and Diagnostic Utility

Postmortem examination is usually carried out in following situations by the Veterinary graduate.

(i) In a veterolegal case to give an expert opinion about the possible cause and time of death.

(ii) For diagnosis and confirmation of disease after death. Accurate diagnosis is very essential in case of contagious disease and poisoning so as to enable taking appropriate preventive measures.

A regular systematic examination should be followed so that every organ and tissue is examined and nothing is missed. Recording of postmortem examination should be objective and fully descriptive.

Veterolegal Postmortem Examination

(i) Remember to read the report and the letter from Police authority carefully.

(ii) Have the police representative present during examination.

(iii) Disallow other unauthorised persons to witness.

(iv) Do not delay the p.m. examination so that putrefactive changes would not spoil the carcass. At the same time do not perform p.m. examination during night hours in artificial light.

(v) Examine every organ even though the cause of death is found in the initial stage of examination.

Take the following with you:

(A) Measuring tape for measuring injuries.

(B) Measuring cylinder for measuring fluids.

(C) Empty wide mouth bottles for collecting Viscera (*if poisoning is suspected*).

(D) Microscopic slides and clean papers for wrapping. Take heart blood smears and impression smears from liver, lungs, and spleen in *all veterolegal* p.m. to rule out other diseases which may be co-existing. These slides be sent to the diagnositic laboratory after fixing the smears with alcohol or spirit.

(E) A small note book and pencil. *Note down every point on the spot and do not depend on your memory.*

Following Points must be Noted:

Date and time of postmortem and at whose request the examination is done. Descriptions of animal with identification marks, colour, species, age, sex, external appearance. Type, nature and location of external injuries with measurements, rigour mortis, putrefactive changes, observed and approximate time of death should be noted.

Examine the natural orifices for discharges and body condition of animal *whether well fed for emaciated and hide bound etc.* Enquire about symptoms observed while the animal was alive and treatment if any was given to the animal before death.

If the animal has died *suddenly with bleeding room natural orifices a quick blood smear from the ear vein be taken and got examined to rule out Anthrax.* If anthrax is confirmed, postmortem is not conducted and carcass is buried in deep soil with salt.

Next step is to skin the animal. For this the body is supported on its back in the dorsal recumbent position. A linear incision be made from the tip of lower jaw and extended in the middle of neck, thorax and abdomen avoiding penis in males and udder in females.

Afterwards, first cut the abdominal muscles and open abdominal and pelvic cavity. See if there is any fluid in peritoneal cavity. Note the character and measure the quantity if there.

Note the position of organs. Note if there are adhesions between various organs and also with diaphragm. It is necessary between various organs and also with diaphragm. It is necessary to examine reticulum and its adhesions in bovines. The fore stomachs and abomasum are removed after ligating thoracic part of oesophagus and duodenum. Contents of *rumen, reticulum, omasum and abomasum* should be examined. Examine duodenum, pancreas, liver and spleen. Examine liver for cysts and parasites (*liver flukes*) by cutting open. Palpate the consistency of these organs and note your observations. Note the size, thickness and consistency of spleen.

The urogential organs, adrenals, kidneys and rectum are removed and examined. Kidneys are grasped and detached from their attachments. In females the ovaries, cornua of uterus are detached and examined. The ureters and bladder are then examined. The diaphragm is cut along its insertion and organs of thoracic cavity are carefully examined.

Examine pericardial sac for fluid/exudates. Examine trachea, heart and lungs together. Examine all seven lobes of lungs by palpation and look for *hydatid cysts*.

Examine values of heart after cutting it open. Note the contents of chambers-full or empty, clotted or unclotted blood etc.

Brain and meninges should be examined for congestion, haemorrhages and clots.

Endocrine glands, mediastinal glands, mesentric glands and musculature should be examined and peculiarities should be noted.

Blood smears and impression smears from cut surfaces of lungs, liver, spleen and kidneys must be collected in every veterolegal postmortem, air dried, fixed with alcohol and forwarded to the diagnostic laboratory after wrapping in clean paper. This is done to rule out other possible causes.

The postmortem report of a veterolegal case by prepared in the printed proforma wherein the observation about every organ is mentioned. While writing the cause of death at end, you should mention your opinion in a guarded language stating as *"From the observations I feel that the death might have been due to............. ...."*.

In case the carcass is putrefied, you should mention about it and state that "no opinion as to the cause of death can be given due to advanced putrefactive changes."

The copy of veterolegal postmortem report be submitted to your superior District Officer for his information and remarks and one copy be kept in your office record.

In case you desire to conduct the histopathological examination, the piece of the tissue (such as from lungs, liver, spleen, kidneys etc.) of the size of one cubic centimeter be collected from the suspected area of lesion in 10% formal saline and sent to the diagnositic laboratory where histopathological reporting is done. Complete history of the case must be informed to the laboratory along with tissue sample sent.

Postmortem in a Dog

Apart from routine reasons, postmortem examination is insisted by some dog owners for confirmation of Rabies. In such a case postmortem examination must be conducted after taking due precautions. Every person conducting postmortem and helping in the procedure must wear protective hand gloves, and face mask and person, having injuries on his fingers or hands must avoid conducting postmortem in suspected case of rabies.

Brain is required to be sent to the diagnositic laboratory as under-

Half vertical section of brain in 50% Glycerine phosphate buffer soln. on ice for virus inoculation tests in mice.

Remaining half vertical section (*containing hippocampus major*) in 10% formal saline in a wide mouthed stoppered bottle for examination of "Negri bodies".

Impression smears (fixed) of hippocampus also may be prepared and sent for examination of "Negri bodies".

The bottles must be properly stoppered, labeled and packed so as to avoid spilling and breakage. The parcel should preferably be sent with a courier with a special note to *"Handle with Care" "Rabies material inside"* etc. should be written in Red ink on the exterior part of the parcel.

Submission of Samples to the Diagnostic Laboratory

The information about symptoms and gross lesions and the material to be collected for submission to the Disease diagnostic laboratory is mentioned in the description of the particular diseases and under poisonings.

Veterolegal Examination of *a Live* Animal.

Usually required to perform examination in case of accidental injuries, weapon injuries, maiming and other offenses:

(i)   Give a correct and complete description of the animal.

(ii) Describe the injuries in details (*age, size, depth, direction, situation etc.*).

(iii) Mention probable cause of injuries.

(iv) Give prognosis of injuries. Postpone giving your final opinion if you would like to observe the animal after treatment.

(v)   Give your opinion as to whether the animals would be rendered permanently useless for the purpose for which it is meant.

Procedure in the Court of Law

One should attend the court on the day and time specified in the summons. If physically unable due to illness or other valid and important reasons, you must inform the court well in advance, about your inability to attend.

(i)   Go through the office-copy of report pertaining to cause and be prepared for probable questions.

(ii) Always stick to the statements that you have made in the report.

(iii) As far as possible avoid use of technical terms.

(iv) Answer the questions with *"yes"* or *"no'* as far as possible. If unable to answer, say *"I am unable to answer"*.

(v) Express opinion from your own knowledge and experience.

(vi) Statement should always be guarded and the replies should be brief and *to the point.*

Common Offenses against Animals

(1) **Mischief-** Killing, poisoning and maiming (*rendering the animal permanently useless*) phooka practice, inducing abortions by hitting or injuries.(*Punishable under section 428 & 249 of I.P.C.*)

(2) **Cruelty against animals-** Beating overloading, using sick or diseased animal for work, starvation, phooka practice etc. are punishable under the prevention of Cruelty to Animals, Act, 1890.

(3) **Bestiality-** Unnatural voluntary sexual intercourse with animals by man or a woman, punishable under *Section 377 of I.P.C.* Examine the genital organs and collect swabs or washing for precipitation test by Forensic lab.

(4) **Frauds:**

(a) Alteration of description.

(b) Bishoping.

(c) Adulteration of milk and meats.

Differentiation of various meats

Physical Examination: Based on anatomical variations and type of flesh. Identification is easy if long bones are available. Sex can be identified if genital organs are available.

(i) **Mutton** (*Sheep Meat*)- Dark red, has ammoniacal odour, rich fat depositions between groups of muscles. Fat is white, hard and not intermixed with muscles, wool fibres usually seen adhering.

(ii) **Goat Meat-** Paler than mutton. Has a peculiar "goaty" smell.

(iii) **Pork-** Consistency soft. Fat intermixed with muscles. Fat is white and granulated. Has ammoniacal odour.

(iv) **Dog meat-** Dark red in colour and fat intermixed with muscles.

(v) **Beef (*Cattle meat*)**- Red in colour with brownish tinge. Fat intermixed with muscles. Fat is yellow in colour. Calf meat is called "Veal", its fibres are fine and bone marrow is pink red in colour. In case of old cattle fat is yellow and bone marrow is pure white to reddish yellow.

(vi) **Horse meat**- Dark to brown red in colour, becomes blackish when exposed to air, fat is golden to dark yellow in colour and bone marrow is greasy.

Other Tests for Differentiation

Chemical Tests: Glycogen test, Iodine values.

Biological Tests: Precipitation tests are very specific. Minced meat (*Kheema*) and even cooked meat can be identified. (Cocto antibody test). Send the meat sample to the Regional Forensic Science Laboratory for getting the report.

Some Important Acts and their Provisions.

(1) Glander and Farcy Act-1899

A graduate Veterinary Officer appointed as an "Inspector" under the provision of the Act and can examine any horse suspected to be suffering from Glanders and if confirmed after "Mallein test" the horse has to be destroyed and premises disinfected compulsorily, as per the provisions of this Act.

(2) Prevention of Cruelty to Animals Act 1890 and amended in 1960

When this act is made applicable to any particular area, all the acts of cruelty such as beating, overloading, starvation, phooka practice, cruel treatment by quacks, using sick animal for work etc. are punishable offenses. The amendment covers the experimental and laboratory animals. It is compulsory to provide proper housing and management to laboratory animals like rabbits, guinea pigs, mice etc. and avoid cruelty. So also, the animals should be not be used for producing experimental disease or for experimental surgery and if at all necessary, then their number should be minimum.

(3) Bombay Animal Contagious Diseases Act, 1948 and C. P. & Berar Cattle Diseases Act, 1934

When any contagious disease is prevailing in any area the same can be declared as *infected area by* approaching the Collector of the district. Under the provisions of this Act, cattle movements, cattle markets, fairs, rallies, exhibitions etc. can be prevented to stop the spread of diseases. Prophylactic vaccination can be made compulsory and sick animals can be detained and/or isolated. (*Similar Acts are existing for every State*).

(4) The Maharashtra Animal Preservation Act, 1976

Has been brought into force with effect from 15th, April, 1976 for the entire State of Maharashtra. The important provisions are as under:

(i) Slaughter of cow is totally banned. The cow includes a heifer or male or female calf or a cow (*male calf upto one year age*).

(ii) The animals included in the schedule for which a certificate can be issued are-*Bull, Bullocks, Female buffaloes, Buffalo calves (Both males and females*). Male buffaloes over one year age are not included in the schedule.

(iii) Only those Veterinary Officers in—charge of dispensaries, whose designations have been notified in the extraordinary gazette published on 15th April, 1978 can issue the certificate as a competent authority. (*Every Veterinary Officer cannot*).

(iv) The officers who have been authorized to declare the place of slaughter are as under:

(A) The Chief officers of all Municipal Councils	All places of slaughter falling in their jurisdiction.
(B) Municipal Commissioners, Bombay/Nagpur/Pune/Solapur/Kolhapur/Amravati etc.	Entire area falling in the jurisdiction of the concerned Municipal Corpn. (*Newly declared Corporations will be included.*)
(C) All District Animal Husbandry Officers in the State.	All places which do not fall within the jurisdiction of any Municipal council or Corporation in their district.

(v) A she buffalo or female buffalo-calf over one year which is likely to be economical for giving milk or bearing off-spring **cannot** be certified. If there is no permanent damage to the udder and reproductive organs such animals **cannot** be passed.

(vi) Bulls which could be useful for breeding, draught or any kind of agricultural operations **cannot** be passed.

Bullocks which could be economical for draught or agricultural operations also **cannot** be passed.

It would be necessary to examine the reproductive system and limbs of all scheduled animals and incapacity of permanent nature should exist so as to pass such animals included in schedule. Deliberate mutilating of animals should be curbed by finding out whether the injury is recent or old and whether deliberately inflicted.

The certificate has to be issued in the following proforma only.

Form of Certificate

This is to certify that I have, this..........................day of 20 .... examined the animal whose description is given below and that I consider the animal to be fit for slaughter:

(1)   Name of the owner............................

(2)   Description of the animal :

Species............................

Breed............................

Sex............................

Age............................

Colour............................

Important distinguishing marks............................

(3)   Reasons for certifying the animal as fit for slaughter............................

(4)   Received rupees one on account of the fee for inspection of the above animal.

Place ....

Date ....

Signature

(Stamp of designation)

Rules Governing Private Practice

(Applicable to Maharashtra vide Govt. Resolution No. VET/1075/5754/4 Dated 18.02.76)

A veterinary graduate who is not getting non-practicing allowance may undertake private practice in his spare time (other than office/hospital hours of duty) and without allowing his office duties to suffer. A practitioner must have registration to practice as per the **State Govt. and Veterinary Council of India** regulation. The rules and circulars issued from time to time by the Govt. department in which he is serving must be followed. These rules differ from state to state, hence recent circulars must be followed.

Schedule of Charges

(The charges may have been revised from time to time. For this the recent circulars of the department may be consulted).

(i)   To attend a case within Municipal limits Rs. 5/-

To attend a case Beyond Municipal limits Rs. 10/-

Attendance during night hours Rs. 2/-extra.

(ii) For the case of Dystokia - Rs. 5/-extra.

(iii) For issuing soundness certificates:

Cattle- Rs.5/-

Horse- Rs.10/-

(iv) Post mortem with certificate (but without chemical analysis): Large animals: Rs.10/-

Small animals: Rs. 5/-

Chapter 25

Common Laboratory Procedures & Their Interpretations

Haematological Examination
- For confirmation or elimination of tentative diagnosis
- As an index to prognosis.
- As a guide to therapy.

Particularly important in haemoprotozoan and bacterial infections.

Collection of Blood

Site: Large animals- Jugular vein.

Dog and Cat: Cephalic vein (foreleg)

or Recurrent tarsal vein (hinge leg)

Containers: Should be dry and chemically clean. Empty vials of antibiotics could be used. For getting serum, use large bottles or one inch. diameter test tubes to collect blood. *Allow blood to clot in t*he slanting position. Keep overnight and decant clear serum. Centrifuse for clearing and transfer to a clean-preferably sterile, rubber capped vial bearing a label. Add *Merthiolate 1:10,000* (a drop of 1 per cent aquious. sol. to 10 ml. serum) or Phenol 0.5% (Add 1 ml. of 5% to 10 ml. serum) Store at 4°C.

Anticoagulants- (Used while collecting blood for haematological and biochemical examination.)

(1) Double oxalate mixt. (10% sol.) @ 0.3 ml

Amm. oxalate 6 parts | dried up in a vial for 10 ml blood.
Pot. oxalate 4 parts |

(2) Sodium citrate 4% sol. @ 1 ml for 10 ml blood.

(3) EDTA 1% soln. @ 1 ml or few grains of EDTA for 10 ml blood.

(4) Heparin 1% soln. .... Rinse the vial or syringe with 0.1 ml soln. for 10 ml. blood.

(5) Sodium. fluoride 1% soln. .... for glucose estimation.

Precautions

In case of large animals, use a wide bore needle and collect blood directly in the vial, while in case of small animals use a *perfectly dry syringes* and a 20 guage needle. It is preferable to use sterile disposable syringe with needle.

(i)   *Do not push* out blood forcefully from syringe.

(ii) *Do not* agitate the vial unnecessarily.

(iii) *Do not* use alcohol or spirit for sterilization of syringe.

(iv) *Do not* freeze or expose the blood sample to high atmospheric temperatures.

Preparation of Blood Smears

Prepare blood smears *preferably* from fresh blood drawn by pricking the ear vein rather than preparing from blood collected in anticoagulant. See that iodine or spirit from the swab does not get mixed with blood at the site of the prick. Use dry, clean greese-free slides previously dipped in 95% alcohol. Select a good slide with smooth edge for drawing the smears. Take a small drop of blood, touch it with the smooth edge of the drawing slide held at an accurate angle and draw a uniform smear. Take at least 2 smears. Dry in air and then fix with methylated alcohol or methylated spirit for 1 minute. Dry and wrap in clean paper, label the smear.

Remember that nicely prepared good smear is essential for getting correct diagnosis. History about symptoms also be preferably given along with the sample.

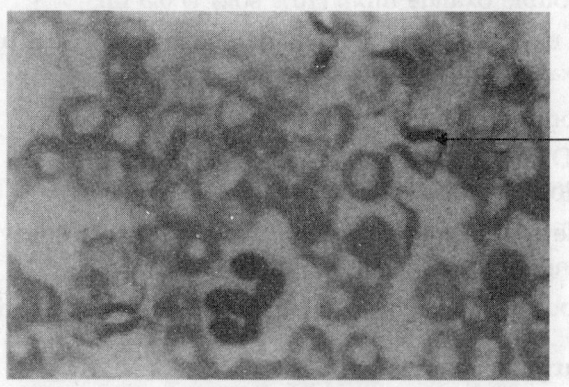

Positive for Trypanosomiasis.
(extra cellular)

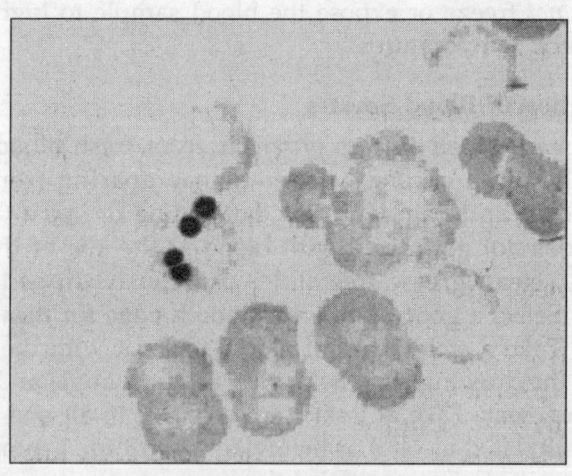

Blood smear
Piroplasms (Babesia sp.) inside red blood cells

(A) Erythrocyte Sedimantation Rate (ESR)

Procedure-Collect 5 ml. blood in anticoagulant. Fill the *Wintrobe-ESR* tube (with mm. divisions) using a Pasteur pipette having a long fine tapering end. Start filling the tube from bottom upwards. Blood should be uniformly mixed and the tube should not have any air bubble. Keep the tube in the straight upright position and read after one hour. Note the upper column of plasma. ESR is expressed as mm/hour.

In Cattle, Sheep, Goat, – – – – 0.2 mm/hr.

Dog & Cat: – – 5 to 20 mm/hr. Horse: 15-30 mm/hr

(B) Packed Cell Volume (PCV) or Haematocrit

This is the volume of packed blood cells recorded by centrifuging whole blood collected with anticoagulant. The Wintrobe tube after recording ESR can be centrifuged for one hour at 3000 rpm. Read the column of packed cell volume *from below, as mm. per cent.* This gives very good idea about degree of haemoconcentration, anaemia and has a direct correlation with hemoglobin and total erythrocyte count. Normal PCV in healthy animals of most species ranges between 30 to 40 mm%.

(C) Haemoglobin Estimation : (*Sahli's Method*)

Procedure: Place a few drops of N/10 or 10 per cent HCL in the graduated haemoglobinomiter tube. Take well mixed blood upto 20 cm. mark in the Sahli pipette; wipe out exterior of pipette and discharge it in 0.5 ml HCL in the tube by rinsing once or twice. Allow the mixture to stand for 15 minutes. Then add either N/10 HCL or dist. water slowly drop by drop, constantly stirring with a glass rod till the colour matches the standard colour of the haemoglobinometer. Read the Hb. conc. in gms. per 100 ml.

Normal values: (per 100 ml blood)

Horse: 9-14 gms. *Cattle* : 8-13 g Dog: 12-16 g

(D) Total Erythrocyte Count (TEC)

Procedure: (i) Use the RBC pipette (with red bead). Fill it with blood upto 0.5 marks, wipe off and fill it with Gower's soln. or Hayem's soln. upto 101 mark (*for composition of reagents,*

337

see under "lab. reagents".)

(i)   Mix well by rotating the pipette for 2 minutes.

(ii) Affix the cover glass over the polished surface of Neubaur haemocytometer slide's counting chamber.

(iii) Shake the pipette, discard 2 drops from the capillary and touch the tip of the pipette, against the edge of cover glass so that the space between cover glass and counting chamber gets filled in by capillary action. Fill the other side of the counting chamber in the similar way.

Do not allow excess fluid to flood over.

(v)   Mount the slide on the microscope stage and focus under low-power objective.

Enumeration- Adjust the central ruled square under high power objective. It has in all 25 small squares in it. Out of these, count RBC in 4-corner small squares and one central small square (total area 1/5 cmm). Total number of cells counted multiplied by 10,000 will give you the TEC per cubic mm. (usually expressed as million/cmm).

Normal Values:

H & C: 6 to 9 million /cmm. *Dog:* 6-8 million /cmm.

(E)   Total Leukocyte Count (TLC)

Use WBC pipette (with a white bead)

(i)   Fill the pipette with blood upto 0.5 mark.

(ii) Wipe off the exterior and fill with N/10 HCL upto 11 mark and mix for about 2 minutes.

Other procedure upto charging the counting chamber is the same as described under TEC.

Enumeration- Focus under low-power objective and count cells in 4 large corner squares (4 sq. mm. area) Total cells counted multiplied by 50 will give the TLC per cubic mm.

Normal values: *H & C* : 6 -12 thousand/cm

Dog: 5-12 thousand/cm.

(F) Differential Leukocyte Count (DLC)

A nicely prepared smear is very essential.

Staining procedure: (Leishman's method)

(i) Pour measured numbers of drops of stain to cover the entire slide so as to cover the smear surface.

(ii) Allow to react for 1-3 minutes.

(iii) Add double number of drops of buffered distilled water (pH 6.8) to the slide and mix with a dropper.

(iv) Allow to react for 15 minutes.

(v) Wash, dry and examine under oil-immersion objective.

Giemsa method- Smear fixed with with alcohol is necessary. Add enough of diluted Giemsa stain to cover the smear completely; or immerse the slide in the staining jar filled with stain. Allow to react for 25-—45 minutes. Keep for longer time if smear is being examined for protozoa. Wash with water, dry and examine under oul-immension objective.

Differentiate 5 different types of leukocytes and count the individual types in a total of 100 leukocytes. Make duplicate count and take average. Individual cell types are expressed in percentages.

Normal values:	Neutro	Eosion	Baso	Lympho	Mono.
Horse:	50-55	2	1	30-35	8
Cattle :	30	5-8	1	60	6
Dog :	70	5	1	20-30	6

Interpretation of Haematological findings

Alternation in ESR, PCV. Hb and TEC.

ESR increases in infective diseases.

In dogs increased ESR is seen in distemper, ICH, accute infections and hypoproteinemia. PCV is a very good index of haemoconcentration. PCV may be as high as 70% when the patient is in critical stage of dehyradation. Fluid administration is necessary till the PCV returns to 45% when the patient could be considered out of danger. If a patient is having pre-existing anaemia, his PCV may appear in normal range even though the

339

patient is severally dehydrated. Hence interpretation of PCV to assess haemoconcentration is proper only when haemoglobin and TEC are within normal limits. Increase in Hb and TEC beyond normal range indicates haemoconcentration, which occurs in dehydration, in case blood is collected immediately after exercise or struggling or if vein is occluded for a long time.

Decrease in Hb and TEC indicates anaemia.

(i) *Haemorrhagic*	(excessive blood loss; blood-sucking parasites).
(ii) *Haemolytic*	(due to haemoprotozoan infections, haemolysis due to toxins etc)
(iii) *Nutritional*	(deficiency of Iron, Copper, Cobalt , etc.)
(iv) *Defective blood formation*	Hypoplastic and aplastic

Alteration in Leukocyte Picture

Leukopenia	*(Reduction in TLC with overall reduction of all types or one cell type)*

DLC in relation to TLC alone would give correct idea whether there is absolute increase or decrease of any single type of leukocyte.

Common Causes of Leukopenia:

(i)   Characteristic in early stage of viral diseases. (Distemper, ICH, Rinderpest, MDC, Bov. malignant catarrh) and certain protozoan diseases.

(ii) Terminal stages in overwhelming bacterial infections. *(unfavourble prognosis)*

(iii) Extreme debility and loss of resistance.

(iv) Physical agents *(ionizing radiation, X-ray exposure)*.

(v)   Effects of drugs *(Antibiotics, Sulpha drugs, analgesics, antihistamines and corticosteroids)*

Leukocytosis : (Increase in TLC-overall or any single type)

Common Cause of Leukocytosis:

(i) Bacterial infections (rise in proportion to severity to infection. Response spectacular in dogs and horse but not so much in cattle).

(ii) Physiological variations (highest in young ones of cattle and dogs whereas low in piglets)

(iii) Localization of infection process produces greater neutrophilic leukocytosis than generalized process (e.g., traumatic reticulitis, pericarditis, peritonitis, metritis)

Shift to the left means increase in immature cells of granulocyte series.

If with leukopenia: A sign of bad prognosis.

If with leukocytosis: A sign of regeneration and a good prognosis. Eosionophlia is observed in parasitic, allergic conditions and rarely in chronic traumatic reticulitis.

SOME HEMATOBIOCHEMICAL TESTS AND THEIR INTERPRETATIONS

It is sometimes necessary to undertake biochemical tests on blood to get additional information about body functions in certain conditions to arrive at correct diagnosis so as to adopt proper line of treatment.

Blood Calcium: (*normal levels: 8 to 12 mg/dl*)

Calcium in blood is in free ionized form and in protein bound form, total blood calcium variations has some diagnositc value. Diagnosis of "milk fever" and "hypogalactia" due to low blood calcium levels can be confirmed. Periodical estimation in high yielding animals is useful and can prevent acute hypocalcaemia by suitable timely measures like oral supplementation, administration of Vit. D_3 etc.

Inorganic Phosphosrus (*normal levels : 4-5 to 7 mg/dl*)

In some areas incidence of post parturient hypophosphatemia (Hemoglobinuria) is common due to deficiency in the soil and fodders. Levels below 3 mg/dl are considered critical and results in severe muscular weakness.

Hyperphosphatemia is associated with renal failure and excessive intake of Vit. D.

Serum Magnesium (*normal levels 2-5 mg/dl*)

Low level produces lactation tetany in high yielder cows after parturition and whole milk tetany in newborn calves. Levels below 1.0 mg/dl are critical in cattle and will cause tetanic spasms, tachycardia, tremors, hyperaesthesia and collapse.

ELECTROLYTES

Imbalances of serum electrolytes are very important to understand for proper assessment of the condition of patient in the state of sever dehydration, hypovolumia and shock.

Serum Sodium (*Normal levels:* Cattle 130-140 mEq/1 Dogs: 141-152 mEq/1)

Sodium ions are extracellular cation and maintain its osmotic pressure. Na^+ is lost in enteritis, diarrhoea and dehydration. More severe losses in infectious diarrhoea of newborns. Results in hypovolaemia, peripheral circulatory failure and ultimate renal failure.

Serum Potassium (*Normal levels : Cattle 4.0 to 5.18 mEq/l Dogs: 4.35 to 5.65 mEq/l*)

Potassium ions are mainly intracellular. They are lost in persistent severe enteritis, intestinal obstruction, abdominal stasis, Hypokalemia results in muscular weakness and decreased neuromuscular activity. *Hyperkalemia is* less common and occurs following severe metabolic acidosis. It is more dangerous and K+ levels above 7-8 mEq/1 has marked action in cardiac function (*bradycardia, arrhythmia and cardiac arrest*). Variations are very significantly reflected in ECG of dogs.

In addition to Na^+ and K^+ the estimation of serum *bicarbonates and chlorides* are also important for proper assessment of conditions.

LIVER FUNCTION TESTS
Serum alkaline phosphatase (AKP)
Cattle : 16 + 8 I.U./L,

Young Dogs: Upto 284 I.U./L

Adult Dogs 44.7 I.U./L

Aspartate aminotranferase (AST) *(formerly* SGOT)

Cattle: 20-34 I.U./L Dog: 15-20 I.U./L Horse: 58.100 I.U./L

Aianine aminotransferase 9 A

Cattle: 10.4 I.U./I Dog: 19/20 I.U./I Horse: 7.3I.U.

The variations in above *three serum enzymes* as indicated by high rise is of great significance in dogs and are indicative of heptic damage. In cattle, the results are variable and should be interpreted with caution.

KIDNEY FUNCTION TESTS:
Blood Urea Nitrogen (BUN)

Normal values: Cattle : 20-40 mg/dl.

Dog : 17-38 mg/dl

Urea is the end product of protein metabolism and is excreted in urine. Levels increase in kidney damage and retention of urine due to any cause. The rise in levels is in proportion to renal damage. BUN levels may increase in animal with very high protein diets and feeding of urea, as feed supplement.

Creatinine:
Normal values: Cattle : 1.0 to 2.0 mg/dl

Dog : 1.0 to 1.7 mg/dl

Creatinine is the product of breakdown of muscle phosphocratine. It is not reutilized and is excreted by kidneys. Increases in creatinine level indicates defective excretion due to kidney damage.

Urinalysis
Use a chemically clean container for collecting urine. Catheterized samples preferred wherever possible. See reaction with litmus paper. Record transparency, colour and smell.

(A) Specific gravity: Fill the urinometer cylinder to within 1 inch of the top. Place the urinometer in urine and spin between, thumb and finger. Read the sp. g. and record it in decimals as 1.020 etc. (*Avoid bubbles in the cylinder*)

(B) Albumin determination:

(i)   Place 2 ml *Robert's reagent* in the test tube.

(ii) With a dropper add 2 ml urine on the reagent slowly as to form a layer.

A white or grey ring at the zone of contact indicates albumin.

Report as : Trace, (+), Moderate (++), Heavy (+++) Conc. Nitric acid can also be used in place of *Robert's Reagent*.

(C) Acetone or Ketone bodies determination

Rothera's test:

(i)   Take 3 ml urine in a test tube.

(ii) Add 1 ml Roterha's Reagent and mix.

(iii) Stratify 1 ml Liqr. Amm. fortis over the solution in the tube.

A strong *permangante colour* at the zone of contact within a minute indicates the positive reaction.

Weak or delayed reactions may be ignored because low levels of ketone bodies in urine are of no clinical significance in ruminants.

(D) Sugar Determination (*Beneficts' test*):

(i)   Take 0.5 ml (7-8 drops) urine in the test tube.

(ii) Add 5 ml Benedict's qualitative reagent.

(iii) Mix well and boil the mixture on spirit lamp for 5 minutes (take care to avoid spurting)

(iv) Allow to cool in a rack.

Interpret as under

Green colour with **slight yellow** sediment: Traces

Green colour with **heavy yellow** sediment : + (1.0%)

Yellows colour with **heavy** sediment : + + (1.5 %)

Yellow colour with **heavy reddish** sediment : +++ (2.0%)

(E) Occult Blood or Haemoglobin

(i) Prepare a saturated sol. of Benzidine powder in 2 ml glacial acetic acid.

(ii) Add 2 ml fresh 3% sol. of Hydrogen peroxide.

(iii) Mix equal parts of urine to above. Development of the colour indicates presence of blood or *haemoglobin*.

Interpretation of Urinalaysis

Specific Gravity

Increased sp. gr.: Observed in reduced fluid intake, dehydration, fever, acute, intersitial, nephritis, cystitis, diabetes mellitus etc.

Decreased sp. gr.: Chr. interstitial nephritis, diabetes insipidus, excessive water intake.

Albuminuria: Transient albuminuria observed in febrile conditions.

Renal causes: Nephritis, toxic nephrosis, effects of chemicals and drops.

Post renal causes: Cystitis, urethritis, urolithiasis, trauma (during catherterization), mixing with vaginal or preputial discharges.

Glycosuria: Emotional, chr. liver diseases, Enterotoxaemia in sheep, excess carbohydrates and sugars in the diet, Diabetes Mellitus.

Ketonuria: Ketosis and hypoglycemia, Diabetes mellitus, Acidosis, Imparied liver functions, starvation.

Haematuria

Renal causes: Acute nephritis, passive congestion of kidneys, pyelonephritis.

Post renal causes: Cystitis, urethritis, urolithiasis, trauma. crystaluria due to the sulpha drugs and certain other drugs.

Haemoglobinuria: Babesiosis, post parturient-hemoglobinuria, Leptospirosis, Anaplasmosis (rarely), certain poisons and toxins.

Faecal Examination

(For identification of parasitic infection and worm-load. Also for coccidiosis)

Methods:

1. Direct Method

This is a quick method when time is short but results are inconclusive.

Procedure: Take a small quantity of faeces and make a uniform suspension with a few ml. water. Take a drop. of suspension on the microscope slide. With a cover slip cover it and examine first under low-power and then under high power objective for details.

2. Concentration Methods

(A) Floatation Method

Make the faecal suspension in sugar solution or sodium nitrate soln. of greater density. (See under Lab. reagents) so that the parasitic ova of lower density float on the surface.

Procedure- Take 2-3 g faeces in a beaker and make a uniform suspension using 20 ml of either sugar soln. of sod. nitrate soln. Remove fibre particles by using tea strainer. Pour the suspension in the centrifuge tube and centrifuge at 600-1000 rmp or keep the tube in the test tube rack of 15-20 minutes. Lift up the surface layer using the headed glass-rod and transfer a drop on the slide. Put a cover slip and examine.

(B) Sedimentation Method

Useful for treated ova and other roperculaed ova which are heavier. Prepare the faecal suspension in water (2 g in 20 ml water) strain and centrifuge at 1000 rpm for 2-3 minutes. Discard the supernatant and examine the sediment.

Interpretation of Faecal Examination

Only a rough estimate can be made by the above qualitative method.

1 to 2 ova per low power field: Indicates only a mid infection which is not usually responsible for clinical signs of diseases.

3 to 4 ova per field: Indicates moderate infection.

More than 5 ova per field: Indicates heavy infection. For more accurate judgment and for evaluation studies with, drugs, egg counting techniques are to be employed (*ex. Stoll's method or McMaster technique*). Identify ova with the help of some standard manual with illustrations.

Rumen Function Tests

(*Tests to asses the ruminal digestion*)

In cases of indigestion that do not respond to routine treatment within 2-3 days. it is desirable to examine the rumen fluid for pH and microflora activity. owners usually permit such investigations when response to treatment is not seen.

Collection of Rumen Fluid

(1) By passing probang

It is possible to collect sufficient quantity of rumen contents by passing a lubricated probang through the mouth gag. With a little practice it is possible to pass a probang in quiet animals it is however difficult in various animals without use of tranquliser. After the probang is in the run, the rumen fluid flows out if the head of the animal is lowered slightly. If an aspirator pump is used then there is more ease in collecting rumen fluid. About 100-200 ml fluid can be easily collected.

(2) By Paracentesis

By using a 4 inch long 14 gauge aspiration needle connected to a syringe it is easy to collect about 5 to 10 ml. rumen fluid. The site (about 2 sq. inch area) on the left side of abdomen below the paralumbar fossa is prepared by shaving and sterilizing with a swab of alcohol. The sterile needle is inserted carefully and conned to the syringe. By little to and fro movement it is possible to aspirate about 5-10 ml rumen fluid unless in some cases the rumen content is very dry and hard. Animal must be properly and securely restrained. While withdrawing the needle some antibiotic solution should be injected and the needle withdrawn quickly in one jerk. This will prevent possible peritonitis. (See figure).

TESTS

Rumen fluid should be transferred to air-tight bottle immediately. The colour and smell should be observed. In normal animal, the colour is yellowish brown and has an aromatic smell.

(1) Estimation of pH

If the quantity is more, the pH can be estimated by using pH meter in the laboratory. In the field, indicator papers of BDH with a pH range of 2-10 are quite satisfactory and fairly accurate results are obtained.

(2) Sedimentation Activity Tests

The rumen fluid is strained to remove the coarse particles. The strained fluid is allowed to stand in a glass jar at body temperature (37°C in incubator or water bath) and the time required for floatation of particles is recorded. In normal animals the time required ranges between 3 to 9 minutes. If the particulate matter settles down it indicates gross inactivity. In less severe cases the time needed for floatation is very long.

(3) Cellulose Digestion Test

This indicates the microbial digestion activity. Time required for the digestion of cotton thread is recorded by suspending one small glass bead with a *thread of cotton in* the rumen fluid in a jar. If the cotton thread is digested the bead will fall down in the jar in incubator at 37°C, if the time required for digestion of cotton thread is more than 3 hours, it indicates gross abnormality.

(4) Microscopic Examination

A drop of freshly collected rumen fluid is taken on the microscope slide and covered by a cover slip and examined under low power objective. If the rumen microflora activity is normal you observe a good number (about 20 per field) of a large (**holotrics**) and small (**oligotrics**) ciliated protozoa swimming across the field vigorously. In case the rumen microflora activity is affected or microflora are destroyed due to any cause the activity considerably reduced or sometimes totally absent.

(5) Examination of Stained Smear

A drop of rumen fluid is spread of the slide and allowed to dry and then fixed. It is stained with *Gram's method and examined.* In normal sample the proportion of *gram negative bacilli* is predominant, whereas in a acid indigestion there is an overwhelming population of *Gram positive loctobacilli* in the sample.

SPECIAL DIAGNOSTIC PROCEDURES

(1) Blood Calcium Estimation
Rapid Semiquantitative test

The test utilizes the whole blood but expresses the calcium concentration in term of serum Ca. The P.C.V. of 33.33% is assumed for this test. The amount of EDTA required for chelating different amounts of calcium in blood is made use of as a principles of this test.

A series of 6 test tubes (75 x 12 mm. size) of uniform size are taken and labeled as control. 6, 7, 8, 9 and 10. (The number indicates the serum Ca as mg/100ml).

(Na$_2$EDTA) Disodium EthyleneDiaminotetraacetic acid solution is prepared so as to have conc. of 5 mEq/litre (Approx 93 mg/litre conc. of pure grade Na2 EDTA). To each tube the EDTA soln. is added by use of miropipette as shown in the table. The solution in the tubes is oven dried and these tubes form a set for one test.

Serum Ca mg/dl	Whole blood Ca mg/dl	EDTA sol. ml
6	40	0.40
7	47	0.47
8	53	0.53
9	60	0.60
10	67	0.67
Control tube	—	—

Take 6 ml blood accurately by a syringe. Add 1 ml of each tube accurately (including the control tube). Keep the tubes at body temp. by holding the tubes in hand for 20 minute after which the test is read.

Tubes are inverted after 20 min.to examine presence of a clot, and those containing clot. the blood remains at the bottom and doesn't flow. The end point is the last tube in the series containing the clot.

For ex. When blood in 7 mg tube clots and in 8 mg. tube does not clot. the serum Ca is read as between 7 and a 8 mg/dl. The blood in the control tube must clot.

(2) Cerebrospinal Fluid (CSF) Examination

Pandy' s Test

This test detects the presence of globulins in the CSF. Normally the CSF contains albumin and a very small fraction of globulins (5 to 40 mg/dl.) The globulin fraction increases in pathological conditions which can be shown qualitatively by this test. Pandy's test is positive in inflammatory diseases of brain and menings.

Procedure- One ml of saturated aqueous solution of Phenol (*Carbolic acid*) is taken in tube and 3 or 4 drops of CSF are added and mixed. Normally there is only a slight or no turbidity.

In case of positive test a clearcut white turbidity occurs due to precipitation and remains for quite some time. The reaction can be graded as +, ++, or +++ according to intensity.

In addition to Pandy's test glucose estimation, cytological and cultural exam., of CSF is done and these tests have very useful diagnostic value.

(3) California Mastitis Test (CMT)

This is considered as the most reliable Indirect test for detection of subclinical mastitis under field conditions, i.e., to detect mastitis before clinical symptoms (swelling, visible alteration in milk like clots, pus, blood etc.) are seen. This test detects increased WBC count in milk which is an early indication of infective process.

Procedure- About 5 ml. CMT reagent (See under reagents) is taken in a clean petri dish or the cup of the plastic paddle and the equal quantity of milk is directly taken from the suspected animal and mixed by rotating movements. Formation of a jelly like clot within 2 minutes is indicative of a positive reaction.

This field test is not conducted in first 21 days after parturition and during the last week of drying off stage; because during this period the cell count is normally high and so may give a false positive reaction.

(4) Diagnosis of Rabies

(*Examination of Negri bodies in impression smear of brain-Hippocampus major*)

The impression smears are made by pressing the clear glass slide on the cut surface of hippocampus major. Two or three impressions can be taken on one slide. The P.M. exam. must be done with great care. Hand gloves and mask must be used. The smears are air dried and fixed with methyl alcohol or spirit for 15 minutes.

Stains Required-

Stock solutions (1) Saturated Basic Fuchsin in alcohol

(*Store in freeze*)

(2) Saturated Methylene blue in alcohol.

Procedure

Prepare the stain as under the time of staining

Basic Fuchsin sol.	2 drops
Methylene blue sol.	7 drops
Distt. water	10 ml

Mix well in a tube.

351

Pour the above prepared stain mixture on the slide and heat gently from below till steam rises. Allow the stain to react for 15 minutes. Wash, dry in air and examine under oil immersion lens.

Findings : *"Negri bodies"* stain bright red and the nerve cells stain blue.

(5) Diagnosis of Brucellosis

Standard tube agglutination test (STAT)

A clear nonhaemolysed, well preserved serum (about 1ml) is required. Plain Brucella antigen, agglutination tubes, steel tube rack, micropipette and incubator are the other requirements.

Procedure- Arrange 6 agglutination tubes in a row in the rack. Add 0.8 ml carbol saline (Normal saline with 0.5% phenol as preservative) in the first tube and 0.5 ml in all the other tubes.

Add 0.2 ml serum (*to be tested*) to the first tube and mix well. First tube thus has total 1 ml volume. Transfer 0.5 ml from first tube to tube number 2 and mix. Transfer 0.5 ml from tube 2 to tube 3. Continue till 6th tube and the last 0.5 ml to be discarded.

Now add 0.5 ml plain antigen to all the tubes and mix well. The serum gets diluted like 1:10, 1:20, 1:40, 1:80, 1:60 and 1:320 in the tubes. Keep one positive control (with known positive serum) and one negative control (with known negative serum or blank).

Incubate the rack with tube at 37°C for 24 hrs. Examine for complete agglutination (clumping of white antigen cells at the bottom of tube). The last tube in which complete agglutination occurs is the titre of serum antibody for the test sample.

Agglutination in 1:40 and above is a positive test.

A Rapid Plate Test:

A rapid plate test using coloured Brucella antigen is performed on whole blood. A drop of blood is taken on a clean slide and drop of coloured antigen is added and mixed with a match stick. In a positive sample the blue particles of antigen form clumps within 2 minutes. This test is only qualitative and does not indicate antibody titre.

Chapter 26

Useful Information for Clinician

Weights and Measures

1 ml	=	16 minims (approx.)
1 g	=	15 grains (") = 1000 mg
1 drachm	=	4 g (")
1 fluid ounce	=	30 ml (")
1 teaspoonful	=	1drachm = 4ml
1 tablespoonful	=	4 drachm = 15 ml
1 Lb	=	450 g (approx.)
1 Pint	=	560 ml (20 ounces)

Average Gestation Periods

Mare	=	340 days
Cow	=	282 days
She Buffalo	=	310 days
Sow	=	116 days
Ewe and she goat	=	148 days
Bitch	=	60 days.
Cat	=	55 days

Estrus Periods of Animals

Animal	Duration of Estrus	Recurrence after
Mare	2 to 11 days	22 days
Cow and Buffalo	4 to 30 hours	21 days
Ewe and Goat	9 to 16 days	Usually once
Cat	7 to 10 days	during the season

354

Average Normal Rectal Temp

Horse	100.6	°F.	38.0 °C
Cattle & Buffaloes	101.6		38.6
Sheep & Goats	101.0		38.4
Poultry	107.0		41.6

To convert °C into °F multiply by 9/5 and add 32.
To convert into °F into °C subtract 32 and multiply by 5/9.

Average Normal Pulse & Respiration (per minute)

Species-	Pulse	Respiration
Horse	28-42	8-16
Cattle	60-80	18-24
Sheep & Goat	68-90	10-20
Dog	80-100	20-30
Cat	100-120	20-30

Age at Weaning and Puberty

Species	Weaning	Puberty
Cow	8-16 weeks	12-18 months
Buffalo	8-16 weeks	12-18 months
Mare	12-16 weeks	12-16 months
Ewe & Doe	8-16 weeks	8-12 months
Sow	6 weeks	4-5 months
Bitch & Cat	4-6 weeks	7-10 months

FORECAST OF CALVING DATE FOR COWS

Date of Service											
1	1	1	1	1	1	1	1	1	1		1
Jan	Feb.	Mar.	Apr.	May	June.	July	Aug.	Sept.	Oct.	Nov.	Dec.
Date of Calving											
7	7	5	5	4	4	6	7	7	7	7	6
Oct..	Nov.	Dec.	Jan.	Feb.	Mar.	Apr.	May	June.	July	Aug.	Sept

355

Homoeopathy in Veterinary Practice

Homoeopathy — a system developed by Dr Samuel Hahnemann has been recognised as very efficient branch of medicine all over the world. It works on the principle that **"Similars are cured by similar"** meaning that if a particular drug, plant or poison produces a particular drug or poison produces a particular set of symptoms in a healthy person those symptoms are cured by a same drug or plant or poison if administerd in homeopathic form i.e., in the minutest dilution. This is confirmed by **"proving"**. The homeopathic system doses not recognize the disease entity or casual organism as such, but is based on the symptomatology.

The drugs are described instead of diseases. The drugs which can produce and alleviate the particular symptoms related to various systems of body are described in homoeopathy materia medica. The symptom and past history, the mental reactions as to *how one feels* (depressed mind, fear, happiness or distress etc.) are considered as very important guidelines for selection of the remedy and may not be effective in all patients suffering from the same symptoms. Selection of drug differs from patient to patient depending on his constitution and such other considerations. **Generalization therefore is not possible in this system, i.e., one particular remedy may not be effective in all patients suffering from a particular disease.** It is therefore not easy to practice homeopathy without adequate study. Difficulty in making generalization and absence of subjective symptoms are the chief constraints in application of homoeopathy in Veterinary medicine. However, several workers including the author have tried homoeopathic remedies in animal treatment with success.

There is quite a number of published reports and books which deal with homoeopathic treatment of animal diseases. an experienced veterinary physician will appreciate that animals do express their feelings, signs of pain, signs of comfort, joy, excitement, fears etc. by their facial expressions and behaviour. Careful observation is necessary. After having tried homoeopathy in a systematic way it has been possible to say that homoeopathy has certainly a good scope and deserves consideration particularly when in many conditions the allopathy has no specific remedies or the treatment becomes financially out of reach of a poor person.

The author was invited to visit Calicut (*Kozikode*) and Bangalore conferences on Ethnoveterinary Medicine when he presented paper on use of Homoeopathy in veterinary practice. He observed that in this area large number of veterinary graduates employed in MILMA and NDDB who are using Homoeopathy in their veterinary practice, particularly mastitis and reproductive disorders for which antibiotic therapy is extremely costly and is facing hazard of resistant strains of bacteria. They are very much satisfied with the use of Homoeopathy.

Based on the experience of author remedies are suggested in tabular form (**See chart IX**) for each disease condition. These should be tried and findings recorded and reported by all veterinary physicians for the benefits of others.

Chapter 27

Ointments - Liniments and Lotions

1. Iodine Ointment (1.25)

(For painful swelling and sprains)

Iodum	4 g
Pot. Iod.	4 g
Glycerin	12 g
Vaseline	80 mg

2. Tr.

	Iodine	**mitis**	**fortis**
	Iodine	5 g	5 g
	Pot. Iodide	3 g	3 g
	Distt. water	5 ml	5 ml
	Rect. Spirit	ad. 200 ml	ad 50 ml

3. Lugol's Solution

Iodum	2 g
Pot. Iodide	3 g
Dist. Water	80 g

4. Blister (Red Ointment)

Hydragyri Iod. rubr	1 part
Vaseline	8 parts

5. Sulphur Ointment (for mange)

Sulphur sublimated	1 part
Vaseline	10 parts

358

6. Golden Lotion (for mange)
Sulphur sublimated 250 gm.
Quick lime   500 g
Water   4 litres
Boil slowly till it takes golden yellow colour.
Keep as it is for 3 days and then decant supernatant.

7. Dressing Oil
Creaosote   10 ml
Oil. turpentine   125 ml
Oil lini   500 ml

8. Carron Oil (*for burns*)
Liquor calcis (lime water) 1 part
Linseed oil   8 parts
mix by shaking

9. B.I.P.P. (*for sinus and fistulae*)
Bimuth subnitrate   1 g
Lodoform   2 g
Liquid Paraffin sufficient to make a paste

10. Salicyclic Ointment (*for Ringworm*)
Acid Salicylic   2 g
Acid Carbolic   2 g
Vasuline   30 g

11. For Moist Eczema
Acid Salicylic   2 g
Acid Tannic   2 g
Spirit   30 ml

12. Eye Drops (*for conjuctivitis*)
Protargol or Acid Boric 1 g
Distt. water   45 ml

(*for granular conjuctivits*)

Silver nitrate	0.5 g
Distt. water	100 ml

13. Liniment Ammonia (*for sprains*)

Liq. amm. fortis	30 ml
Ol. turpentine	30 ml
Aqua	30 ml
Simple oil	250 ml

Note: *mix by shaking and store in a tightly corked bottle. Protect eyes and face while opening bottle.*

14. White Lotion

(*Astringent and cooling lotion for sprainted tendons*)

Lead acetate	30 g (1 part)
Zinc sulphate	24 g (3/4th part)
Aqua	600 ml (20 parts)

15. Refrigerant Lotion (*cooling lotion for application over sprained and painful parts*)

Amm. chloride	1 part
Lead acetate	1 part
Alum	1 part
Vinegar	40 parts
Water	20 parts

Soak the bandages in the Lotion No. 14 or 15 and apply to the affected limbs.

16. Antiseptic Powder (*Astringent powder for dressing of unhealthy wounds and ulcerated surfaces*)

Boric Acid	2 parts
Iodoform	1 part
Zinc oxide	2 parts

Chapter 28

Laboratory Reagents

1. Benedict Qualitative Reagent (*for sugar in urine*)

Copper sulphate	17.3 g
Sodium citrate	173.0 g
Sodium carbonate	100 g
Distilled water to make	1000 ml

2. Gower's Solution (TEC *Count*)

Sodium sulphate anhydrous	12.5 g
Glacial Acetic acid	33.3 ml
Distilled water	200 ml

3. Hayem's Solution (TEC *Count*)

Mercuric chloride	0.5 g
Sodium sulphate	0.5 g
Sodium chloride	1.0 g
Distilled water	200 ml

4. HCL Solution (*for Haemoglobin and TLC*)

Conc. HCL	1.0 ml
Distilled water	100 ml

5. Robert's Reagent (*for albumin in urine*)

Saturated aqueous sol. of Magnesium sulphate 100 ml.

Conc. Nitric acid	20 ml

6. Rothera's Reagent (*for Ketone bodies in urine*)

Ammonium nitrate	30 g
Sodium nitroprusside	2 g
Distilled water	80 ml

7. Sugar Solution (*for faecal exam. by flotation*)

Sugar	1280 g
Water	1000 ml
Phenol (as preservative)	20 ml

8. Sodium Nitrate Sol. (*for faecal exam.*)

Sod. nitrate	850 g
Water	1000 ml

9. Lactate Ringer's Sol. (*for use in severe dehydration*)

Sodium chloride	0.60 g
Sodium lactage	0.27 g
Potassium chloride	0.04 g
Calcium chloride	0.02 g
Distilled water (*pyrogen free*)	100 ml

Autoclave at 20 lb pressure for 30 min. for parenteral use.

10. Mastitis Test Reagent (*for CMT test*)

(a) Sodium Lauryl sulphate	30 g
Bromocresol purple	5 g
Distilled water	1000 ml
or	
(b) Sod. Hydroxide	15 g
Teepol	5 g
Bromothymol	1 g
Distilled water	1000 ml

Chapter 29

List of Biological Products Manufacturers

Various centres from where veterinary biological products can be indented.

1   Indian Vety. Res. Institute, IZATNAGAR.

2. Institute of Animal Health & Vet. Biological Products, (IAH & VB) BANGALORE.

3. Institute of Vety. Preventine Medicine, RANPET (Chennai).

4. M.P. Vaccine and Research Institute, Huzrat Road, GWALIOR (M.P.) (for Anti Rinderpest Serum).

5. Madhya Pradesh Vaccine & Research, Instt. MHOW (M.P.).

6. Biological Products Section, A.H. Deptt. U.P., LUCKNOW.

7. Institute of Vety. Biological Products, PUNE-7 (M.S.).

8. Serum Institute, CUTTAK (Orissa).

9. Biological Products Section HISSAR (Haryana).

10. Serum Institute, HYDERABAD (Andhra Pradesh).

11. Biological Products Section, GAUHATI (Assam).

12. Bengal Vety. College, Belgachia CALCUTTA (W.B.).

13. Bihar Vety. College, PATNA (Bihar).

14. Biolgical Prod. Section, JAIPUR (Rajasthan).

15. Haffkin Institute, MUMBAI (M.S.).

16. Bio Med» Pvt. Ltd. C-96, Site Not 1. Industrial Area, GHAZIABAD (U.P.).

17. Institute of Viraml Vaccine (P) Ltd, Parivazhy, ULLANPUR (Kerala).

18. Serum Institute of India, Hadapar, PUNE (M.S.).

19. Venkateshwariya Hatcheris (*for poultry vaccines*) "Ventri Biologicals", 13/6 Milestone, Panshet Road, PUNE-25 (M.S.).

20. Indian Immunologicals, Rakshapuram, HYDERABAD-1.

Chapter 30

New Developments in
Veterinary Sciences

Embryo-Transfer-Technology

Efforts have been constantly made to improve the breed of cattle with an aim to increase production in the country. Importance of cross breeding has long been appreciated as one important tool to achieve the goal of increasing production. Cross breeding started as upgrading by use of better Indian cattle breeds which initially started as key village centres by locating breeding bulls of improved breeds for natural breeding, was replaced by artificial insemination with liquid semen, followed by introduction of exogenous cattle breeds like Jersey and Holstein Frezian and use of frozen semen straws to the door step of the owner. This procedure had the limitation of getting one calf per insemination of a cow and we could get only 8-10 calves from a high yielding cow in her lifetime. This gave an idea of getting more than one ovum from the cow in one oestrus, fertilizing and harvesting the fertilized ova by the collection technique. These fertilized ova if transferred to the uterus of indigenous cows, could yield more number of calves from a high yielder cow at a time. This is called *Embryo Transfer Technology* (ETT). This consists of selection of high yielder cow (a donor cow), inducing multiovulation in her by giving injections of hormones, inseminating the donor cow by using semen of a high pedigree breeding bull and then recovering the fertilized ova from the uterus of this donor cow. It is possible to cause ovulation of about 15-20 ova from ovary of a donor cow in a single heat. Recovered fertile ova could be implanted in the uterus of any healthy cow in oestrus so that the fertilise ovum could attach itself(nidation) inside uterus and develop into foetus under natural uterine environment. These fertilized ova however need uterus of any healthy cow in heat period.

So, the problem came up as how get, so many number of cows in heat at one time? This was solved by hormonal stimulation (*Prostaglandins*) of heat (*Heat Synchronization*) so that the fertilised ova could be transferred in many cows within a reasonable time without any loss of fertilized ova. Further techniques were developed for preservation of these fertilzed ova in liquid Nitrogen. Now it is possible to preserve the fertilised ova for a reasonable time till suitable cow is available for transfer of the ovum during heat period.

This could yield 10-15 improved breed pedigree calves from a donor cow during a single heat period provided these fertilzes ova could be implanted in healthy uterus indigenous cows. However, it is not possible to forecast as to the how many of them could be females? So, now a technique is being developed to do sexing of the fertilized ova and to retain only females to transfer. If this technique of embryo sexing is achieved, then there could be **"embryo bank"** where embryo of high pedigree could available. Although this technique is presently costly and sophisticated, it will be the major break through in animal science and will be popular in times to come.

Country's First Blood Bank for Animals and the **Veterinary Nuclear Medicine Centre (VNMC)** are being started under MaharashtraAnimal and Fishery Sciences University (MAFSU) at Nagpur and Mumbai Veterinary college respectively. The ICAR, New Delhi has agreed to give grants Blood Bank and Bhodba Atomic Research Centre (BARC) is governing collaborate for Nuclear Centre Bank Prime Minister's Jai Vighyan Programme.

MAFSU starts PASHU-SOOCHANALAYA to desseminate information to users

The city based Maharashtra Animal and Fishery Science University (MAFSU) will soon be launching a new concept as "Pashu-Soochanalaya". Information will be disseminated to the end users through the two-way interaction between farmers and the experts in the university through which all querries related to day to day management of animals, their diseases, fodder preparation, manure preparation, etc. will be answered, through information centres at village Panchayat offices and veterinary colleges in the state.

(i) Differential Diagnosis of Common Disorders in Bovines

Symptom	Duration	Probable Cause	Points of Differential Diagnosis
Loss of Appetite (Anorexia)	(a) of short duration	Simple Indigestion *With Impaction/tympany*	History of change in the feed and overeating *Afebrile*. Ruminal movements reduced and weak. Usually responds to purgatives, ruminotorics, carminatives and correction of ruminal pH and microflora. Rule out acute acidic indigestion if animals are fed on rice, wheat or sweets from human food
(A Symptom in almost every disease in animals and in febrile conditions)	(b) for a long duration	(1) Abomasal displacement	Usually in females with history of recent parturition. Distension on left side, anterior to flank with splashing sounds. Rumen displaced, slightly to the right side. Partial anorexia. Confirmation by exploratory puncture (*Liptik test*) and pH exam
		(2) Traumatic reticulitis	Recurrent indigestion with tympany, grunt and signs of pain on pressure at reticular region (*bamboo test*), leucocytosis and mild fever. Animal sits with caution. Females urinate frequently in the small quantities due to pain during urinating posture. No response to treatment. Facial expression of pain. Confirm by metal detector, radiology and exploratory rumenotomy

		(3) Liver dysfunction and anaemia	General debility, pale, icteric m.m., Symptoms of deficiency of Co., Cu., Fe., malnutrition. Good response to appropriate treatment. Slow recovery. Confirmation by exam. of blood, faeces and liver function tests
		(4) Ketosis	Usually in a high milk yielder and at the time of peak yield. Selective appetite (takes roughage but rejects concentrates). Confirm by *Rotheri's test on urine* and good response to appropriate treatment
		(5) Actinobacillosis *involving rumen & reticulum*	Irregular and progressive loss of appetite. No fever, No pain or grunt, obstinate indigestion. Slight response to the course of Streptopenicillin

(ii) Differential Diagnosis of Common Disorders in Bovines

Symptom	Duration	Probable Cause	Points of Differential Diagnosis
Distension of Abdomen	*Sudden* Left Side	(i) Ruminal Tympany	History of feeding on fermentable feed stuff. Left side distended and left flank bulged out due to free gases accumulated in the dorsal sac. Drum-like resonance on percussion. Respiratory distress due to pressure on diaphragm. Confirm by trocarization
	"	(ii) Frothy bloat	Gases mixed with ingesta with froth formation. Distension and bulge of left flank not so marked. Moderate resonance on percussion. Rumen movements present. Confirm by trocarization
	"	(iii) Ruminal Impaction	Distension marked only in acute impaction due to engorgement on grains. Dull resonance on percussion. Contents hard on palpation. Rumen atonic, animal dull and toxaemic
	Sudden Right side	(iv) Distension of Abomasum with gases or feed	Not a very common condition Examine at a proper site (*see fig. on page 12 on the right side*)

(v)	Strangulation of intestines or paralytic ileus	Distension anterior to point of obstruction. Posterior part of intestines and rectum empty. Rectal exam. may evince pain. Animal may go in shock due toxaemia
(vi)	*Gradual* **Right side** Advance Pregnancy	Only in *females*, history of conception. No discomfort or sign of disease. Confirmation easily possible by P.R. exam. Critically examine if hydrops amnii, mummified foetus or twin pregnancy is suspected
(vii)	*Gradual* **Lower side** Ascites (accumulation of fluid)	Not very common in adult bovines. Hypoprotinemia due to Chr. parasitic infection, liver-fluke disease and other liver disorders. Congestive cardiac failure etc. are common causes. Abdomen pendulous. Confirm by test puncture
(viii)	*Duration of* **3 to 4 days** Rupture of Urinary bladder	Usually in untreated case of urolithiasis in male bovine. Has a history of retained urine. Symptoms of uraemia and shock. Confirm by rectal exam. of bladder and exploratory puncture of lower abdomen. Blood urea levels highly increased

371

(iii) Differential Diagnosis of Common Disorders in Bovines

Symptom	Duration	Probable Cause	Points of Differential Diagnosis
Diarrhoea *Watch for dehydration and loss of electrolytes*	*Aucte in young calves*	White Scours (*Colibacillosis*)	Seen in newborn calves below 3 months age. shooting white diarrhoea with offensive smell. Rapid dehydration, toxaemia. Mortality heavy in colostrum deprived calves. Overcrowding & unhygienic conditions are predisposing factors
	-	Coccidiosis	Faeces contain *blood and mucus*. Confirmation by faecal examination
	-	Worm infestation	Diarrhoea not very severe. Round worms seen in faeces. Poor condition of calf. Convulsions and fits. Faecal exam. for confirmation
	-	Dietetic Scours	In newborn calves due to overfeeding of milk, unhygienic condition. Diarrhoea with white faeces, without toxaemia. Responds to astringent mixture. Death rate low
	Acute in Adults	H.S. Anthrax	Accompanied with high fever and other symptoms of specific diseases. *Blood in faeces and urine in Anthrax.* Short course and high mortality rate

		Acute in Adults	Poisonings	Poisoning with Arsenic, Lead, Mercury and other corrosives. Other specific symptoms present. Afebrile, symptoms of shock. Confirmation by submitting materials to Forensic laboratory
			Rinderpest, M.D.C. Virus diarrhoea: Boving Malignant Catarrh	Specific viral diseases characterized by *initial high fever.* Leucopenia followed by diarrhoea. Buccal m.m. shows ulcers typical of each disease. No response to treatment. Confirmation by C.F. test, virological studies, morbidity-mortality patterns
		Subacute and persistent in adults	Tuberculosis	Enteric T.B. usually in adults. Chronic fever emaciation in spite of normal appetite. Confirm by herd history, exam. of faecal smear and *Tuberculin test*
			Johne's Disease	Age group 2-6 years. Persistent incurable diarrhoea and wasting. Confirm by exam. of faecal smear, rectal pinch, Johnin Test
			Parasitic cause	Srongyles sp. and other round worms. Liver fluke infection. Faeces black with offensive smell. Rough coat, anaemia. — Submandibular oedema. Confirmation by faecal examination

(iv) Differential Diagnosis of Common Disorders in Bovines

Symptom	Duration/Intensity	Probable Cause	Points of Differential Diagnosis
Symptoms of Respiratory system Involvement (*e.g.*, Cough, Nasal discharge Adventitious sounds, change in rate and character of respiration. Fever in infectious condition.)	Recent origin and mild	Upper Resp. Tract infections	Febrile reaction moderate, nasal discharge, cough, lacrymation, lungs clear. Good response to treatment
	Sudden and severe	Pneumonia CBPP and H.S.	Pneumonia (*Bacterial, Viral or Verminous*) common in young calves. High fever, initial congestion of lungs, followed by moist rales, consolidation, dyspnoea. Toxaemia seen in bacterial pneumonia. T.I.C. increased with neutrophilia

		CBPP & H.S. Clinically similar. Acute pneumonia. High fever, dyspnoea, toxaemia. Mortality rates very high. Both lungs simultaneously involved. T.L.C. increased with neutrophilia. Blood smear positive in H.S.
Chronic and moderate	Chr. Bronchitis, Emphysema	Dry crackling sounds over bronchial regions, dry cough, mild febrile reaction sometimes seen. Animal cannot sustain exercise, Jugular vein prominent. *Lungworm (Dictyocaulus)* infection common in some areas, should be confirmed by faecal exam. Rule out T.B.
Sudden and severe	Aspiration Pneumonia	History of faulty drenching or regurgitation due to casting or lying recumbent for long time. Rattling sounds over trachea and bronchi. Copious nasal discharge and froth with offensive smell, toxaemia. *Usually has fatal termination*
Chronic and persistent	"Panting"	After effects of foot and mouth disease occurs in about 5 per cent recovered animals due to endocrine damage. Chronic dyspnoea, overgrowth of hair and poor heat tolerance. Bullocks get easily fatigued and are unable to work. Cows become uneconomical milk producers. *Condition is incurable*

(v) Differential Diagnosis of Common Disorders in Bovines

Symptom	Duration/Range	Probable Cause	Points of Differential Diagnosis
High Fever	*Sudden onset 104-106°F* *in young calves*	(1) Bacterial/Viral Pneumonia	Acute Resp. symptoms, rapid progress. Toxaemia in bact. pneumonia
		(2) Colisepticemia	Colisepticemia : Sudden deaths, short duration. Confirmation by blood culture
	All age groups *Sudden onset 104-106°F*	Bacterial Diseases	H.S. Respiratory involvement, oedema of throat, tongue, pneumonia, death in 24-28 hrs. Confirmation by B.S. exam. and rabbit inoculation
		H.S., B. Q., Anthrax CBPP, Listeriosis	B.Q.: Disease of young bovines. Huge crepitating swelling on muscular parts with toxaemia
			Anthrax : Peracute disease, blood from natural orifices. Confirmation by B.S. exam. and guinea pig inoculation.
			CBPP : Resembles H.S. clinically. Course of disease 3-4 days. Marbled lungs are characteristic. Confirm by lung smears on P.M.
			Listeriosis: CNS involvement, circling. Response to penicillin in heavy doses
	106°F and above	Viral diseases	Rinderpest : High morbidity and mortality, ulcers, typical (like wheat bran) followed by diarrhoea, exhaustion and death, C.F. test for confirmation

Rinderpest, M.D.C. F.M.D. Ephermeral fever	M.D.C. : Low morbidity, high mortality, young animals more commonly affected, ulcers on buccal m.m. shallow and typical. Confirmation by C.F.T.
	F.M.D.: High morbidity, spreads very fast; No mortality in adults. Foot lesions and mouth lesions very typical
	Ephemeral fever: High morbidity, pain and lameness with one of the limbs. Recovery without treatment on 4th day. No mortality except in secondary complications
Protozoan Diseases Babesiasis Theileriasis, Anaplasmosis, Surra	Babesiasis: Haemoglobinuria, anaemia and jaundice. Ticks on body, confirmation by B.S. exam.
	Theileriasis: Persistent fever, Lymph nodes enlarged, ticks, severe hemolytic anaemia. Confirmation by B.S., exam. and lymph node smear
	Anaplasmosis: Similar to Theileriasis. No swelling of lymph nodes, jaundice may be seen. B.S. exam. to confirm
	Surra: Signs of CNS involvement, circling, blindness, head pressing. Confirmation by B.S. examination
Chr. Fever of low grade (adults) — Tuberculosis, Metritis, Mastitis, Reticuloperitonitis	Specific history and clinical symptoms are characteristic

(vi) Prophylactic Vaccination Schedule *(Cattle, Sheep, Goats and Swine)*

Animals	No.	Diseases	Vaccine	Dose/Route	Immunity
CATTLE & BUFFALOES	1.	RINDERPEST (This vaccination is abandoned due to successful eradi-cation of disease)	* F.D. G.T.V. *(for Indian Breeds)* * Tissue culture R.P. Vaccine (TCRP) *(for exotic, crossbred cattle, sheep and goats)*	1 ml sc 1 ml s/c (can be used in very young calves also)	* 14 years * 2 years *(even more as recently reported)*
	2.	F.M.D.	* Tetravalent *(including A-22 Strain)* I.V.R.I. Bangalore, B.A.I.F. and Intervet Vaccines - Intervet *(Concentrated)* - Raksha *(Ind Immunol)* - Raksha OVAC (" ")	-10 ml subcut. - 5 ml subcut. - 3 ml im Cattle - 2 ml im Sheep/goat- 1 ml im	* First vaccination at 3 months age *(even earlier)* * Booster : after 3 months * Afterwards : at 6 monthly intervals
	3.	H.S.	* Alum - precipitated * Oil adjuvant (IVBP) Pune	5 ml sc 2.5 to 3 ml im	* 6 months * 1 month
	4.	B.Q.	* Alum - precipitated Combined H.S. , B.Q., vaccine also available with BAIF	5 ml sc	* 6 months

No.	Group	Disease	Vaccine	Dose	Remarks
5.		ANTHRAX	* Spore Vaccine (IVBP Pune & BAIF)	1 ml sc	* 1 year
6.		BRUCELLOSIS	* Cotton-19 " strain. Handle the vaccine with care (IVBP Pune)	5 ml sc.	Vaccination of calves be done at 4-8 month of age only if incidence of disease is more than 25% in the herd
7.		THEILERIASIS	NDDB-Raksha-T (*Ind. Immunol.*) Animals in adv. pregnancy **not vaccinated.** Vaccine stored in liquid nitrogen	3 ml sc	* 1 year
8.	SHEEP	ENTEROTOXEMIA	* Multicomponent clostridial vaccine (I.V.R.I. & IVBP)	5 ml sc (2 doses. 3 weeks apart)	* 1 year
9.		SHEEP POX	* Tissue culture vaccine (BAIF, I.V.R.I., IVBP)	0.5 ml sub cut (*inside ear*)	* 1 year
10.	GOATS	C.C.P.	* I.V.R.I. Vaccine	0.2 ml (*at ear tip*)	* 1 year
11.		P.P.R.	* T.C.R.P. Vaccine	1.0 ml sub cut.	* 1 year
12.	PIGS	SWINE FEVER	* Freeze dried Tissue culture vaccine (I.V.B.P. Pune & BAIF)	1 ml sc (*inside thigh*)	* 1year

(vii) Prophylactic Vaccination Schedule (Poultry)

No.	Disease	Type of Vaccine	Age of Vaccination	Dose/Mode of Administration	Immunity
1.	Rainkhet (ND) (Newcastle)	• F₁ or Lasota strain	2-6 days	Intra ocular/nasal drops	6-8 weeks.
		• Avinew (Glaxo-Virbac) VG/.GA strain	Day Old	Individual-Intranasal/occular	
		Live modified Freeze dried vaccine	First Booster 5-6 days	Mass-oral (through/ drinking water spray)	6-8 weeks
			Second Booster 6-7 weeks.	"	
		○ Freezed dried Mukteswar or R2B Strain Live Vaccine	6-8 weeks	"	
		• IMOPEST (Inactivated N.D. Virus)	16 weeeks Booster	.05. ml sc or intra muscular	12-18 months
			17 weeks	0.3 ml sc or intra muscular	" "
2.	FOWL POX	• Live Vaccine (IVBP or Ventri)	6 weeks.	Scarificatin or puncture on wing web	6 months
		• Pigeon Pox virus	Young chicks & during outbreak	Feather follicle by brush	3-6 months
		• BM Strain (BioMed) for all ages	All ages	Intra muscular	1 year
3.	MAREK'S DISEASE	• HVT Strain- Living cell associated vaccine (Biomed). (Ventri) LYOMAREX (Glaxo-Virbac) and IVBP Pune	1-14 days	0.2 ml. sc to be vaccinated only once.	Lifelong (?)
4.	INFECTIOUS BRONCHITIS (IB)	• Massachuetts strain live attenuated (BioMed)	3-4 weeks.	Oral drops or in drinking water and repeat at 13-15 weeks age.	
		• Mass type Live attenuated (Ventri)	4-6 weeks	as above and repeated at 16 weeks.	
		• BORAL - H120 (Glaxo-Virbar) Live freeze dried	day old for broilers	oral/ or intra occluar/intranasal.	Lifelong (?)
		• Also combined IB-ND (Binewvax), IB- ND-IBD (Bigopest) vaccines	32 days with booster at 9 - 10 weeks	To be given 0.3 ml sc or im at 21-22 wks age.	

5.	GUMBORO DISEASE (IBD)	• Live, attenuaed (BAIF/Ventri)	(Primary) at 2-3 weeks. Booster at 18-21 weeks.	Oral drop/drinking water method	Lifelong (?)
		• GUMBORIFFA (Glaxo-Virbac) inactivated vaccine in oil adjuvant	21-22 weeks and 45th weeks.	0.5 ml sc as booster after primary 0.3 ml sc or intramuscular	"
		• BUR-706 Modified Live IBD strain vaccine Freeze dried	12-14 day Booster on 28 day	Individual-Intraocular/intranasal-mass-oral (through drinking water)	"
		• Also in combination with IB and ND (BIGOPEST) and ND (GUMBOPEST) (Glaxo-Virbac)	21st to 22 weeks and at 45 weeks	0.3 ml sc/intramuscular	"
6.	INFECTIOUS CORYZA	• Inactivated vaccine (*Ventri*)	8 weeks, again at 12 weeks	0.5 ml sc on the neck.	1 year
		• Inactivated vaccine HAEMOVAX (Glaxo Virbac)	4-6 weeks 12-14 weeks	0.3 ml sc or intramuscular	" "
7.	FOWL CHOLERA	• Killed vaccine (IVRI) and inactivated vaccine Ventri	6 weeks	1 ml sc above 6 weeks. age	1 year
8.	SPIROCHETOSIS IS	• Killed, freeze dried vaccine IVRI, I.V.B.P. (Ventri)	6 weeks	1 ml/intramuscular	1 year
9.	EGG DROP SYNDROME (EDS)	• Killed vaccine (BioMed)	15-18 weeks	0.5 ml/intramuscular	1 year

(viii) Differential Diagnosis of Common Condition & Lab. Diagnostic Tests Recommended (*for Dog*)

Predominant Symptom	Age Group	Typical Symptoms	Possible Diagnosis	Laboratory Tests Recommended
FEVER	Pups below 6 months	Cough & Colds with Nasal Discharge and severe dullness	Distemper (if not protected) Respiratory distress Bronchitis / Pneumonia	Blood for TLC (*Leukopenia*) and DLC (*Lymphopenia*) Blood for T.L.C. (*Leukopenia*) and DLC (*Neutrophilia*)
		Jaundice & tenderness on liver site	Infectious Canine Hepatitis (if not protected)	Blood for TLC (Initial Leukopenia) & Clotting Time (*increased*) & Liver function tests
		Diarrhoea & Vomiting	Parvo-viral gastro enteritis (if not protected)	Blood for T.L.C. (*Initial leukopenia*) and D.L.C. (*Secondary leukocytosis*) Serum Sodium, Potassium & Chloride, E.C.G.
	Above 6 months	Jaundice & abortion in females	Leptospirosis (if not protected)	Blood for T.L.C. (*Leukocytosis*) & D.L.C. (*Neutrophilia*)
		Jaundice and severe anaemia. Ticks on the body	Babesiosis and Trypanosomiasis	Blood smear for Haemoglobin & Liver Function Tests
		Nervous Signs, epilepsy, convulsions, tremors	Meningitis or Encephalitis	Blood for T.L.C. (*Leukocytosis*) D.L.C. (*Neutrophilia*) C.S.F. for culture

		Foul smelling uterine discharge (in females associated with whelping)	Metritis or Pyometra	T.L.C. (*Leukocytosis*) D.L.C. (*Neutrophilia*) uterine swab for culture & sensitivity test
		Summer	Sunstroke	High rise in P.C.V. (Increased in severe dehydration) serum *Na, K*
DIARRHOEA	Pups below 6 months	Severe diarrhoea with yellow/white coloured faeces	Bacillary Diarrhoea	P.C.V. (increases in dehydration) Faeces for bact., culture. Serum *Na, K and Chlorides*
		Black & reddish Feces with occasional mucus and itching with alopecia.	Hookworm infection	Faeces for Parasitic Ova.
	Above 6 months	Persistent, non responding to routine treatment. Presence of fats & undigested food particles	Maldigestion or Malabsorption Syndrome	Special tests for Amylase, Lipase and Pancreatic enzymes, Liver Function Tests
		Persistent diarrhoea with inflammation & swelling of rectum.	Inflammation of anal glands.	Examination of anal glands & their gentle squeezing with sterile mop
		Black Faeces, itching of skin & wasting.	Hookworm infection and other worms.	Faeces exam for parasitic ova

383

(ix) Homoeopathic Remedies in Some Animal Diseases

(Some remedies are already mentioned under respective diseases in the text.)

No.	Diseases Condition	Clinical Signs	Remedies recommended	Mode of administration
1.	Traumatic injuries, contusious, Haemorrhagic shock. Post parutrient bleeding. Injuries to prolapsed uterus etc.		Arnica mont	200 potency tincture 2 to3 drops directly in mouth with plastic dropper at one hourly interval, 3 to 4 doses
2.	Suppurating wound, ulcers and fistule	Having no tendency of early healing	Calendula mother tincture mixed with equal parts of glycerine.	Dress the wound with gauze soaked in saturated soln. of Mag. sulph. on the first day followed by calendula soaked gauze daily afterwards
3.	Sudden high fever	(a) Breath hot, eyes red and rapid respirations *(viral fevers)* (b) Sunstroke	(a) *Aconite &Belladona very good for young animals and pups)* (b) Glonine	30 to 200 potency tincture or globules at three hourly interval. "
4.	Prolapse of vagina, uterus or rectum.	Pre or Post partum prolapse with straining (tenesmus)	*Pulsatilla, Podophyllum & Sepia*	30 to 200 potency tincture or globules at two hourly interval after reducing the prolapsed mass
5.	Sub-clinical mastitis	CMT reaction positive to ++ and +++ grade, with pathogenic Staphylocci and blood tinge to milk	Phytolacca 200 C	Tincture @ 5 drops twice a day for 3–4 days effected complete cure in 67% cases

			Merc. Sol. & Cantheris or Khurinol (a prop. preparation)	
6.	Foot & Mouth Disease	Typical lesions (initially blister followed by ulcers) on buccal m.m. and interdigital space.		Tinctures of 200 potency. In alternation 2-3 drops twice a day for 6 to 7 days
7.	Acute impaction and constipation	Rumen, completely atonic. Faeces very hard and scanty. Abdomen slightly distended, Animal dull.	*Opium*	200 potency tincture 2-3 drop thrice daily
8.	Warts	Pedenculated cauliflower like growths on any part of body as well as buccal m.m. and around mouth.	*Thuja*	Tincture of 30 potency twice daily for 15-20 days

Also apply Thuja ointment locally |
9.	Skin Diseases	Scabies, with severe itching and bad smell particularly in dogs.	*Sulphur and Hepar sulph.*	6 potency globules twice a day for 1 week. Also use ointment of sulphur
10.	Vomiting & Diarrhoea	Haemorrhagic gastroenteritis in dogs.	*Ipicac*	30 potency globules 3-4 times a day
11.	Corneal Opacity	Cornea becomes white and opaque (most commonly due to some injuries)	*Euphrasia*	30 potency globules for 10-15 days. Dilute tincture instilled as eyedrops also effective

Diagnostic Workup

Bacterial Diseases

Name of the Disease	Etiological agents	Sp. Affected	Diagnosis	Prophylaxis	Treatment
1. Anthrax	*Bacillus anthrasis*	Buff., horse, cattle, sheep and goat	Blood smear. Biological test. Cultural tests. Ascolis test	Attenuated spore vaccine cattle 1 ml sc. Sheep and Goats 0.3-0.5 ml.	Penicillin in massive doses, till recovery. Streptomycin 8-10 g daily in 2 doses im Antiserum iv in 100/200 ml. with antibiotics
2. Black quarter	*Cl. Clauvoei*	Exudate Smear Exam. Biological test	Buff., Cattle, Sheep and goats	Formalised Vaccine cattle 5 ml sc. Sheep and Goat 2 ml	Penicillin 5000 units per lb b. wt.
3. Pasturellosis	*Pasturella septica*	Buff. Cattle, Sheep and Goat	Blood smear exam. Biological tests Cultural tests	Adjuant vaccine upto 300 lb, 2 ml above 300 lb, 3 ml	Streptomycin 5-10 mg per lb, b.wt. Sulphameathine 33 1/3 per cent. sc. or iv gives good results.
4. Brucellosis	*Br. abortus*	Buff. Cattle, Sheep and Goat	Serum agglutination test, Tube method and Quick method Biological test	Cotton 19 Female calf hood Vaccination 5 ml. sc.	Treatment not undertaken. Streptomycin and Auromycine used in the human beings

Various Information Charts

Name of the Disease	Etiological agents	Sp. Affected	Diagnosis	Prophylaxis	Treatment
5. Tuberculosis	*Mycobacterium tuberculosis var. bovine*	Buff., Cattle, Sheep and Goat and Dogs	Pus smear from the affected parts stainted with Z-N method. Acid fast organism are seen. Biological test in G. pigs. Tuberculin test	B.C.G. Vaccination 50-100 ml, sc, calves are vaccinated as soon as birth, not much used because animals remain as reactors	Not much used
6. Johne's disease	*Mycobacterium para tuberculosis*	Buff., Cattle, Sheep and Goats	Rectal mucus membrane smear examination Biological test Johnin test	Rinjard and Valle Vaccine. Living animal react to tuberculin test	Not much used Streptomycin 25 mg per lb b.wt. daily gives transient improvement
7. Glanders diseases	*Malleomyces*	Horses	Pus smear Exam, Biological test Strau's reaction in G. pigs. Mullein test	No vaccine	Sodium sulphadiazine is effective and is tried in hamsters
8. Contagious Caprine Pleuro pneumonia	*P.P.L.O.*	Goats	Symptoms cultivation and isolation of the agent. Goats experimentally infected.	Attenuated vaccine 2 ml sc	Terrymycine has been found to be effective

387

Name of the Disease	Etiological agents	Sp. Affected	Diagnosis	Prophylaxis	Treatment
9. Mastitis	*Streptococcus Staphylococcus*	Buff, Cattle, Sheep and Goat.	Milk sediment smear exam. Strip cup method Whiteside test Cultural exam	No vaccine, Toxoid against Staphylococcus tried but not much useful	Penicillin intramammary is very useful in early stage. Dihydro Streptomycin is also effective Use antibiotic after A.S. test
10. Fowl Cholera	*Pasteurella septica.*	Birds	Blood smear exam. Isolation and identification of the organism	Killed broth Culture is used. Not much useful	Sulphamezathine and Sulphadimidine orally by injection are useful
11. Leptopirosis	*Leptospim pomona and canicula*	Dogs, Buffalo, Cattle	Demonstrate the organism in the urine under the dark ground illumination. Cultivation of the agent in the chicks	Killed bacterin	Vaccine is still doubtful

Virus Diseases

Name of the Disease	Etiological agents	Sp. Affected	Diagnosis	Prophylaxis	Treatment
1. Foot and mouth	Virus O.A.C. types. SAT-1, SAT-2, SAT-3 ASIA-1	Buffalo, Cattle, Sheep, Goats and Pigs.	Symptoms and the nature of the epidemic. Isolation of the virus in the G. Pigs and calves	Crystal violet vaccine, not much used. It is costly to prepare	Symptomatic Treatment (see Homoeopathic remedies in Table IX)

388

Name of the Disease	Etiological agents	Sp. Affected	Diagnosis	Prophylaxis	Treatment
2. Pox	Virus	Cattle, Buffalo, Sheep, Goat and Birds	Symptoms-Isolation of the virus in the eggs	Low virulent Pigeon Pox vaccine is available and it is rubbed on the legs with brushes	Symptomatic treatment
3. Rinderpest	Virus	Cattle, Buffalo, Pigs, sheep and goat	Symptoms and the history of the epidemic, biological test. Serum neutralisation test	Goat adopted tissue vaccine is used TCRPV	Hyperimmune serum. Disease has been eradicated from India
4. Hog Cholera	Virus	Pigs	Symptoms serum neutralisation test	Modified, live vaccine and crystal violet vaccine. Not yet prepared in our State	Hyperimmune serum is the only available treatment
5. Canine distemper	Virus	Canines	Symptoms Biological in Ferrets	Distemper virus vaccine s/c, dose from 6-9 weeks age are protective	Symptomatic treatment
6. Ranikhet Disease	.Virus	Birds	Symptoms and history of the epidemic. Isolation of the Virus in the egg. H.I. test	Attenuated Vaccine 0.5 ml sc (See table VII)	Symptomatic treatment

Name of the Disease	Etiological agents	Sp. Affected	Diagnosis	Prophylaxis	Treatment
7. S.A.H.S.	Virus	Equines	Symptoms and history of the epidemic Isolation of the virus in suckling mice. Serum Neutralisation test	Attenuated live vaccine	Symptomatic treatment
8. Contagious respiratory (C.R.D.) disease	Bacteria and P.P. L.O.	Birds	Symptoms, quick agg. test. Isolation of the casual agents	No effective vaccine	Symptomatic treatment
9. Rabies	Virus	Dogs, Cattle, Buffaloes, Sheep and Goats	Symptoms Fluorescence antibody coating test. Biological test mice	Attenuated Flury strain (L.E.P.) killed vaccine	No treatment

Parasitic Infection

1.	Fasciola *hepatica*	*Trematode*	Cattle, Sheep and Goats	Clinical symptoms	Avlothane; 1, C.I. Hexachlorethane
2.	*Schistosoniasis*	*S. insalis*	Cattle	Clinical symptoms	Control of snails by ducks and geese and CuSO₄. Treatment of water tanks. Antimony preparations
3.	Surra	*T. evansi*	Cattle	Symptoms, Blood smear examination, M.B. 693 test.	Naganol Bayers 205 Antripol Antricide, Diaminazine aceturate
4.	Babesiosis	*B. canis* *B. bigemina.*	Cattle Buffaloes and Dogs.	Symptoms blood smears examination.	Acapirin Babosan, Diaminazine aceturate
5.	Anaplasmosis	*A. marginale*	Cattle, Birds	Symptoms, blood smear examination C.F. test.	Tetracyline 3-5 mg. per lb b.wt. one injection
6.	Coccidiosis	*Emieria*	Cattle, Birds	Symptoms and faecal matter examination	Sulpha drugs-Sulphonamide Nitrofurazone 1 per cent, and in food Atebrine

Fungal Diseases

1.	Aspergillosis	*A. fumigatus*	Birds	Symptoms Isolation of the fungus, and identification	
2.	Epizoatic lymphangitis	*Cryptococcus farciminiosis*	Equines.	Pus smear examination	
3.	Ringworm	*Fungus*	Cattle, Buffaloes, Dogs, Sheep and Goats.	Lesion on the affected part, Wood's light, scrapings examination	Salicylic ointment, Resorcine, Griesofulvin.

Diagnosis of Respiratory Diseases

Symptoms	Nasal Catarrh	Pharyngitis	Bronchitis	Lobular Pneumonia	Interstitial Penumonia	Chronic Alveolar Emphysema	Pleurisy 1st Stage	Pleurisy 2nd Stage
Nasal discharge	1. Serous 2. Mucoid 3. Purulent	May be Mucoid or purulent	May be Mucoid or purulent	May be Mucoid or purulent	-------	-------	-------	-------
Swelling	-------	May be difficult.	-------		-------	-------	---?---	-------
Cough	Absent	1. Dry and Harsh 2. Moist and soft	1. Dry and Harsh. 2. Moist and soft May be paroxysms	Copious Expectorate ------- cough may be very frequent	-------	Deep hollow cough	-------	-------
Respirations	Normal	Normal	Dyspnoea may be severe	Dyspnoea may be severe	Rapid Shallow	Double expiratory effort Dyspnoea on exertion	Mainly abdominal pleuritic line	Dyspnoea exudate voluminous
Fever	Usually slight.	Only May be marked	May be marked	May be marked	Slight	Absent	Present	Present
Regional (Throat) lymphatic glands	May be swollen	May be swollen	-------	-------	-------	-------	-------	-------

Chest, Vesicular sounds	May be exaggerated	May be exaggerated	-----	increased in volume, Crackling noises	-----	-----
Bronchial sounds	Sonorous and sibilant bronchi. Present.	Sonorous and sibilant bronchi Present	Loud	-----	-----	-----
Moist sounds	Present.	Present	-----	-----	-----	-----
Crepitation	-----	Present	May be crackling due to emphysema	No true Crepitation	-----	-----
Friction sounds	-----	-----	-----	-----	Are present	Absent dull area in lower part of chest
Percussions	Normal	-----	General reduction in resonance. May be dull	Loss of reasonance develops in upper third	May be an increase in resonance and size of area	-----

393

Subject Index

394

References

1. Anon, (1999) Food Outlook,
   Food & Agriculture Organisation of the United Nations,
   Rome, Nov. 1999

2. Blood, D. C. Radostitis, O.M. and Henderson, A.J.
   "VETERINARY MEDICINE"
   6th Edition, 1983, Bailliere Tindall, London.

3. Boddie, G.F.
   "Diagnostic Methods in Veterinary Medicine"
   6th Edition 1970, Oliver & Boyd. Edinburgh

4. Boericke, William (1981)
   "Homoeopathic Materia Medica"
   9th Ed., Jain Publishers, New Delhi

5. Concannon, C.W.
   "Physiology & Endocrinology of Canine Pregnancy"
   D. W. Morrow's "Theriogenology" 2nd Ed. 1986

6. Dakshinkar, N. P. (1999)
   "Personal Communication" and
   "Handbook of Animal Husbandry"
   Mangesh Prakashan - 2001

7. "Handbook of Animal Husbandry" (1962)
   I.C.A.R. Publication, New Delhi

8. "Indian Journal of Veterinary Medicine"
   (Relevant Issue)

9. "Indian Veterinary Journal"
   (Relevant Issues)

10. Kadu, M. S. (1999)
    "Personal Communication"

11. Kelly, W.R. (1984)
    "Veterinary Clinical Diagnosis"
    3rd Ed., Bailliere Tindall, London.

12. Kent, J. T. (1969)
    "Lectures on Homoeopathic Materia - Medica"
    2nd Ed. Roy Publishing House, Calcutta

398

13. Kirk, Robert W. & Bistner S.I.
    "Handbook of Vety. Procedures & Emergency Treatment"
    W. B. Saunders & Co.,
    Philadelphia / London / Toronto

14. Lander, P. E. (1949)
    "Feeding of Farm Animals in India"
    MacMillan & Co. Ltd.,
    Calcutta, Bombay, Madras, London

15. Macleod, G. (1983)
    "The Treatment of Cattle by Homoeopathy"
    Jain Publishing Co., New Delhi

16. Paikne, D. L. (1999)
    "Personal Communication"

17. Rosenberger, G. (1979)
    "Clinical Examination of Cattle"
    Verlag Paul Parey, Berlin & Haemburg

18. Rush, John (1959)
    "The Handbook to Veterinary Homoeopathy"
    Economic Homoeo Stores, Calcutta

19. Sapre, V. A. (1974)
    "Management of Foot & Mouth Disease Outbreak in a Herd"
    Maha Vet-I : 5-7

20. Sapre, V. A. (1977 - 1997)
    Unpublished Research Data and Personal Experiences in
    Practice

21. Shastri, Ganti, A. (1976)
    "Veterinary Clinical Pathology"
    (T. V. Press, Tirupati)

22. Shrivastava, D. N. & Soni, J. L. (1987)
    "Clinical Vety. Toxicology & Jurisprudence"
    Anubha Prakashan, Jabalpur

23. Dr. Shirish Gode
    Vyankatesh Emu Farms,
    (Information Leatlet)
    Kharangna, Distt : Wardha

24. Emu Production in the United States
    (Information Leaflets of American Emu Association)

Notes

_____

_____

_____

_____

_____

_____

_____

_____

_____

_____

_____

_____

_____

_____

_____

_____

_____

_____

_____

_____

_____

_____

_____

Notes

Notes

Notes

Notes